Strategies to Protect the Health of DEPLOYED U.S. FORCES

Medical Surveillance,

Record Keeping, and

Risk Reduction

Lois M. Joellenbeck, Philip K. Russell, and
Samuel B. Guze, *Editors*

Medical Follow-Up Agency

INSTITUTE OF MEDICINE

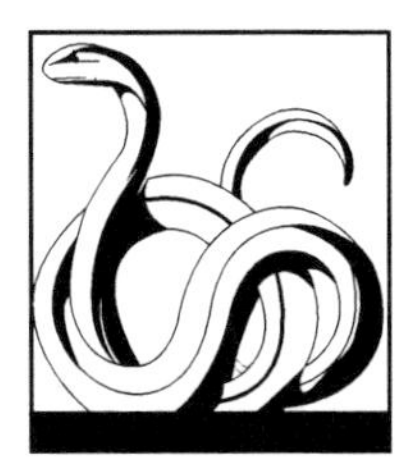

NATIONAL ACADEMY PRESS
Washington, DC

NATIONAL ACADEMY PRESS • 2101 Constitution Avenue, N.W. • Washington, DC 20418

NOTICE: The project that is the subject of this report was approved by the Governing Board of the National Research Council, whose members are drawn from the councils of the National Academy of Sciences, the National Academy of Engineering, and the Institute of Medicine. The members of the study team responsible for the report were chosen for their special competences and with regard for appropriate balance.

The Institute of Medicine was chartered in 1970 by the National Academy of Sciences to enlist distinguished members of the appropriate professions in the examination of policy matters pertaining to the health of the public. In this, the Institute acts under both the Academy's 1863 congressional charter responsibility to be an advisor to the federal government and its own initiative in identifying issues of medical care, research, and education. Dr. Kenneth I. Shine is president of the Institute of Medicine.

Support for this project was provided by Contract No. DASW01-97-C-0078 between the National Academy of Sciences and the Department of Defense. The views, opinions, and/or findings contained in this report are those of the authors and do not necessarily reflect the view of the organizations or agencies that provided support for the project.

International Standard Book Number 0-309-06637-9

Additional copies of this report are available for sale from National Academy Press, 2101 Constitution Avenue, N.W., Lock Box 285, Washington, DC 20055. Call (800) 624-6242 or (202) 334-3313 (in the Washington metropolitan area), or visit the NAP's online bookstore at **www.nap.edu.** The full text of this report is available online at: **www.nap.edu/readingroom.**

For more information about the Institute of Medicine, visit the IOM home page at: **www.iom.edu.**

Printed in the United States of America

The serpent has been a symbol of long life, healing, and knowledge among almost all cultures and religions since the beginning of recorded history. The serpent adopted as a logotype by the Institute of Medicine is a relief carving from ancient Greece, now held by the Staatliche Museen in Berlin.

STRATEGIES TO PROTECT THE HEALTH OF DEPLOYED U.S. FORCES: MEDICAL SURVEILLANCE, RECORD KEEPING, AND RISK REDUCTION

Principal Investigators

SAMUEL B. GUZE, Spencer T. Olin Professor of Psychiatry, Washington University School of Medicine
PHILIP K. RUSSELL, Professor Emeritus, Department of International Health, Johns Hopkins School of Hygiene and Public Health

Advisory Panel

ARTHUR J. BARSKY, III, Professor, Department of Psychiatry, Harvard Medical School, Brigham and Women's Hospital
DAN BLAZER, II, Dean of Medical Education and J.P. Gibbons Professor of Psychiatry, Duke University Medical Center
GERMAINE M. BUCK, Associate Professor, Department of Social and Preventive Medicine, University at Buffalo, State of New York
CHARLES C. J. CARPENTER, Professor of Medicine, The Miriam Hospital, Brown University
JOHN A. FAIRBANK,* Associate Professor, Department of Psychiatry and Behavioral Sciences, Duke University Medical Center
KENNETH W. GOODMAN, Director, Forum for Bioethics and Philosophy, University of Miami
SANFORD S. LEFFINGWELL, HLM Consultants, Atlanta, Georgia
BRUCE S. McEWEN, Professor and Head, Harold and Margaret Milliken Hatch Laboratory of Neuroendocrinology, Rockefeller University
G. MARIE SWANSON, Director, Cancer Center, and Professor, Department of Family Practice and Medicine, Michigan State University
PAUL C. TANG, Medical Director, Clinical Informatics, Palo Alto Medical Foundation, and Vice President, Epic Research Institute
FRANK W. WEATHERS, Assistant Professor, Department of Psychology, Auburn University
NEIL D. WEINSTEIN, Professor, Department of Human Ecology, Cook College, Rutgers University

Study Staff

LOIS JOELLENBECK, Study Director
RAJESH VENUGOPAL, Research Assistant
AIMEE BOSSE, Project Assistant
RICHARD MILLER, Director, Medical Follow-Up Agency

---

*Through September 1998.

REVIEWERS

This report has been reviewed in draft form by individuals chosen for their diverse perspectives and technical expertise, in accordance with procedures approved by the National Research Council's Report Review Committee. The purpose of this independent review is to provide candid and critical comments that will assist the Institute of Medicine in making the published report as sound as possible and to ensure that the report meets institutional standards for objectivity, evidence, and responsiveness to the study charge. The review comments and draft manuscript remain confidential to protect the integrity of the deliberative process. The study team wishes to thank the following individuals for their participation in the review of this report:

JOHN F. AHEARNE, Ph.D., Sigma Xi Center, Research Triangle Park, N.C.
MARION J. BALL, Ed.D., School of Nursing, Johns Hopkins University, and First Consulting Group, Baltimore, Md.
RUTH BERKELMAN, M.D., Centers for Disease Control and Prevention, Atlanta
DONALD L. CUSTIS, M.D., Potomac, Md.
JAMES D. EBERT, Marine Biological Laboratory, Woods Hole, Mass.
HAROLD M. KOENIG, M.D., San Diego, Calif.
KATHLEEN A. McCORMICK, Ph.D., SRA International, Fairfax, Va.
ENRIQUE MENDEZ, Jr., M.D., Stafford, Va.
CHARLES E. PHELPS, Ph.D., University of Rochester
MICHAEL C. SHARPE, M.D., University of Edinburgh and Royal Edinburgh Hospital, Scotland
GUTHRIE L. TURNER, Jr., M.D., Division of Disability Determination Services, State of Washington

Although the individuals listed above have provided constructive comments and suggestions, it must be emphasized that responsibility for the final content of this report rests entirely with the principal investigators and the Institute of Medicine.

Preface

Protecting the health of military service members during deployments is vitally important to the accomplishment of the military mission as well as to the welfare of the service members. Deployments present unique and difficult challenges in preventive medicine, but through many years of research and progress in military medicine, military medical departments have made tremendous strides in the medical protection and care they can now offer soldiers, sailors, airmen, and marines.

The medical consequences of the Gulf War have made it clear, however, that some threats remain poorly understood and inadequately addressed. Despite very low levels of combat casualties and disease and non-battle injuries during both the buildup to the war and the war itself, many veterans have since reported health problems that they attribute to their service in the war. Many of these are unexplained illnesses that have proved to be frustrating to diagnose and treat.

Since the Gulf War, our military has seen an increasing tempo of deployments and demands, including operations in Haiti, Somalia, Bosnia, Southwest Asia, and Kosovo. What lessons have been learned from these operations as well as the Gulf War, and how can forces in future deployments best be protected? A 3-year National Academies study has been charged with addressing these questions.

The first part of the 3-year study has been carried out as four parallel 2-year tasks. The four tasks were to (1) develop an analytical framework for assessing the risks to deployed forces; (2) review and evaluate improved technologies and methods for the detection and tracking of exposures to those risks; (3) review and evaluate improved technologies and methods for physical protection and decontamination, particularly for chemical and biological agents; and (4) review and evaluate medical protection, health consequences management and treatment, and medical record keeping.

Now at the close of the 2-year efforts, the group responsible for each task is providing a report to the U.S. Department of Defense and the public on its findings and recommendations in these areas. These documents will serve as the starting point for the work of a new committee that will prepare a synthesis document for the U.S. Department of Defense in the third year of the project. The committee will consider not only the topics specifically raised by the four 2-year studies but also overarching issues relevant to its broader charge.

The study presented in this report has focused upon the fourth task described above. Our broad charge (found in Appendix B and discussed further in Chapter 1) includes almost all aspects of military medicine: both prevention of adverse health outcomes from exposures to deployment risks and treatment of the health consequences of prevention failures, including battle injuries, disease and non-battle injuries, acute management, and long-term follow-up. The charge also specifies seven other areas including medical surveillance, medical record keeping, risk communication, reintegration, vaccines and other prophylactic agents, predeployment screening, and active-duty retention standards.

Unlike the typical National Academies study, this effort was carried out not by consensus committee but by ourselves as principal investigators with the help and guidance of a panel of experts in the range of topics covered by the study. We held five workshops to gather information on topics within the study charge.

No single study team or series of workshops could do justice to the entire breadth of topics included in our study charge. We therefore decided to focus on topics in which we felt outside consultants could provide particularly helpful advice to the military in light of lessons from recent deployments. We did not address topics such as management of battle injuries or prevention of well-known infectious disease threats with which the military has a depth of expertise. We had little additional to offer on such topics, and therefore were silent.

This study team did not take up issues of the etiologies of illnesses in Gulf War veterans, as it was not part of our charge. Considerable effort and expertise have been and continue to be applied to these issues by several expert panels and researchers, and their work is likely to continue for many years to come.

However, we believe that there are clear lessons from the Gulf War experience, and these are reflected in our report's focus on medically unexplained symptoms, medical surveillance, and medical record keeping. With medically unexplained symptoms, there is a growing body of evidence that they can be managed and treated, even though their cause or pathogenesis is not fully understood. A signed paper provided in Appendix A of the report was particularly helpful in informing our deliberations on this topic.

We emphasize medical surveillance and medical record keeping because they are crucial tools for providing optimum population-based and individual medical care for service members and providing the basis for future population-based epidemiologic studies of deployment-related illnesses. The two topics are necessarily interrelated. Complete and accessible medical records are an essential component of effective medical surveillance as well as a critical element of optimal health care.

Risk communication is another important component of the responsibility that the military has to its service members, as is supportive reintegration of service members back to their nondeployed status. We dwelt on these topics at some length because they are important tools for the care of service members. Ready formulas for carrying them out well are not available, so concerted effort and research are needed.

In many of these areas, the U.S. Department of Defense has already made important progress. New programs have been implemented and others have been planned. One particularly encouraging event was the release by the Executive Office of the President of *A National Obligation: Planning for Health Preparedness for and Readjustment of the Military, Veterans, and Their Families after Future Deployments.* This document presents a strategic plan prepared by an interagency working group with representatives of the U.S. Departments of Defense, Veterans Affairs, and Health and Human Services. The plan includes many excellent goals, objectives, and strategies for protecting the health of service members and veterans and providing reintegration support for them and their families. It is a very positive sign that these goals have been recognized at the highest levels, and we hope that implementation of these goals similarly finds high-level support. A tool to help with aspects of the plan requiring interagency coordination is the establishment of the Military and Veterans Health Coordinating Board. As this report enters review this group is being constituted, and we hope that they are effective champions of implementing the strategic plan outlined in *A National Obligation.*

We are grateful to our panel of advisors who gave their time and talents to this project. We are similarly indebted to the members of the public health, military preventive medicine, and military and veterans health care communities who offered their insights to this project. A list of these people, no doubt incomplete, is found in Appendix G.

Improving the ability of the armed services to protect and maintain the health of service members remains a challenging endeavor. We hope this study will assist the U.S. Department of Defense with carrying out its responsibilities to the military men and women who serve our nation.

Philip K. Russell, M.D.
Samuel B. Guze, M.D.
Principal Investigators

Acronyms

AVIP	Anthrax Vaccine Immunization Program
BT	botulinum toxoid
CBT	cognitive behavior therapy
CDC	Centers for Disease Control and Prevention
CFS	chronic fatigue syndrome
CHCS	Composite Health Care System
CORBA	Common Object Request Broker Architecture
CPR	computer-based patient record
CSC	combat stress control
DEERS	Defense Eligibility Enrollment Record System
DHHS	U.S. Department of Health and Human Services
DMED	Defense Medical Epidemiologic Database
DMSS	Defense Medical Surveillance System
DNBI	disease and non-battle injury
DoD	U.S. Department of Defense
FDA	U.S. Food and Drug Administration
GCPR	Government Computer-Based Patient Record
HEAR	Health Evaluation and Assessment Review
HIPAA	Health Insurance Portability and Accountability Act
HIV	human immunodeficiency virus

ICD-9	International Classification of Diseases, version 9
IND	investigational new drug
IOM	Institute of Medicine
ITM	Immunization Tracking Module
JCS	Joint Chiefs of Staff
JPO-BD	Joint Program Office for Biological Defense
JTF	Joint Task Force
JVAP	Joint Vaccine Acquisition Program
MFUA	Medical Follow-Up Agency
MI	mass immunization
NBC	nuclear, biological, and chemical
NCHS	National Center for Health Statistics
NSTC	National Science and Technology Council
Operation READY	Operation "Resources Educating About Deployment and You"
PAARTS	Patient Accounting and Reporting Real-Time Tracking System
PB	pyridostigmine bromide
PHCA	Preventive Health Care Application
PIC	personal information carrier
PPMs	personal protective measures
PTSD	post-traumatic stress disorder
RAP	Recruit Assessment Program
RCS	Readjustment Counseling Service
TMIP	Theatre Medical Information Program
USARIEM	U.S. Army Research Institute of Environmental Medicine
VA	U.S. Department of Veterans Affairs
WRAIR	Walter Reed Army Institute of Research

Contents

Executive Summary

Nine years after Operations Desert Shield and Desert Storm (the Gulf War) ended in June 1991, uncertainty and questions remain about illnesses reported in a substantial percentage of the 697,000 service members who were deployed. Even though it was a short conflict with very few battle casualties or immediately recognized disease or non-battle injuries, the events of the Gulf War and the experiences of the ensuing years have made clear many potentially instructive aspects of the deployment and its hazards. Since the Gulf War, several other large deployments have also occurred, including deployments to Haiti and Somalia. Major deployments to Bosnia, Southwest Asia, and, most recently, Kosovo are ongoing as this report is written. This report draws on lessons learned from some of these deployments to consider strategies to protect the health of troops in future deployments.

In the spring of 1996, Deputy Secretary of Defense John White met with leadership of the National Research Council and the Institute of Medicine to explore the prospect of an independent, proactive effort to learn from lessons of the Gulf War and to develop a strategy to better protect the health of troops in future deployments.

The study presented in this report developed from those discussions. The U.S. Department of Defense (DoD) sought an independent, external, and unbiased evaluation of its efforts regarding the protection of U.S. forces in four areas: (1) assessment of health risks during deployments in hostile environments, (2) technologies and methods for detection and tracking of exposures to a subset of harmful agents, (3) physical protection and decontamination, and (4) medical protection, health consequences and treatment, and medical record keeping. Studies that have addressed topics 1, 2, and 3 have been carried out concurrently by the Commission on Life Sciences and the Commission on Engineering and Technical Systems of the National Research Council.

The study presented here, carried out with staff support from the Medical Follow-up Agency of the Institute of Medicine, addresses the topics of medical protection, health consequences and treatment, and medical record keeping. The study team was charged with addressing the following:

> • Prevention of adverse health outcomes that could result from exposures to threats and risks including chemical warfare and biological warfare, infectious disease, psychological stress, heat and cold injuries, unintentional injuries;
> • Requirements for compliance with active duty retention standards;
> • Predeployment screening, physical evaluation, risk education for troops and medical personnel;
> • Vaccines and other prophylactic agents;
> • Improvements in risk communication with military personnel in order to minimize stress casualties among exposed, or potentially exposed personnel;
> • Improvements in the reintegration of all troops to the home environment;
> • Treatment of the health consequences of prevention failures, including battle injuries, disease and non-battle injury (DNBI), acute management, and long-term follow-up;
> • Surveillance for short- and long-term outcomes, to include adverse reproductive outcomes; and
> • Improvement in keeping medical records, perhaps using entirely new technology, in documenting exposures, treatment, tracking of individuals through the medical evacuation system, and health/administrative outcomes. (Statement of Task, Appendix B)

Within the breadth of this charge, the study team chose to emphasize areas in which greatest needs were evident from the lessons learned from the Gulf War and other recent deployments and to treat other areas (those areas where the study team believed that it had little to offer the military) less thoroughly. Since an important motivating force for the study was the health and reproductive concerns of veterans after the Gulf War, the study team chose to focus on the major challenges for prevention and data needs indicated by the health problems widely reported by deployed forces after the Gulf War and the efforts to better understand them.

What were the lessons of the Gulf War? Briefly, one of the lessons was that even in the absence of widespread acute casualties from battle, war takes its toll on human health and well-being long after the shooting or bombing stops. Although military preventive medicine programs have developed reasonably effective countermeasures against many of the discrete disease and non-battle injury hazards of deployment, they have not yet systematically addressed the medically unexplained symptoms seen not only after the Gulf War but also after major wars dating back at least to the Civil War. The health problems reported by veterans after the Gulf War also brought out two other major and interrelated needs for improvements in preventive care for deployed forces. One is for a health surveillance system with documentation so that health events in the field are noted and responded to. Closely allied is the need for an automated medical record that can provide information about a service member's health events over his or her service career and into civilian life after military service. These three topics of medically unexplained symptoms, medical surveillance, and medical record keeping form the critical areas of emphasis of the report.

Although the study team considered the service member's life cycle of recruitment, predeployment, deployment, and postdeployment to include separation from the service, the postdeployment period appeared to be a time when, in particular, additional effort could be crucial in attending to the health of the deployed forces. The report discusses needs and opportunities for improved surveillance, special focused health care, and assistance with reintegration into the home environment during this time.

Two other major issues emerged as the study group went about its work. One serious challenge to the protection of deployed U.S. forces is that of providing the National Guard and Reserve components with the preparation and health surveillance afforded the active-duty component. The reserves play an increasingly important role in military deployments. Yet, their lack of access to the military health care system while they are inactive places serious limitations on the routine health care that they receive and the ability to monitor their health status over both the short and long term after a deployment. This problem for the reserves highlights a challenge for many active-duty service members after they separate from military service. To the extent that they receive their health care in the civilian sector and not through the U.S. Department of Veterans Affairs (VA), the capture of any data on their health care is problematic, as is the concept of a true lifetime medical record as promised by President Clinton in 1997 (White House, 1997).

A second issue that the study team came to recognize as a serious concern was that although there have been encouraging changes in DoD policy with new emphasis on what is termed Force Health Protection, these changes have not yet been reflected in the structural and cultural changes that will be needed within the services and DoD so that they may carry out the laudable new policies. Effective application of an improved health surveillance system and an integrated computer-based patient record will require concerted leadership and coordination to prevent the inexorable tendency toward "stovepiping"—that is, the development or continuation of an array of independent task- or service-specific systems that cannot meet the current needs for information exchange and follow-up.

High-level leadership and coordination are also needed to effect changes in the way in which medically unexplained symptoms are addressed in military populations. Although the problem is not unique to the military, it is regularly seen in populations who have participated in major deployments and will likely be observed after future deployments. Efforts to intervene to try to prevent or ameliorate medically unexplained symptoms are needed, as are careful evaluations of these efforts and a related research program.

Need for additional high-level leadership and coordination for military public health and preventive medicine run counter to current momentum within DoD. The medical structure of DoD is focused on the delivery of health care and the operation of the Tri-Care program (the military health maintenance organization). The costs of the health care delivery system are enormous, and management of the health care delivery system has come to dominate the DoD's medical leadership. High-quality health care is crucial to recruitment and retention of good service members, but in the current environment, the practice of military preventive medicine and military medicine appears to compete very poorly for personnel, funding, and leadership resources.

Nevertheless, DoD has made considerable efforts in several areas relevant to this study since the Gulf War. An important step occurred in November 1998, when the National Science and Technology Council (NSTC) released a plan in response to a Presidential Review Directive (National Science and Technology Council, 1998). Developed by an interagency task force with representatives from DoD, VA, and the U.S. Department of Health and Human Services (DHHS), the plan is entitled, *A National Obligation: Planning for Health Preparedness for and Readjustment of the Military, Veterans, and Their Families after Future Deployments*. The plan describes many laudable goals related to health during deployments, record keeping, research, and health risk communication that the government should implement to better safeguard military forces. Taking those efforts into account, with this report the study team proposes additional and complementary strategies to more effectively address medically unexplained symptoms, medical surveillance, and medical record keeping for future deployments, as well as other aspects of prevention such as risk communication and reintegration. The report emphasizes the need to extend medical surveillance and record keeping and other protections to the reserve components.

MEDICALLY UNEXPLAINED SYMPTOMS

Medically unexplained symptoms is the term used in this report to refer to symptoms that are not clinically explained by a medical etiology and that lead to use of the health care system. They are increasingly recognized as prevalent and persistent problems among civilian populations, in which they are associated with high levels of subjective distress and functional impairment with extensive use of health care services (Hyams, 1998; Engel and Katon, 1999). In military populations, similar medically unexplained symptom-based conditions have been observed after military conflicts dating back to the Civil War (Hyams et al., 1996) and are anticipated after future deployments (Presidential Advisory Committee on Gulf War Veterans' Illnesses, 1996b).

Clinicians and other persons working in medical surveillance must recognize that medically unexplained symptoms are just that; namely, there are no current explanations for them. Therefore, communicating the limits of modern medicine coupled with a compassionate approach to patients with medically unexplained symptoms is essential to the management of such patients. Until clear etiological factors are identified, the health care professional relies upon a body of knowledge about the management of these symptoms that has proven to be effective in many cases. Although a program of primary prevention is not feasible given the current state of knowledge, enough is known to recommend the implementation of a secondary prevention strategy. Good clinical evidence indicates that medically unexplained symptoms are much harder to treat and ameliorate once they have become chronic. It is thus important to identify the patient with medically unexplained symptoms early, when there may be a greater opportunity to restore the patient to his or her previous level of function. Providers with the clinical skills needed for medical management of these patients can then work with them toward a mutually agreed upon set of therapeutic goals that include striving to cope with residual symptoms and rehabilitation in the absence of a definitive diagnosis.

Recommendations[1]

The study team recommends that the U.S. Department of Defense develop an improved strategy to address medically unexplained symptoms, involving education, detection, evaluation, mitigation, and research. (Recommendation 6-9[2])

- **Undertake a program of continuing education for military primary care providers to improve their clinical ability to diagnose, treat, and communicate with patients with medically unexplained symptoms.** Incorporate the topic into the curricula of military graduate medical education programs such as the Uniformed Services University of the Health Sciences and the service schools for medical personnel. To the extent possible, make information about medically unexplained symptoms available and accessible to service members and to civilian health care providers for members of the reserves.
- **Carry out a pilot program to identify service members in the early stages of development of medically unexplained symptoms through the use of routinely administered self-report questionnaires (examples are noted in Chapter 6) and through informed primary care providers.**
- **Evaluate the efficacy of the pilot secondary prevention and treatment program, including the ability of screening questionnaires to detect early stages of medically unexplained symptoms.**
- **Treat medically unexplained symptoms in the primary care setting whenever possible, with referral to more intensive programs as necessary.**
- **Carry out a research program with prospective studies to assess the role of predisposing, precipitating, and perpetuating fac-**

---

[1]Because of the large number of recommendations in this report, a subset are presented in this Executive Summary.

[2]Recommendation 6-9 is Recommendation 9 in Chapter 6.

tors in medically unexplained symptoms. As feasible, involve academic health centers in the research efforts.

MEDICAL SURVEILLANCE

The military has launched many medical or health surveillance initiatives in the last several years in response to the problems highlighted by the Gulf War illnesses. Pre- and postdeployment questionnaires and blood draws, periodic health assessments, baseline health surveys for recruits, and improved systems for the tracking of inpatient and ambulatory care visits during deployments have all been planned or implemented to various degrees.

The multiplicity of medical surveillance-related tools that have developed reflects a genuine effort on the part of DoD and the individual services to better track and document the health of deployed forces. However, with no central authority for military public health, the tools lack coordination as part of an overall plan for achieving public health goals.

Recommendation

Clarify leadership authority and accountability for coordination of preventive medicine and environmental and health surveillance across the U.S. Department of Defense and the individual services. (Recommendation 4-16)

Part of the work of such a body would be to coordinate and potentially consolidate the surveillance tools referred to above, such as the Recruit Assessment Program to gather baseline data from incoming recruits, the Health Evaluation and Assessment Review (HEAR) and other sources of pre- and postdeployment self-reported health status data, surveillance systems for use during deployments, exposure assessment and environmental surveillance measures, and laboratory-based surveillance. Since these tools and systems were developed independently, they do not necessarily work toward shared purposes. The study team makes the following recommendations in considering these surveillance tools as part of an armamentarium of surveillance means.

Recommendations
(additional recommendations are in Chapter 4)

- **The Recruit Assessment Program should be implemented to collect baseline health data from all recruits (active-duty, National Guard, and Reserve), and should be periodically reassessed and revised in light of its goals. Its data should be used prospectively to**

test hypotheses about predisposing factors for the development of disease, injury, and medically unexplained symptoms. (Recommendation 4-1)

• **Annually administer an improved Health Evaluation and Assessment Review (HEAR) to reserve as well as to active-duty personnel to obtain baseline health information. Refine the Health Evaluation and Assessment Review by drawing on additional survey instrument and subject matter expertise.** (See full Recommendations 4-2a and 4-2b.)

• **Reinforce the laboratory capability for public health surveillance within the military. Mandate central reporting of laboratory findings of reportable conditions.** Continue to provide increased resources to overseas laboratories for surveillance in regions of military interest. (See full Recommendation 4-6.)

• **Discontinue pre- and postdeployment health (versus readiness) questionnaires unless they are warranted for military reasons other than gathering baseline and postdeployment health status information.** (See full Recommendation 4-7.)

• **As quickly as possible, implement a deployment disease and non-battle injury surveillance system that is integrated with the patient care information system and that automatically reports information to a central medical command.** Continue efforts to capture data at the individual level as well as at aggregate levels during deployments. (See full Recommendation 4-8.)

• **Integrate the efforts of environmental surveillance, preventive medicine, clinical, and information technology personnel to ensure the inclusion of medically relevant environmental and other exposures in the individual medical record.** (Recommendation 4-9)

Given the experiences after the Vietnam and Gulf wars, the postdeployment period is crucial for carrying out medical surveillance and providing appropriate care for returning service members. The Veterans Benefits Improvement Act of 1998 (P.L. 105-368) provides that service members will be eligible for medical care for a period of 2 years after their return from service in a theater of combat operations during a period of war or hostilities. The provision of this care without the need for establishing service-connection provides a valuable opportunity to ascertain the health needs of this population, including those related to medically unexplained symptoms. Rather than naming a special deployment-specific registry, veterans should be able to receive care as needed from the designated sources. It will be important to determine who uses this care and how well data surrounding this care can be captured from DoD and VA providers and their contractors. To gather postdeployment health status information from a more representative sample of veterans after deployments, a self-report survey could be used.

Recommendations

- **Carry out studies to evaluate the data captured from the 2 years of care provided after a deployment.** Try to determine the extent to which the data are representative of the population of service members who deployed and whether they could be used to indicate the health of service members after a deployment. (Recommendation 4-10)
- **Annually administer Health Evaluation and Assessment Review (HEAR) to a representative sample of service members who have been separated from the service for 2 to 5 years after a major deployment to track health status and identify health concerns including medically unexplained symptoms.** Also administer the HEAR to those separated service members who seek health care during the 2 years after a deployment. Evaluate the validity and usefulness of the information collected. (Recommendation 4-11)
- **Avoid whenever possible the creation of deployment-specific registries. Depend, instead, on the data provided by routine medical care under the Veterans Benefits Improvement Act of 1998 (P.L. 105-368) and the annual Health Evaluation and Assessment Review.** (Recommendation 4-12)

POSTDEPLOYMENT REINTEGRATION

The changing demographics of deployed forces, increased operational tempo, and increased reliance on the reserve component bring heightened needs for support services for service members and their families both during and after deployments. It is crucial that service members returning from deployments have seamless access to health care and support services and be made aware of the resources available to them. Since the Gulf War, the service components have made progress in providing support services to service members and families during reintegration, but the programs have not been adequately evaluated.

Recommendations

- **Planning and operational documents for military deployments should be required to include plans for supporting the return and reintegration of active-duty and reserve service members involved in the deployment and should specify the strategies that should be used to address anticipated problems, the resources needed to carry them out, and proposals for how the resources will be made available.** (See full Recommendation 7-1.)
- **Carry out research into the needs of service members and their families during deployments and upon reintegration into the**

home environment. Use the findings to reevaluate programs and policies. (See full Recommendation 7-3.)

MEDICAL RECORD KEEPING

Previous studies have cited deficiencies in medical record keeping as a major impediment to understanding and treating the health effects associated with deployment to the Gulf War (Institute of Medicine, 1996a; Presidential Advisory Committee on Gulf War Veterans' Illnesses, 1996b). The study team and other health information experts consider the computer-based patient record essential for DoD to meet the health care needs of service members before, during, and after deployments. In 1996, the Presidential Advisory Committee on Gulf War Veterans' Illnesses directed the NSTC to develop an interagency plan to address health preparedness for and readjustment of veterans and families after future conflicts and peacekeeping missions (Presidential Advisory Committee on Gulf War Veterans' Illnesses, 1996b). NSTC subsequently recommended that DoD "implement a fully integrated computer-based patient record available across the entire spectrum of health care delivery over the lifetime of the patient" (National Science and Technology Council, 1998, p. 23). To serve the military health system needs, the computer-based patient record (CPR) system must meet several needs simultaneously:

1. provide access to an individual's health data anytime and anywhere that care is required,
2. support record keeping for the administration of preventive health services,
3. facilitate real-time medical surveillance of deployed forces and timely medical surveillance of the total force,
4. provide comprehensive databases that support outcomes studies and epidemiological studies, and
5. maintain longitudinal health records of service members beginning with recruitment and extending past the time of discharge from the military.

During the course of the study, the team heard briefings on several military health information system projects. In general, each need for health data has been addressed by a separate data-gathering activity at the individual service level. No central oversight authority common to all three services was apparent to ensure that independent efforts are coordinated or, better yet, consolidated into a single activity that serves the needs of all three services. The military health system has adopted a "best of breed" approach, in which task-specific software applications are interfaced together. This strategy takes advantage of multiple niche products, but it presents a significant challenge to the integration of data because of the lack of a common data model or a common database. To the extent possible, the needs of all three services should be considered concurrently to maximize the reuse of data and software programs.

In addition to the development of technical plans for data integration, organizational plans need to be developed to standardize policies and practices related to medical record keeping. Currently, guidelines for medical record documentation vary on the basis of the type of data involved (e.g., outpatient, inpatient, and immunization information), the location of the service member (e.g., garrison, deployed, and location of deployment), and the branch of service. Policies, procedures, and practices should be standardized to store consistent and comprehensive data in the computer-based patient record (CPR) throughout the military.

Recommendations
(additional recommendations are in Chapter 5)

- **Clarify leadership authority and accountability for establishment of an integrated approach to the development, implementation, and evaluation of information system applications across the military services. Establish a top-level technical oversight committee responsible for approving all architectural decisions and ensuring that all application component selections meet architecture and data standards requirements.** (Recommendation 5-1)
- **Coordinate the evaluation of information needs for maximum reuse of data elements, data-gathering instruments (e.g., surveys), and software systems across the military health system.** (See full Recommendation 5-2.)
- **Develop standard enterprisewide policies and procedures for comprehensive medical record keeping that support the information needs of those involved with individual care, medical surveillance, and epidemiologic studies.** (Recommendation 5-3)
- **Develop methods to gather and analyze retrievable, electronically stored health data on reservists.** (See full Recommendation 5-6.)

There are many challenges to the development, implementation, and maintenance of a health information system to serve the diverse needs of the military. It is not surprising that there are separate activities in each of the services. In some cases these separate activities are driven by immediate needs, and in other cases they arise out of a lack of awareness of existing solutions or projects under way elsewhere. To meet the needs of U.S. forces deployed abroad, however, a unified CPR system is essential. The study team recommends that a comprehensive review of the military health information systems strategy be undertaken to enumerate the information needs; define an expedient process for development of an enterprisewide technical architecture, common data model, and data standards; identify critical dependencies; establish realistic time lines; assess the adequacy of resources; and perform a realistic risk assessment with contingency plans.

The process of developing an integrated CPR for the military health care system is complex yet essential to ensuring military readiness and a healthy force. It involves a tremendous expenditure of money and resources and requires extensive expertise. With so much at stake, the study team recommends that an external advisory board participate in the effort by providing ongoing review and advice regarding the military health information systems strategy. Composed of members of academia and industry, this group would provide synergy and potential leverage between the military and civilian sectors in information systems. The study team believes that this partnership will increase the likelihood of success of the overall endeavor.

Recommendations

Conduct an independent risk assessment of the military health information systems strategy and implementation plan. Establish an external advisory board that reports to the Secretary of Defense and that is composed of members of academia, industry, and government organizations other than the Department of Defense and the Department of Veterans Affairs to provide ongoing review and advice regarding the military health information system's strategy and implementation. (Recommendation 5-4)

Given the mandatory nature of medical data collection in the military, including sensitive information (e.g., human immunodeficiency virus infection status and mental health status), stringent regulations, policies, and procedures are necessary to maintain system security and protect the confidential medical information of all service members and their dependents.

Recommendation

Make available to service members the regulations, policies, and procedures regarding system security and protection of individually identifiable health information for each service member. (See full Recommendation 5-7.)

RISK COMMUNICATION

Risk communication has come to describe a process of concerted information and opinion exchange among individuals, groups, and institutions (National Research Council, 1989). The study team believes that a clear commitment to improvements in risk communication is needed from DoD. Responsibility should be designated to attempt a change in the culture within DoD and the military services so that dialogue and exchange about risks are facilitated at all levels. Aspects of risk communication need to be incorporated into the training programs for line commanders and health care providers. Furthermore, discussion is needed within DoD and the services about what problems the tool of risk communication may be used to try to solve. Such a discussion can lead to goals for reducing those problems and means of evaluation and improvement.

The risk communication efforts associated with the vaccination against anthrax, the risk communication goal articulated in Presidential Review Directive 5, the guide developed in response to recommendations from earlier independent advisory bodies, and the *Comprehensive Risk Communication Plan for Gulf War Veterans* (Persian Gulf Veterans Coordinating Board, 1999) are encouraging signs that the importance of risk communication has been acknowledged within some quarters at DoD. An additional indication of commitment to a cultural change throughout the entire system is needed from the top.

Recommendation

Although responsibility for risk communication must permeate all levels of command, the U.S. Department of Defense (DoD) should designate and provide resources to a group within DoD that is given primary responsibility for developing and implementing a plan to achieve the risk communication goal articulated in the National Science and Technology Council's Presidential Review Directive 5. (Recommendation 6-1) **Such a plan should**

- **Involve service members, their families, and outside experts in developing an explicit set of risk communication topics and goals. In other words, decide what information people need to know and when they need to know it.**
- **Consider how to deliver the information, including the intensity of communication needed for different types of risks. Some topics will necessitate full, ongoing dialogue between the involved parties, whereas others will require less extensive efforts. Incorporate procedures to evaluate the success of risk communication efforts and use these evaluations to revise the communication plan as needed.**
- **Include a response plan to anticipate the inevitable appearance of new risks or health concerns among deployed forces. The plan should include a process for gathering and disseminating information (both about the risks themselves and about the concerns of the troops) and for evaluating how communications about these issues are received and understood by service members and their families.**
- **Educate communicators, including line officers and physicians, in relevant aspects of risk communication.**

- **Carry out the interagency applied research program described in Presidential Review Directive 5, Strategy 5.1.2.**

RESERVES

Several of the most important components of a strategy to protect the health of deployed forces (improved medical surveillance and care that is responsive to medically unexplained symptoms, record keeping, risk communication, the use of preventive measures, and reintegration into the home environment) pose particular challenges for the reserve component because of their quasicivilian status and geographically dispersed situation. Since the Ready Reserve now constitutes almost half of the total force and is a significant component of deployed forces, the needs of the reserves cannot be ignored or postponed. Although their special circumstances make it impossible to mandate a health protection strategy identical to that for the active-duty forces, a coherent strategy should be developed to provide similar programs working toward the same ends that are provided with adequate resources.

Recommendation

Include the reserves in the planning, coordination, and implementation of improved health surveillance, record keeping, and risk communication. Develop a strategy for the reserve forces that takes into consideration their limited access to the military health care system before and after deployments but that recognizes their particular needs for health protection and that provides adequate resources to meet those needs. (See full Recommendation 8-1.)

CONCLUSIONS

Since the Gulf War, DoD has demonstrated much greater awareness of the importance of medical surveillance and record keeping in protecting the health of its deployed forces. It has launched or planned a variety of initiatives to address acknowledged shortcomings in these areas. These efforts suffer from a lack of the concerted planning required for efficient use of systems and resources. For medical surveillance this might be addressed with leadership and coordination in the area of military public health. With medical record keeping, outside expert review is needed to provide ongoing input into the challenging effort of implementing a successful CPR for the military.

The medically unexplained symptoms reported by veterans after the Gulf War have motivated many of DoD's constructive changes in medical surveillance and medical record keeping, but these initiatives cannot be anticipated to prevent them after future deployments. Indeed, it is not yet known how medically unexplained symptoms can be prevented. Better medical surveillance and record keeping can lay the foundation so that similar questions can be more readily answered in the future, however, and permit better insights into questions of etiology. The study team urges a research effort to obtain a better understanding of predisposing, precipitating, and perpetuating factors for these conditions. In the meantime, steps should be taken to identify those suffering from medically unexplained symptoms and intervene with management and treatment of symptoms to mitigate them and prevent chronicity. The efficacies of these steps should be evaluated.

1

Introduction

Nine years after Operations Desert Shield and Desert Storm (the Gulf War) ended in June 1991, uncertainty and questions remain about illnesses reported in a substantial percentage of the 697,000 service members who were deployed. Even though it was a short conflict with very few battle casualties, the events that occurred during the Gulf War and the experiences of the ensuing years have made clear many potentially instructive aspects of the deployment and its hazards. Since the Gulf War, several other large deployments have also occurred, including deployments to Haiti and Somalia. Major deployments to Bosnia, Southwest Asia, and, most recently, Kosovo, are ongoing as this report is written. This report draws on lessons learned from some of these deployments to consider strategies for improved preventive measures to protect the health of troops in future deployments.

By the spring of 1996, at least six different expert panels had reviewed or were in the process of reviewing various aspects of the illnesses reported by Gulf War veterans or programs developed in response to the illnesses (National Institutes of Health Technology Assessment Workshop Panel, 1994; U.S. Department of Defense, 1994b; Institute of Medicine, 1996a; Institute of Medicine, 1996c; Presidential Advisory Committee on Gulf War Veterans' Illnesses, 1996b; U.S. Department of Veterans Affairs, 1996). Deputy Secretary of Defense John White met with leadership of the National Research Council and the Institute of Medicine to explore the idea of an independent, proactive effort to learn from lessons of the Gulf War and to develop a strategy to better protect the health of troops in future deployments.

The study presented in this report developed from those discussions. The U.S. Department of Defense (DoD) (acronyms used in this report are found in front of the Table of Contents) sought an independent, external, and unbiased evaluation of its efforts regarding the protection of U.S. forces in four areas: (1)

assessment of health risks during deployments in hostile environments, (2) technologies and methods for detection and tracking of exposures to a subset of harmful agents, (3) physical protection and decontamination, and (4) medical protection, health consequences and treatment, and medical record keeping. Studies that have addressed topics 1, 2, and 3 have been carried out concurrently by the Commission on Life Sciences and the Commission on Engineering and Technical Systems of the National Research Council, and have resulted in three companion reports (National Research Council, 1999a,b,c).

The study presented here, carried out with staff support from the Medical Follow-up Agency of the Institute of Medicine, addresses the topics of medical protection, health consequences and treatment, and medical record keeping. The charge to the study team was included in the contract between the Department of Defense and the National Academies and became central to the Statement of Task:

> The [*overall*] project will advise DOD on a long-term strategy for protecting the health of our nation's military personnel when deployed to unfamiliar environments. Drawing on the lessons of previous conflicts, it will advise the DOD with regard to a strategy for managing the health and exposure issues faced during deployments: these include infectious agents, vaccines, drug interactions, and stress. It also will include adverse reactions to chemical or biological warfare agents and other substances. The project will address the problem of limited and variable data in the past, and in the development of a prospective strategy for improved handling of health and exposure issues in future deployments.
>
> This study concerns medical protection, health consequences and treatment, and medical record keeping. Specific issues to be addressed include:
>
> Prevention of adverse health outcomes that could result from exposures to threats and risks including chemical warfare and biological warfare, infectious disease, psychological stress, heat and cold injuries, unintentional injuries;
>
> Requirements for compliance with active duty retention standards;
>
> Pre-deployment screening, physical evaluation, risk education for troops and medical personnel;
>
> Vaccine and other prophylactic agents;
>
> Improvements in risk communication with military personnel in order to minimize stress casualties among exposed, or potentially exposed personnel;
>
> Improvements in the reintegration of all troops to the home environment;
>
> Treatment of the health consequences of prevention failures, including battle injuries, disease and non-battle injury (DNBI), acute management, and long-term follow-up;
>
> Surveillance for short- and long-term outcomes, to include adverse reproductive outcomes; and
>
> Improvement in keeping medical records, perhaps using entirely new technology, in documenting exposures, treatment, tracking of individuals through the

medical evacuation system, and health/administrative outcomes. (Statement of Task, Appendix B)

EMPHASIS AND IMPLICIT ASSUMPTIONS

The charge to the study team is very broad. Its different specific components roughly include all of military preventive medicine. With this broad scope, the study team members chose to emphasize areas in which they saw the greatest needs or needs of a systemic nature and to treat other areas with a necessarily broader brush. A brief review of many of the risks to the health of deployed forces is found in Chapter 2. Since an important motivating force for the study was the health concerns of veterans following the Gulf War, the study team chose to focus on the major challenges for prevention and data needs pointed out by the health problems widely reported by deployed forces after the Gulf War and the efforts to better understand them.

What were the lessons of the Gulf War? Briefly, one of the lessons was that even in the absence of widespread acute casualties from battle, war takes its toll on human health and well-being long after the shooting or bombing stops. Although military preventive medicine programs have developed reasonably effective countermeasures against many of the discrete disease and non-battle injury hazards of deployment, they have not yet systematically addressed the medically unexplained symptoms seen not only after the Gulf War but also after major wars dating back at least to the Civil War. Medically unexplained symptoms are described and discussed in Chapter 3.

The health problems reported by veterans after the Gulf War also brought out two other major and interrelated needs for improvements in preventive care for deployed forces. One is for a health surveillance system with documentation so that health events in the field are noted and responded to. This is discussed in Chapter 4. Closely allied is the need for an automated medical record that can provide information about a service member's health events over his or her service career and into civilian life after military service. Chapter 5 discusses DoD plans for electronic medical record keeping.

Although the study team considered the service member's life cycle of recruitment, predeployment, deployment, and postdeployment to include separation from the service, the postdeployment period appeared to be a time when, in particular, additional effort could be crucial in attending to the health of the deployed forces. The report discusses needs and opportunities for improved surveillance, special focused health care, and assistance with reintegration into the home environment during this time.

Two other major issues emerged as the study group went about its work. One serious challenge to the protection of deployed U.S. forces, discussed in Chapter 8, is that of providing the National Guard and Reserve components with the preparation for deployment and health surveillance afforded the active duty component. As active-duty forces have been reduced, the reserves play an increasingly important role in military deployments. Yet, their lack of access to the military health care system while they are inactive places serious limitations on the routine health care that they receive and the ability to monitor their health status over both the short and long term after a deployment. This problem for the reserves highlights a challenge for many active-duty service members after they separate from military service. To the extent that they receive their health care in the civilian sector and not through the U.S. Department of Veterans Affairs (VA), the capture of any data on their health care is problematic, as is the concept of a true lifetime medical record promised by the President in 1997 (White House, Office of the Press Secretary, 1997).

A second issue that the study team came to recognize as a serious concern was that although there have been encouraging changes in DoD policy with new emphasis on what is termed Force Health Protection, these changes have not yet been reflected in the structural and cultural changes that will be needed within the services (the Army, Navy, and Air Force; the Marines are a part of the Navy, and the Coast Guard is part of the Navy only in wartime) and DoD so that they may carry out the laudable new policies. Effective application of an improved health surveillance system (Chapter 4) and integrated computer-based patient record (Chapter 5) will require concerted leadership and coordination to prevent the inexorable tendency toward "stovepiping"—that is, the development or continuation of an array of independent tasks or service-specific systems that cannot meet the current needs for information exchange and follow-up.

High-level leadership and coordination are also needed to effect changes in the way in which medically unexplained symptoms are addressed in military populations. Although the problem is not unique to the military, it is regularly seen in populations who have participated in major deployments and will likely be observed after future deployments. Efforts to intervene to try to prevent or ameliorate medically unexplained symptoms are needed, as are careful evaluations of these efforts and a related research program. The needs in this area are further described in Chapter 6.

Need for additional high-level leadership and coordination for military public health and preventive medicine run counter to the current momentum within DoD. The medical structure of DoD is focused on the delivery of health care and the operation of the Tri-Care program (the military health maintenance organization). The costs of the health care delivery system are enormous, and management of the health care delivery system has come to dominate DoD's medical leadership. High-quality health care is crucial to recruitment and retention of good service members, but in the current environment, the practice of military preventive medicine and military medicine appears to compete very poorly for personnel, funding, and leadership resources.

RELATED EFFORTS

As the study took place, several relevant efforts were under way at DoD and VA. In response to recommendations from the Presidential Advisory Committee on Gulf War Veterans' Illnesses, an interagency task force with representatives from DoD, VA, and the U.S. Department of Health and Human Services prepared a plan to protect the health of service members and their families. Released in November 1998, the plan, entitled *A National Obligation: Planning for Health Preparedness for and Readjustment of the Military, Veterans, and Their Families after Future Deployments*, articulated many goals that the study team found laudable (National Science and Technology Council, 1998). The document is referred to several times throughout the report, frequently with the hope that the strategies described to meet the goals stated in the plan are actually implemented.

As the present study was under way, the U.S. Congress passed legislation that required the VA to contract with the National Academies to carry out a critical review of their proposed plan for a National Center for War-Related Illnesses. Presumably, such a center would coordinate research related to several of the areas of focus in this report. DoD has also recently named several of its research institutions as centers for clinical and epidemiologic studies of war-related illnesses. Finally, a recent DoD Broad Agency Announcement invited proposals for research related to war-related illnesses (Commerce Business Daily, 1999).

STUDY PROCESS AND INFORMATION SOURCES

The study presented in this report was led by two principal investigators: an infectious disease specialist and a psychiatrist. To provide additional breadth of expertise to match the breadth of the charge to the study, a panel of expert advisors was convened. Members of the panel had expertise in the fields of medical record keeping, epidemiology, reproductive health, toxicology, infectious diseases and vaccines, psychology, psychiatry, chemical warfare agents, risk communication, biomedical ethics, and neurobiology.

The principal investigators and advisors (the study team) gathered information through several means. Four public workshops and a discussion meeting were held to collect relevant information. At the workshops, members of the military services, DOD, and representatives of other relevant agencies such as VA provided briefings and participated in discussions about ongoing and planned programs related to protecting the health of deployed forces. Outside (non-military) experts were also invited to provide relevant information from the civilian sector. The information provided in workshop presentations and discussions formed an important basis of this report. The dates and agendas from these workshops, including names and affiliations of speakers, are provided in Appendixes D and E, respectively.

The study team sought additional inputs from experts through commissioned papers. Focused questions related to various study topics were directed to 11 distinguished people who wrote background papers for the study team. The papers served as useful bases for the workshop discussions and study team considerations. These papers and their authors and affiliations are listed in Appendix F. One paper in particular was integral to the evolution of the report. Chapter 3 draws much of its information from that paper, which is included as a signed contribution in Appendix A. Institute of Medicine staff gathered journal articles, DoD documents, and material from the World Wide Web and other sources to supplement information from the workshops and commissioned papers. Finally, Institute of Medicine staff gathered information and carried out a literature review to augment the information available to the study team on the topic of reintegration into the home environment.

THE FUTURE MILITARY

Joint Vision 2010 is a document prepared by the Joint Chiefs of Staff in 1996 to describe the nature of warfare envisioned in the near future (U.S. Department of Defense, 1996b). Revised operational concepts of dominant maneuver, precision engagement, focused logistics, and full-dimensional protection provide a framework for planning in the future. At the foundation of the vision are quality forces who are better trained and more highly skilled than they were in the past. Active and passive protection measures are anticipated to provide better protection against opponents at all echelons. At the same time, service members will use higher-technology equipment to carry out their missions. Forces will be increasingly dispersed and mobile, with less continuous support from a smaller logistics "footprint" (the size of the deployed presence). The document notes a first priority of recruiting and retaining dedicated high-quality people. For reserve components, less startup time between employment and deployment is anticipated, with the need for rapid integration into joint operations.

The implications of this vision for strategies to protect the health of deployed forces are several. The deployment of smaller, more mobile units means that each service member is more crucial to the success of the mission, but fewer medical resources are available to him or her. Preventive tools will be crucial for the prevention of disease and injury.

Accordingly, this report focuses on prevention measures for future deployments. Lessons learned from the past and from public health suggest that surveillance coupled with record keeping will be crucial. Medical surveillance permits the identification of problems and opportunities for intervention, and the associated record keeping permits additional benefit from retrospective analysis. Coupled with these, research and intervention efforts directed towards medically unexplained symptoms will provide important tools for the future military.

2

Risks to Deployed Forces

War by its nature is a tremendously hazardous endeavor. Clearly, it entails risks to life and limb from weapons and battle. At least up through World War I, however, non-battle-related disease and injury have taken an even greater toll upon the health of deployed forces than have battle injuries (Garfield and Neugut, 1997).

The non-combat-related risks to deployed forces include an array of different threats to health. Infectious diseases, non-battle-related injuries, injuries from heat and cold exposures, and psychological stress have been large contributors to casualties in war after war. Chemical and biological weapons are increasingly seen as threats to deployed forces, as are environmental contaminants and toxic industrial chemicals.

The military has responded to these threats with military medical research programs and the subsequent implementation of doctrine and protective measures that have reduced the impacts of disease and non-battle injury (DNBI) to the very low levels observed in Operations Desert Shield and Desert Storm (the Gulf War) and in Bosnia. Many infectious disease threats have largely been eliminated by use of vaccines, prophylactic drugs, vector control, insect repellents, and protected food and water supplies. Improved clothing, footwear, and military doctrine have greatly reduced the impacts of injuries from heat and cold exposures. The strategies now in place for countering the traditional acute diseases and injury threats to military operations are fundamentally sound. This report has addressed these traditional concerns of military medicine in a very limited fashion and focused on improved medical surveillance to better assess and respond to traditional and emerging threats, record keeping to permit appropriate care and retrospective analysis, and the complex issue of medically unexplained symptoms in returning service members.

INFECTIOUS DISEASES

Throughout history infectious diseases have been the single greatest threat to the health of those involved in military operations. Epidemics of contagious diseases such as influenza, food- and waterborne illnesses such as hepatitis, typhoid fever, and shigellosis, and vector-borne diseases such as typhus, yellow fever, malaria, and dengue have caused entire armies to become militarily ineffective (Zinsser, 1935). Tropical and subtropical regions have been especially hazardous because of vector-borne diseases. As recently as the Vietnam War, infectious diseases took a heavy toll on the U.S. military population. Disease was listed as the cause of 56 to 74 percent of active-duty Army patient admissions to hospitals in Vietnam from 1965 to 1970 (Ognibene, 1982). Until 1967, the total number of lost days of duty by active-duty Army personnel initially admitted for medical care from DNBI outpaced those from battle injury. From 1968 to 1970, DNBI contributed nearly half of the lost days of duty (Ognibene, 1982).

Because infectious disease has long been recognized as a serious threat, the military has, through painful lessons, developed effective strategies to address these threats. At least in the most recent declared war, the Gulf War, the strategies used to reduce risks from infectious disease and severe climate proved successful. In contrast to previous experiences, infectious diseases were not a major cause of lost personnel, even though many infectious diseases that pose serious health threats are endemic to the region of deployment (Hyams et al., 1995).

Although diarrheal disease was common during the rapid buildup of Gulf War troops from August to September 1990, the majority of troops experienced mild traveler's-type diarrhea that resolved spontaneously (Hyams et al., 1995). Gastroenteritis rates also dropped dramatically when fresh produce was eliminated from troops' diets (Hyams et al., 1995). No cases of sandfly fever were observed in Gulf War troops, and only seven cases of malaria were reported, and these were among troops who had crossed into southern Iraq. Twelve cases of visceral leishmaniasis and 20 cases of cutaneous leishmaniasis were diagnosed. In general, careful control of the water and food supplies, inspection of food preparation facilities, and use of insecticides and medical prophylaxes through immunizations seem to have been good defenses against infectious disease. This protection was facilitated by the isolation of the troops and the fact that most troops were deployed during the cold winter months, when sandfly and other arthropod activity is limited.

Infectious diseases remain among the serious threats to deployed military forces. Although the military has exerted tremendous effort in countering these threats and understands them well, the ever-changing and evolving nature of infectious diseases will require continued vigilance and development of preventive methods. Multidrug-resistant malaria, increasingly widespread dengue epidemics, hantavirus infections, and other hemorrhagic fevers are among the current diseases that may be encountered during future deployments, for which vaccines are not available, and against which complete protection may be difficult or impossible to achieve by current methods.

NON-BATTLE INJURIES

Non-battle injuries (injuries sustained in non-combat aspects of a deployment, such as in motor vehicles accidents and during training) have historically been a significant hazard for deployed troops. In past conflicts, rates of such injuries have frequently rivaled those from battle injuries and wounds (Table 2-1) (F. D. Jones, 1995b). In the Gulf War, 55 of the 65 non-battle-related deaths resulted from accidental injuries, including two helicopter crashes and an accident involving a light armored vehicle (Helmkamp, 1994).

Although total DNBI rates have fluctuated slightly between 5 and 10 per 100 soldiers per week during the major deployments in the last decade (Table 2-2), injury has been among the top contributors in all of these deployments. In the Gulf War, 18.4 percent of all DNBI were injuries, whereas in the Somalia and Bosnia deployments, 25.2 and 27 percent of DNBI were injuries (McKee et al, 1998; U.S. Army Center for Health Promotion and Preventive Medicine, 1998). In Southwest Asia since 1996, orthopedic injuries, both sports-related and other, have contributed 23.1 percent of DNBI cases (Thompson, 1999).

TABLE 2-1. Battle Injury and Wound Rates per 1,000 Troops per Year During Various U.S. Wars

War	Year	No. of Non-Battle-Related Injuries	No. of Battle-Related Injuries and Wounds
U.S. Civil War	1861–1865	—	97
World War I	1917–1918	—	238
World War II			
Pacific	1942–1945	122	39
Europe	1942–1945	101	108
Mediterranean	1942–1945	131	80
Korea	1950	242	460
	1951	151	170
	1952	102	57
Vietnam	1965	67	62
	1966	76	75
	1967	69	84
	1968	70	120
	1969	63	87

SOURCE: F. D. Jones, 1995b.

TABLE 2-2. Average Disease and Non-Battle Injury (DNBI) Rates for Recent Deployments

Deployment	Service	Person-weeks	Rate (%/week)
Operation Desert Shield/ Storm (Gulf War)[a]	Army	1,242,300	5.8
Operation Desert Shield/ Storm (Gulf War)[a]	Marine Corps	787,310	6.5
Somalia[a]	Tri-Service	163,093	10.6
Operation Joint Endeavor (1995–1996)[a]	Tri-Service	495,528	7.1
Operation Joint Guard (1997)[a]	Tri-Service	453,002	8.1
Southwest Asia Operations (1996–)[b]	Tri-Service	1,576,738	5.2
Operation Allied Force (1999)[b]	Air Force	63,483	8.1

SOURCES: [a]McKee et al., 1998; U.S. Army Center for Health Promotion and Preventive Medicine, 1998; McKee, 1999. [b]Thompson, 1999. Data are as of May, 1999.

Military rates of hospitalization for injuries, independent of deployments, are quite high and well above the goal specified in *Healthy People 2000* (Bray et al., 1999; Public Health Service, 1991). The high rates have recently prompted interest from the Injury Prevention and Control Work Group of the Armed Forces Epidemiologic Board. The group identified sports-related injuries, motor vehicle-related injuries, and falls or jumps as major causes of hospitalization for injury among military personnel and recommended research focused upon prevention (Injury Prevention and Control Work Group, 1996).

Heat and Cold Injuries

Injuries from exposure to heat, cold, and other environmental factors can constitute important components of non-battle injuries. Injuries that occur as a result of exposure to excessive heat include heat rash, sunburn, heat cramps, heat exhaustion, and heat stroke. They made up less than 1 percent of DNBI during the Gulf War deployment, 2.3 percent during the Somalia deployment, and less than 1 percent during the Bosnia operations (U.S. Army Center for Health Promotion and Preventive Medicine, 1998; McKee et al., 1998). In Southwest Asia Operations, they have contributed roughly 1 percent of overall DNBI cases since 1996 (Thompson, 1999). Commanders have the most critical role in prevention of heat injuries through enforcement of physical fitness requirements, heat acclimation procedures, work and rest schedules, the appropriate use of clothing and equipment, and adherence to proper nutrition (U.S. Army

Research Institute of Environmental Medicine and Walter Reed Army Institute of Research, 1994; Withers et al., 1994).

Among the many cold exposure-related injuries of military significance, trenchfoot, frostbite, and hypothermia are the most common in the military. Although injuries due to cold exposures were not recorded in detail until World War I, historically, many U.S. Army personnel who were exposed to cold environments during a deployment experienced cold-related injuries. For example, 10 percent of the U.S. wounded Army personnel in both World War II and Korea suffered from cold-related injuries (Hamlet, 1987). Commanding officers of every Army unit were responsible for making sure that the soldiers wore dry socks, changed their shoes or boots regularly, rubbed their feet with animal fat at least once a day, and exercised their feet to provide proper circulation (Whayne and DeBakey, 1958). As with heat-related injuries, aggressive leadership will continue to be required for prevention of cold-related injuries in cold climates.

PSYCHOLOGICAL STRESS

Psychological stress is an important potential source of military casualties both during combat and in the years that follow. Especially since the Vietnam War it has been recognized that the stress accompanying combat can have both acute and chronic effects. Acute or short-term stress reactions have gone by many names, as noted below. Posttraumatic stress disorder (PTSD) is the name formalized in 1980 for long-term reactions to war-zone exposure (American Psychiatric Association, 1980).

Acute psychiatric casualties were first recognized as a significant source of personnel loss in battle in World War I. Most neuropsychiatric casualties in World War I were given the popular label "shell shock." By 1917, one-seventh of all discharges for disability from the British Army had been due to mental conditions. Of 200,000 soldiers on the pension list of England, one-fifth suffered from war neurosis (Salmon, 1929). Soon, physicians discovered the importance of forward and rapid treatment, that is, that patients with war neuroses improved more readily when they were treated near the front and were more likely to improve if they were treated quickly (Salmon, 1929). Eventually, three principles became the critical elements of combat psychiatric casualty treatment: proximity, immediacy, and expectancy. The most effective procedure was found to be the treatment of the combat psychiatric casualty in a safe place as close to the battle scene as possible (*proximity*), as soon as possible (*immediacy*), and with explicit understanding that he was not ill and would soon be rejoining his comrades (*expectancy*) (Artiss, 1963). The treatment was to be simple, such as rest, food, and maybe a warm shower.

Once it became clear that shell shock was not caused by the concussion of shelling, "war neurosis" was used as the diagnosis for the acute psychiatric casualty in World War I. Eventually, medical personnel were told to identify such casualties as "N.Y.D. (nervous)," for "not yet diagnosed (nervous)," which did not suggest that it should be incapacitating or require hospital treatment. In World War II, the term "combat fatigue" came to be preferred (F. D. Jones, 1995a).

In World War II, planners operated on the belief that preinduction screening could minimize potential psychiatric casualties (Glass, 1966a). Draft registrants with any significant history of psychiatric disturbance, especially those with anxiety symptoms, were not selected for service. Soldiers who showed symptoms after induction were discharged. Manifestation of psychiatric symptoms provided an honorable way of avoiding induction, producing a massive loss of potential personnel (F. D. Jones, 1995a). Yet, even though the disqualification rate of registrants was about 7.6 times as high as that in World War I (1.6 million registrants were classified as unfit because of mental disease or educational deficiency in World War II), separation rates for psychiatric disorders were 2.4 times as high (Glass, 1966b).

In addition to proving to be ineffective in preventing breakdown, the liberal separation policy for those with neurotic symptoms led to major personnel losses. Glass (1966b) noted that in September 1943, more soldiers were being eliminated from the U.S. Army than were being brought in and most of those separated were for psychoneuroses (35.6/1,000/year). Military psychiatrists concluded that reliance on psychiatric screening was ineffective, with studies indicating more similarities than differences between acute psychiatric casualties and their fellow soldiers (Glass, 1973; F. D. Jones, 1995a).

Epidemiologic studies of World War II combat stress casualties indicated that they had a direct relationship to the intensity of combat and were modified by physical and morale factors (Beebe and DeBakey, 1952). A notable study by Beebe and Appel (1958) indicated a breaking point for the average rifleman in the Mediterranean Theater of Operation of 88 days of company combat—days in which the company sustained at least one casualty. Noy's review of that work found that psychiatric casualties had remained in combat duties longer than medical and disciplinary cases and that their breakdowns were related to exposure to battle trauma more than medical and disciplinary cases were (Noy, 1987).

The importance of group cohesion in possibly preventing and treating psychiatric breakdown was another lesson of World War II. In his summary of lessons learned in neuropsychiatry in World War II, Glass writes,

> Perhaps the most significant contribution of World War II military psychiatry was recognition of the sustaining influence of the small combat group or particular members thereof, variously termed "group identification," "group cohesiveness," "the buddy system," and "leadership." This was also operative in noncombat situations. Repeated observations indicated that the absence or inadequacy of such sustaining influences or their disruption during combat was mainly responsible for psychiatric breakdown in battle. These group or relationship phenomena explained marked differences in the psychiatric casualty rates of various units who were exposed to a similar intensity of battle stress. The frequency of psychiatric disorders seems to be more related to the characteristics of the group than to the character traits of the involved individuals. Thus, WWII clearly showed that interpersonal relationships and other social

> and situational circumstances were at least as important as personality configuration or individual assets and liabilities in the effectiveness of coping behavior. (Glass, 1973, p. 995)

The overall incidence of combat stress casualties in modern warfare has ranged from 10 to 25 percent of all combat casualties (Mareth and Brooker, 1985), but the incidence has been much higher in certain instances. In the 1973 Yom Kippur War, Israel suffered acute combat stress casualties at rates estimated to be from 30 to 50 percent (F. D. Jones, 1995a). The rate of combat stress casualties was highest among support personnel, probably responding to the trauma of seeing dead and mutilated comrades. In the 1982 Lebanon War, the rate of casualties from acute stress was estimated at 23 percent (F. D. Jones, 1995b).

The experiences of Vietnam veterans brought the first widespread recognition of delayed or chronic PTSD in deployed forces. People diagnosed with PTSD are characterized by symptoms of increased arousal, sudden reliving of a traumatic event through recurrent and intrusive recollections or dreams, and avoidance of stimuli associated with the trauma (American Psychiatric Association, 1994).

The National Vietnam Veterans Readjustment Study (NVVRS) was a comprehensive national study of the postwar psychological problems of Vietnam veterans, mandated by the U.S. Congress in P.L. 98-160 (Kulka et al., 1990). The study indicated that 15.2 percent of all male Vietnam theater veterans and 8.5 percent of female Vietnam theater veterans had current cases of PTSD. Among men and women with high levels of war-zone exposure, current PTSD was higher: 35.8 percent among men and 17.5 percent among women. An additional 11.1 percent of male and 7.8 percent of female veterans suffered from "partial PTSD"—symptoms that are of insufficient intensity or breadth to qualify as PTSD but that may still warrant professional attention. NVVRS analyses of the lifetime prevalence of PTSD indicated that almost one-third of male and more than one-fourth of women Vietnam theater veterans had PTSD at some time during their lives (Kulka et al., 1990).

Deployed populations in earlier wars also experienced the chronic effects of combat stress. Futterman and Pumpian-Mindlin (1951) reported a 10 percent prevalence of "war neurosis" in a series of 200 psychiatric patients seen in 1950. Another study observed "gross stress syndrome" in World War II veterans up to 20 years after combat (Archibald and Tuddenham, 1965). After PTSD was recognized in the 1980s, additional studies were carried out to assess PTSD in World War II and Korean War veterans. Although the prevalence of PTSD in older veterans is unknown, World War II veterans were similar to Vietnam veterans in their reactivity to stimuli reminiscent of their war trauma (Orr et al., 1993). An additional study indicated current PTSD prevalences of 37 percent among World War II veterans and 80 percent among Korean War veterans among those who had previously sought psychiatric treatment (Blake et al., 1990; Friedman et al., 1994). In a sample of 1,210 veterans of World War II and the Korean War, the prevalence of PTSD ranged from 0 to 12.4 percent depending on the PTSD measure (Spiro et al., 1994).

During the Gulf War, acute psychiatric casualties were rare. Only 6.5 percent of all medical evacuations from Southwest Asia during the Gulf War were classified as being for psychiatric reasons (Stretch et al., 1996). Since the Gulf War, many different studies have been carried out to estimate the prevalence of PTSD in various groups of Gulf War veterans, with a range of PTSD prevalence reported from 4 to 36 percent (Sutker et al., 1993; Wolfe et al., 1993) (several studies have been critiqued and summarized by Haley [1997]). A telephone survey of a large population-based sample of Gulf War veterans found that 1.9 percent reported symptoms of PTSD, whereas 0.8 percent of the military population deployed elsewhere during the same time reported symptoms of PTSD (Iowa Persian Gulf Study Group, 1997).

Military personnel on peacekeeping as well as combat deployments are at risk of long-term effects from psychological stress. A survey of a large cohort of military personnel deployed to Somalia for peacekeeping duty found that 8 percent met the diagnostic criteria for PTSD roughly 5 months after their return (Litz et al., 1997).

Even when deployment stress does not result in PTSD, it appears to result in increased levels of general psychological distress among deployed forces. Psychological symptom measures for samples of soldiers during deployments to operations in the Persian Gulf, Somalia, and Bosnia indicated that they had significantly elevated levels of psychological distress compared with those for non-deployed soldiers (Stuart and Halverson, 1997).

The deployment missions (combat, peacekeeping) themselves are not the only sources of stress for deployed military personnel. In a recent health survey of Department of Defense (DoD) personnel, the most frequently cited source of stress for both men and women was being away from family (reported by 19.5 percent of both men and women) (Bray et al., 1999). Chapter 7 discusses further some of the varied sources of stresses relating to deployment and separation from family as well as reintegration into the home environment.

Strategies for protecting forces from combat and deployment stress in future deployments must take into account the range of missions and environments that they will likely encounter. Clearly, these stresses cannot be eliminated, but some of their effects may be mitigated. High-intensity warfare, low-intensity warfare, peacekeeping, and humanitarian deployments each pose different challenges and mixes of psychological stressors (F. D. Jones, 1995c), so the preventive response requires flexibility, adaptability, and improvisation (Belenky and Martin, 1996a). As with other risks to the health of deployed troops, commanders must be aware of them and must be prepared to address and prevent them to the extent possible.

TOXIC INDUSTRIAL CHEMICALS

Historically, preventive measures for deployed forces have focused on the prevention of acute risks to health that will affect the mission. Growing awareness of the potential long-term risks posed by environmental and occupational exposures in the United States has been accompanied by recognition that such hazards may be present during military deployments as well. The burning of oil wells in Kuwait during the retreat of the Iraqi Army during the Gulf War made clear that local industrial sources can create hazards for deployed forces. Troops may be exposed to hazardous chemicals through inadequate environmental protection in the area of operations, industrial accidents, sabotage, or the intentional or unintentional actions of other forces (Life Systems Inc. and GeoCenters Inc. for U.S. Army Center for Environmental Health Research, 1997). Since military attention to these exposures is recent, their toll on deployed forces from previous wars is unknown. Improved environmental surveillance and exposure assessment are planned to provide a better understanding of the risks for deployed forces (National Research Council, 1999b). At the same time, improvements in medical surveillance and record keeping after deployments (discussed in Chapters 4 and 5) will be needed to note any long-term effects from environmental exposures.

CHEMICAL WEAPONS

The proliferation of chemical warfare capability among potential adversaries in recent years and the potential effects of chemical warfare agents on U.S. military forces are causes of serious concern. During future deployments, U.S. military forces are increasingly likely to confront opponents with chemical weapons capability. Other sections of this study (National Research Council, 1999a,b,c) address the overall threat and risk assessment and the capability of the military to detect the agents used in chemical weapons and to protect military personnel using avoidance, protective masks, and clothing. Potential exposure to chemical weapons will have medical consequences that must be recognized and managed even if protective measures are used appropriately and minimal or no acute casualties result. The combined effects of low-level exposures, whether suspected or confirmed, and the stress of dealing with a chemical attack will create a need for risk communication, intensive long-term surveillance, careful analysis of medical outcomes, and skillful medical management of the affected personnel.

BIOLOGICAL WEAPONS

Like chemical weapons, biological weapons are an increasing concern because of their intensive development by the former Soviet Union and Iraq and their proliferation to other potential adversaries. The list of potential agents includes bacteria such as those that cause anthrax, plague, and tularemia; viruses, such as smallpox and neurotropic alphaviruses; rickettsiae; and biologic toxins. Although protection against aerosols is afforded by current equipment (masks), the difficulty of detecting and identifying biologic agents in aerosols has limited the effectiveness of detection equipment (National Research Council, 1999b). For the foreseeable future DoD must rely heavily on prophylactic vaccines and drugs and must be prepared to deal with the long- and short-term medical effects experienced by casualties exposed to biological weapons. Immunization of all military personnel with the currently licensed anthrax vaccine has greatly reduced the threat of anthrax which has widely been regarded as the most effective and imminent biologic threat.

PROTECTIVE MEDICATIONS

Some of the potential risks to deployed forces include the protective medications themselves. Although protective medications are selected because they can help protect service members in dangerous environments, they can have risks of their own. In many cases, the benefits have been thoughtfully and thoroughly weighed against these risks. The use of DEET (diethyl *m*-toluamide) as a mosquito repellent is an example. DEET carries a slight risk of neurotoxicity when used at high doses and has been associated with rare deaths in susceptible people. It is considered safe enough for over-the-counter sale to civilians, however, and is far less hazardous to service members than mosquito bites in areas where malaria is endemic. One of the studies carried out concurrently with this study further addresses a framework for assessing risks to deployed forces (National Research Council, 1999a).

INTERACTIONS

In addition to the separate risks posed by each of the exposures described above, the potential for additive or synergistic effects of such exposures has become a source of concern. During deployments, military personnel are exposed to combinations of drugs, biologics, and chemicals to which civilians are not exposed. As in civilian settings, the health effects of exposures to these mixtures are poorly characterized, but the diversity and number of agents preclude testing of all possible combinations or the development of reliable predictors of all possible interactions that could result in increased toxicity (Institute of Medicine, 1996b). The Institute of Medicine Committee to Study the Interactions of Drugs, Biologics, and Chemicals in U.S. Military Forces included in its recommendations enhanced surveillance systems, a battery of experimental studies, and careful epidemiologic studies (Institute of Medicine, 1996b).

The risks described in this chapter are ones that have been recognized to various degrees by the military leadership and preventive medicine community. The next chapter discusses another aspect of health risks to deployed forces that is a particular focus of this study because it has not yet been addressed by the military with a prevention or mitigation strategy.

3

Medically Unexplained Symptoms

The hazards described in Chapter 2, such as infectious disease, psychological stress, chemical and biological warfare agents, and injuries, remain among the serious threats to deployed military forces. The military has exerted tremendous effort in countering these hazards through preventive medicine. Continued effort and an emphasis on preventive measures against these hazards are required, but the study team does not believe that it can provide additional expert advice about them.

In contrast, the experiences of the Gulf War and the illnesses reported in its wake point to an area where additional effort is needed: medically unexplained symptoms. Such symptoms are not new, but the many health problems reported after the Gulf War have brought new recognition of their tremendous effects on both military and civilian populations. It has become clear that there remain many unresolved issues related to the causes of symptoms and how they might be prevented and treated.

After wars dating back at least to the Civil War, soldiers have reported clusters of symptoms that have not been satisfactorily explained medically (Hyams et al., 1996). These symptoms have included fatigue, shortness of breath, headache, sleep disturbance, memory problems, and impaired concentration (Hyams et al., 1996). However, no single demonstrable disease is apparent. Multiple studies in Gulf War veterans have not found a unique illness to account for the multiple symptoms experienced (Fukuda et al., 1998; Iowa Persian Gulf Study Group, 1997; Gray et al., 1996). Unexplained illnesses reported by veterans of the Gulf War have led large numbers of veterans and their family members to be concerned about their health and have led to the expenditure of millions of dollars in research into causal factors.

At the same time, research in the civilian health care system has elucidated similar unexplained symptoms in the general population (Hyams, 1998; Barsky and Borus, 1999). The study team believes that increased attention to prevention and treatment of the medically unexplained symptoms among military populations during and after deployment is warranted because of their prevalence and attendant potential disability.

The section that follows draws heavily upon the paper, Unexplained Physical Symptoms in Primary Care and the Community: What Might We Learn for Prevention in the Military?, which was written for this study under commission by Charles C. Engel, Jr., and Wayne J. Katon. A condensed version of the paper is found in Appendix A.

This report uses the term *medically unexplained symptoms* to refer to symptoms that are not clinically explained by a medical etiology and that lead to use of the health care system. Many common diagnoses are not based on etiologically defined factors but are based on clusters of medically unexplained symptoms for which a more satisfactory designation cannot be found (Jablonski, 1991; Hyams, 1998). The terms *symptom-based diagnosis* or *symptom-based condition* can be used to describe such health problems diagnosed almost exclusively by using patients' verbal descriptions or observed behaviors, when no clinically demonstrable alterations in normal physiology or biological structure can be found. Symptom-based diagnoses tend to provide a label for clinicians and patients without providing any clear explanation of the reason for the symptoms. Indeed, some symptom-based diagnoses most likely involve underlying and measurable alterations in physiology that are as yet poorly characterized or understood (Engel and Katon, 1999). There is some evidence that the prognosis, treatment, and factors that determine disability are similar across different symptom-based diagnoses (Buchwald and Garrity, 1994; Gomborone et al., 1996; Plesh et al., 1996; Clauw et al., 1997; Hyams, 1998; Engel and Katon, 1999).

EPIDEMIOLOGY

Surveys of the general population indicate that 85 to 95 percent of community respondents experience at least one physical symptom every 2 to 4 weeks, although few of these symptoms are reported to physicians (White et al., 1961). Analysis of the population-based Epidemiologic Catchment Area Study found that more than 4 percent of people had a lifetime history of multiple, chronic, unexplained complaints with at least one episode in the past year (Escobar et al., 1987; Swartz et al., 1991). Similarly, in the general population the prevalence of a history of at least six bothersome medically unexplained symptoms during one's lifetime in women and at least four medically unexplained symptoms in men is about 4 percent (Escobar et al., 1987, 1989). These criteria were associated with significant functional impairment and high levels of use of the health care system.

Unexplained symptoms are common in the population of people who seek health care. According to the 1989 National Ambulatory Medical Care Survey, such symptoms account for 57 percent of the roughly 400 million ambulatory care visits per year in the United States (Schappert, 1992). A third or more of these symptoms remain unexplained after a routine medical evaluation. Research by Kroenke and colleagues similarly indicated that a large component of primary care involves the management of medically unexplained symptoms (Kroenke and Mangelsdorff, 1989; Kroenke et al., 1990).

Studies of patients with medically unexplained symptoms indicate high rates of major depression and panic disorder (Katon et al., 1985, 1991a; Goldenberg, 1987; Black et al., 1990; Simon et al., 1990; Hudson et al., 1992; Clauw and Chrousos, 1997). Several mechanisms might account for this correlation. Physical illness may cause psychosocial distress through a direct biological link such as through neurotransmitters involved in both pain and mental disorders. Physical symptoms may cause emotional distress by overwhelming an individual's ability to cope. Distress may increase unhealthy behaviors that increase the risk of such symptoms. The disordered sleep and changes in autonomic nervous system functioning associated with stress may cause these symptoms. Finally, both mental disorders and medically unexplained symptoms may be found together in some people simply by chance.

Studies indicate that increasing numbers of physical symptoms are accompanied by an increasing likelihood of experiencing anxiety and depressive disorders (Katon and Russo, 1992; Kroenke et al., 1994; Russo et al., 1994; Kisely et al., 1997). For example, in a study using self-reports from a sample of more than 1,000 health maintenance organization enrollees, increasing numbers of pain complaints were strongly associated with elevated levels of anxiety, depression, and physical symptoms that did not cause pain (Dworkin et al., 1990). In a separate study, the percentages of people with anxiety and depressive disorders increased with increasing numbers of physical symptoms (both medically explained and unexplained from the perspective of the interviewer) (Kroenke et al., 1994). Indeed, depression and anxiety are consistently associated with medically unexplained symptoms across many studies that have used several different methods and that have had cross-sectional (Simon and VonKorff, 1991), case-control (Katon et al., 1988, 1991a; Sullivan et al., 1988; Walker et al., 1988, 1990b), and longitudinal designs (Leino and Magni, 1993; Von Korff et al., 1993) designs. Katon and colleagues have found that the relationship of physical symptoms to common anxiety and depressive disorders is linear. As the number of anxiety and depressive symptoms or lifetime episodes of these disorders increases, so does the prevalence and number of medically unexplained symptoms (Katon et al., 1991b).

These data suggest that medically unexplained symptoms may sometimes be a marker of psychosocial distress (Engel and Katon, 1999). In occupational medicine settings, like the military, with a younger and medically healthier population than the general population, this effect is probably amplified. With a lower base rate of most diseases, there is a higher likelihood that unexplained symptoms are due at least in part to more common and less easily recognized psychiatric disorders like anxiety and depressive disorders (Engel and Katon, 1999).

Medically unexplained symptoms are important not only because of their prevalence but also because of the loss of functioning, impaired quality of life, and high levels of health care utilization that accompany them. Consistent evidence suggests that those with medically unexplained symptoms report poor functioning and diminished quality of life (Escobar et al., 1987; Katon et al., 1991b; Schweitzer et al. 1995; Anderson and Ferrans 1997; Gureje et al. 1997, 1998; Piccinelli and Simon 1997). Health care utilization is also increased among those with medically unexplained symptoms. In one study, patients with somatization disorder had a six-fold per capita increase in hospital service expenditures, a 14-fold increase in physician costs, and a nine-fold increase in personal health costs compared with national averages (Coryell and Norten, 1981; Smith et al., 1986a). Escobar et al. (1987) found that multiple medically unexplained symptoms (four or more for men and six or more for women) were significantly related to use of general medical services. Medically unexplained symptoms also frequently lead to dissatisfaction with health care because most patients believe that finding a medical explanation for the symptoms is the physician's job.

Understanding the natural history of medically unexplained symptoms is important to considering routes of prevention and treatment. Engel and Katon (1999) described predisposing factors, precipitating factors, and perpetuating factors that play a role in the natural history of medically unexplained symptoms. Rather than being empirical in nature, these categories are part of a heuristic model used to provide a framework for understanding individual variation in medically unexplained symptoms. Predisposing factors are characteristics of individuals that make them more vulnerable to distress, physiological arousal, and bothersome physical symptoms. Precipitating factors are events or factors that send vulnerable asymptomatic individuals into a physically symptomatic episode or that increase levels of disability or distress among those who are already symptomatic. Perpetuating factors are those that maintain symptoms, distress, and disability and that extend their period of duration (Engel and Katon, 1999).

PREDISPOSING FACTORS

There is a large body of literature about predisposing factors for medically unexplained symptoms. These factors fall into categories of hereditary differences, physiological differences, adversity in early life, chronic medical illness, and chronic or recurrent psychiatric illness. Although many of these factors are difficult or impossible to modify (for example, genetic predisposition or childhood experiences), there may be approaches to mitigating the influences of these factors on the subsequent risk of symptom onset, symptom persistence, impaired coping, psychosocial distress, and diminished functional capacity (Engel and Katon, 1999). Each of the predisposing factors is discussed at greater length by Engel and Katon (1999).

Physiological Differences and Susceptibilities

Physiological differences in the susceptibilities of individuals to medically unexplained symptoms are not yet well understood, but it is likely that they are the result of both genetic predisposition and developmental influences and experiences. The following section describes some hypothesized physiological bases of some of the previously unexplained symptoms. Other hypotheses are presented by Engel and Katon (1999).

One of the critical physiological control systems of the body is the hypothalamic-pituitary-adrenal (HPA) axis, which mediates the neuroendocrine stress response. This system is an important common pathway through which responses to the range of physical, psychological, or immune and inflammatory stimuli are mediated. When the HPA axis is activated by a stimulus, the hypothalamus secretes corticotropin-releasing hormone, which in turn stimulates the pituitary gland to secrete adrenocorticotropic hormone and the adrenal glands to produce glucocorticoids. Glucocorticoids feed back at every step to contain and ultimately shut off this response. The HPA axis is also regulated by an internal biological clock entrained to the light-dark cycle. Sleep and activity are related to troughs and peaks in HPA function, respectively, but these are unrelated to external life stress. Sleep deprivation and depression are associated with elevated and flattened diurnal HPA function, and "burn out" from job or other intense experiences is associated with a flattened and lower HPA function.

Activation of the HPA axis and the sympathetic nervous system during acute stress is linked to behaviors and physiological responses, including increased heart rate, sweating, focused attention, and decreased vegetative functions, such as feeding and reproductive behavior (Sternberg, 1998b). With exposures to stressors of moderate intensity for a relatively short duration, activation of the HPA axis and sympathetic nervous system activation enhance performance with increased attention, more efficient muscular activity and energy metabolism, and readiness for response to threat or attack (Sternberg, 1998b), including enhanced immune function (Dhabhar and McEwen, 1999). With exposures of longer durations or with exposure to higher-intensity stressors, some of these responses may fail or may be suppressed (Dhabhar and McEwen, 1997; Sternberg, 1998b).

The HPA axis regulates the immune system systemically, generally playing an immunosuppressive role through the actions of glucocorticoids. Evidence from animal models suggests that genetic differences in the reactivity of the HPA axis system result in differences in susceptibility or resistance to inflammatory and infectious diseases (Sternberg et al., 1989a,b; Sternberg, 1998b). Differences between the Lewis and Fischer rat strains indicate that blunted or underactive HPA axis responses predispose the rats to enhanced susceptibility to inflammatory disease, whereas overactivity of the HPA axis predisposes the rats to enhanced susceptibility to infectious disease (Sternberg, 1998b). However, similar levels of HPA activity do not mean that the immune responses are also similar. Genetic traits determine the optimal level of HPA function required to maintain the proper balance of immune function, and these genetic traits have not yet been identified in animals or in humans (Mason, 1991; Sternberg, 1998b).

These findings have interesting implications for humans. Inherent or developed differences in the responsiveness of the HPA axis could underlie some of the differences in symptoms or illnesses that individuals experience, including thus far medically unexplained symptoms. Although studies of the relationship between differences in the responsiveness of the HPA axis and human disease are not as far advanced as they are for animals, associations have been observed between a blunted or relatively low HPA axis response and rheumatoid arthritis (Neeck et al., 1990; Cash et al., 1992), atopic dermatitis and asthma (Buske-Kirschbaum et al., 1997), chronic fatigue syndrome (Demitrack et al., 1991), fibromyalgia (Crofford et al., 1994), atypical depression (Joseph-Vanderpool et al., 1991), posttraumatic stress disorder (PTSD) (Resnick et al., 1995; Yehuda et al., 1995), and burnout (Sternberg, 1998a,b).

The degree to which individual differences in the responsiveness of the HPA axis are genetic or environmental is not yet known. However, powerful developmental effects are recognized. In rats, early stress and neonatal handling are believed to set the level of responsiveness of the HPA axis and autonomic nervous system. The HPA axis overreacts in animals subjected to early unpredictable stress and underreacts in animals exposed to neonatal handling (Meaney et al., 1994). A factor that determines the activity of the stress hormone axis and the overall allostatic load is early life experience. This has been shown in animal models (Meaney et al., 1988; Higley et al., 1991; Dellu et al., 1994).

In humans, a growing body of data suggests a relationship between developmental or other experiences and physiological changes in the HPA axis. Recent studies raise the possibility that organic changes in the brain may be linked both to early life events, adult trauma, and disorders such as depression and PTSD and to the regulation of the stress hormone axis (Bremner et al., 1995, 1997; Gurvits et al., 1996). How does all of this relate to medically unexplained symptoms? At this point one can only speculate whether the connections exist. By definition there is no clear mechanistic understanding of the medically unexplained symptoms described in this report. However, the studies with animals and humans described above suggest the possibility of systemic effects mediated by neuroendocrine stress response dysregulation. Answers to such questions for humans will require time and additional study, including prospective studies of potential markers for HPA axis hypo- and hyperreactivity.

Early Life Adversity

There is some evidence that traumatic experiences in childhood might be related to health in adulthood. Cross-sectional and case-control studies have shown consistent associations between childhood maltreatment and irritable bowel syndrome (Walker et al., 1990a,b; Irwin et al., 1996) fibromyalgia (Walker et al., 1997; Alexander et al., 1998), back pain in women (Linton, 1997), and chronic pelvic pain in women (Walker et al., 1988; Walker and Stenchever, 1993). A 2-year prospective cohort study examining the natural history of medically unexplained symptoms found that persistent unexplained symptoms were significantly associated with patient reports of poor parental care in childhood, chronic parental medical illness, and chronic medical illness (Craig et al., 1993).

Chronic Medical Illness

Social learning theory holds that people learn behaviors and patterns of communication from those around them beginning very early in life. Some aspects of illness-related behavior may be influenced by behaviors modeled by chronically ill family members. Children of patients with low back pain chose more pain-related responses to situations than children of healthy parents or diabetic parents (Richard, 1988). These children's teachers also rated them as manifesting more illness-related behaviors than the children of healthy control parents. In a prospective study in the United Kingdom, parental health complaints, physical illness during childhood, and teachers' assessments of the behavior and personality of subjects at age 15 predicted medically unexplained physical symptoms in adulthood (Hotopf et al., 1997). The complex contributions to illness-related behavior of parenting roles as well as intrinsic genetic factors passed from parent to child remain to be sorted out.

PRECIPITATING FACTORS

Precipitating factors are those related to the acute onset of medically unexplained symptoms. They include biological stressors, psychosocial stressors, acute psychiatric disorders, and epidemic unexplained illness. A biological stressor might be a concurrent medical illness. Conversion disorder can cause the amplification of a symptom primarily caused by a coexisting medical disorder (Sharma and Chaturvedi, 1995; Silver, 1996). For example, some individuals with diagnosable seizure disorders also experience pseudoseizures of apparent behavioral rather than neurological origin (Lelliott and Fenwick, 1991; Blumer et al., 1995).

Psychosocial events can frequently lead to the start of medically unexplained symptoms in susceptible individuals. Several studies indicate a higher percentage of traumatic life events in patients who seek health care or who are about to undergo surgery and who were found to have nonspecific or unexplained pain compared with the percentage of traumatic life events among those with identifiable disease (Creed, 1981; Craig and Brown, 1984; Craufurd et al., 1990). For example, Creed (1981) interviewed patients with undiagnosed abdominal pain for stressful life events just before they underwent appendectomy, so that during the interview he did not know the eventual pathological diagnosis for the removed appendix. Of individuals with a normal appendix, 60 percent reported that a severely threatening life event had occurred in the previous 38 weeks, whereas 25 percent of those later diagnosed with appendicitis and 20 percent of a healthy control group reported that such an event had occurred.

The acute onset of psychiatric disorders, particularly depressive and anxiety disorders, can also lead to the onset of medically unexplained symptoms. Existing evidence suggests that recognition and successful treatment of panic disorder also reduces physical symptoms and physical health concerns (Kellner et al., 1986; Noyes et al., 1986). Early interventions for patients with panic disorder and major depressive disorder may prevent exposure to perpetuating factors that increase the likelihood of acute medically unexplained physical symptoms becoming chronic with associated disability (Engel and Katon, 1999).

Epidemiclike outbreaks of medically unexplained illness occasionally occur, often in industrial or workplace settings. The controversial sick building syndrome involves the development of symptoms among many individuals living or working in the same building. Although microbial contamination may play a part in some of these outbreaks, they may also be associated with psychosocial factors including job-related stress (Menzies and Bourbeau, 1997; Kroenke, 1998a; Menzies, 1998). Outbreaks of chronic fatigue syndrome are known to occur (Chester and Levine, 1997), and epidemic unexplained illness has been reported to occur in military settings (Struewing and Gray, 1990). Such illnesses often occur after some environmental trigger, after a significant emergency response to a threat, and with the belief of those with symptoms that the environmental event was the cause of their illness or anxiety (Small et al., 1994; Boss, 1997).

PERPETUATING FACTORS

Perpetuating factors, sometimes referred to as illness maintenance systems, are those that may sustain or prolong medically unexplained symptoms once they have occurred (Katon et al., 1982a,b). Personal beliefs about the causes of one's symptoms can sustain or prolong medically unexplained symptoms. For example, the belief that physical activity produces debilitating fatigue may begin a cycle of decreasing activity that further promotes fatigue (Irish Times, 1999). However, a program of regular physical activity is an essential element of successful treatment in most multidisciplinary approaches to chronic pain and fatigue (Engel and Katon, 1999). Misinformation from others, such as health care providers, may also be a perpetuating factor. Continued diagnostic testing, regardless of the physician's reasons for it, sometimes perpetuates patients' beliefs that a disease may yet explain their symptoms and lead to a cure (Kouyanou et al., 1997).

Support groups may also perpetuate medically unexplained symptoms. Although they can reduce the sense of isolation many sufferers experience, they can also encourage a struggle for the medical legitimacy of the illness and reinforce beliefs that a quick fix is possible (Abbey and Garfinkel, 1991). Other sources of social support can also reinforce illness-related behavior. Well-meaning friends or loved ones can enhance disability by urging unnecessary relaxation and relief from undesirable responsibilities (Block et al., 1980; Jamison and Virts, 1990; Engel and Katon, 1999).

Although frequently helpful, diagnostic labeling can sometimes have negative effects by unnecessarily causing patients to define themselves as ill (Meador, 1965). Haynes and colleagues (1978) found that steelworkers participating in hypertension screening and diagnosed with hypertension, an asymptomatic illness, missed 80 percent more days of work after screening than before screening, whereas there was a 9 percent increase among workers who were screened but who did not receive a diagnosis of hypertension. For symptom-based conditions, it has been suggested that the iatrogenic effects of labeling may outweigh the potential for clinical and societal benefits (Hadler, 1997). Furthermore, embedding the putative cause of a new condition into its name or diagnostic criteria may preclude the acceptance of findings that indicate other explanations for the symptoms (Feinstein, 1998).

Workplace factors have been associated with illness-related behavior, in that dissatisfaction with job tasks and elevated scores on the Minnesota Multiphasic Personality Inventory, a psychological test, were the best predictors of subsequent back pain in a prospective study of more than 3,000 aircraft workers (Bigos et al., 1991).

Although disability compensation fulfills a critical role in helping people with occupational injuries or impairments, it can also perpetuate illness by requiring continuing symptoms and disability for the worker to be eligible for benefits. The worker cannot attempt an assertive recovery without risking the loss of a legal settlement or needed benefits (Engel and Katon, 1999). As noted by Hadler, "It is hard, if not impossible, to get well if you have to prove that you are sick" (Sullivan and Loeser, 1992, p. 1834). The period of "proving" the illness can also be protracted, sometimes lasting even years in the military system (Engel and Katon, 1999). Nevertheless, caution is indicated in applying such thinking to any individual.

PROGNOSTIC INDICATORS

Although the predisposing, precipitating, and perpetuating factors described above as influencing the natural history of medically unexplained symptoms are based on theory to provide a heuristic model, prognostic indicators are developed empirically. Prognostic indicators are characteristics of individuals or populations that clinicians, epidemiologists, and policy makers can use to estimate the future burden of illness and the magnitude of future treatment and resource needs (Engel and Katon, 1999). Empirically tested prognostic indicators for medically unexplained symptoms include indicators of prior level of use of the health care system, psychiatric manifestations, physical symptoms, and levels of functioning (Engel and Katon, 1999).

The prognostic spectrum of medically unexplained symptoms includes acute, recurrent, and chronic subtypes. Acute medically unexplained symptoms occur in the absence of a previous pattern or history of medically unexplained symptoms and last a few months at most, and the associated disability is often temporally associated with an acutely stressful life event. Recurrent medically unexplained symptoms are characterized by alternating symptomatic, asymptomatic, and mildly symptomatic periods. Chronic medically unexplained symptoms are a pattern of persistent unexplained symptoms associated with chronic disability, high levels of use of the health care system, and persistent problems with coping. Chronic coping problems are often associated with large numbers of physical symptoms (Russo et al., 1994, 1997). Individuals with chronic medically unexplained symptoms also often describe the occurrence of adversity during childhood (Walker et al., 1992).

Recognition of the importance of medically unexplained symptoms after wars going back at least as far as the Civil War and their importance in civilian populations makes clear the need to consider strategies to prevent and ameliorate them after future deployments. Throughout the chapters that follow, an emphasis is placed on the early recognition of medically unexplained symptoms and steps that might be taken to try to address them early, as well as the research effort that is needed to better understand their natural history and treatment.

4

Medical Surveillance

Even within a public health or medical context, the term *surveillance* can have different meanings to different people. The Centers for Disease Control (CDC; now called the Centers for Disease Control and Prevention) defines *epidemiologic surveillance* as:

> the ongoing and systematic collection, analysis, and interpretation of health data in the process of describing and monitoring a health event. This information is used for planning, implementing, and evaluating public health interventions and programs. Surveillance data are used both to determine the need for public health action and to assess the effectiveness of programs. (Centers for Disease Control, 1988, p. 1)

Similarly, Benenson, writing in the context of communicable diseases, defines *disease surveillance* as:

> the continuing scrutiny of all aspects of occurrence and spread of a disease that are pertinent to effective control. Included are the systematic collection and evaluation of 1) morbidity and mortality reports; 2) special reports of field investigations of epidemics and of individual cases; 3) isolation and identification of infectious agents by laboratories; 4) data concerning the availability, use and untoward effects of vaccines and toxoids, immune globulins, insecticides and other substances used in control; information regarding immunity levels in segments of the population; and other relevant epidemiologic data. A report summarizing the above data should be prepared and distributed to all cooperating persons and others with a need to know the results of the surveillance activities. The procedure applies to all jurisdictional levels of public health from local to international. (Benenson, 1995, p. 543)

Crucial components in these definitions are the continuing and systematic nature of surveillance activities and the fact that they are related in some way to facilitating the control of disease or certain health events in a population. Reporting of selected conditions and laboratory-based surveillance are both part of disease surveillance. The routine collection of medical data does not constitute disease surveillance per se, but when that information is assembled and used for disease prevention or control, it can play an important role in a health surveillance system. Epidemiologic investigations to determine etiology are not surveillance but are part of the appropriate and necessary response to surveillance information (Halperin, 1992). Overseas laboratories have a critical role in carrying out relevant disease surveillance in areas where troops are likely to deploy.

Carrying out an effective medical surveillance program in the military is challenging, as it is in the civilian sector. It is important that it be carried out not as an end in itself but considered in the context of a larger plan for public health within the military. During its investigation, the study team has learned of a variety of different health surveillance initiatives and efforts that are planned or under way. Although each has its own justifiable goals, the disjointedness of the efforts makes it less likely that the goal of keeping the force healthy during a deployment will be reached efficiently. As articulated in the three pillars of the Department of Defense's (DoD) current effort of Force Health Protection, reaching this goal entails (1) promoting wellness and sustaining health to deliver a healthy and fit force; (2) preventing acute and chronic casualties during training, deployment, and war, and (3) providing high-quality health care in peacetime and on the battlefield (Bailey, 1999a).

Professional personnel are needed to evaluate data needs over time as well as to analyze the information and respond to emerging trends and events. A reliable record keeping system will be crucial (this is addressed in Chapter 5). The push to develop and implement a policy and system for medical surveillance has been strong since the Gulf War. There might be some tendency to think or hope that such a system, when fully functional, would preclude or prevent health problems such as those that have been reported in many Gulf War veterans. This is unlikely. What such a system should be able to do, however, is to help identify high- and low-risk populations to permit the implementation of appropriate preventive measures for the array of known and well-understood hazards to deployed forces, as well as provide early alerts about new or emerging health problems in the population. It will also provide data to permit retrospective analysis when future problems arise.

The following sections describe aspects of the medical surveillance system under development by DoD and the military services, and evaluate them on the basis of their apparent objectives and the needs and definitions discussed above.

DoD POLICIES ON MEDICAL SURVEILLANCE

Since the Gulf War, and particularly from 1996 to 1999, DoD and the military services have placed new emphasis on the importance of medical or health surveillance. This emphasis has been encouraged by outside organizations such as the Presidential Advisory Committee on Gulf War Veterans' Illnesses (1996a,b) and the Institute of Medicine (1996a). A DoD joint directive and instruction have been published on the topic, as has a more recent DoD joint memorandum. Coinciding with these has been the development of the concept of Force Health Protection.

Force Health Protection

Force Health Protection is a campaign to place greater emphasis on protecting the health of service members. Its goal is "a unified strategy that protects service members from all health and environmental hazards associated with military service" (Clines, 1998). In November 1997, President Clinton directed DoD and the U.S. Department of Veterans Affairs (VA) to create a new "Force Health Protection Program" to help provide a military force fully protected from preventable and avoidable health threats throughout military operations and deployments (White House, Office of the Press Secretary, 1997). The four critical elements of the Force Health Protection Strategy are threat analysis, countermeasures, medical surveillance in the area of operations, and analysis (National Science and Technology Council, 1998).

DoD Joint Directive

In August 1997, DoD released the directive Joint Medical Surveillance (U.S. Department of Defense, 1997b) (Appendix H) as well as an instruction on its implementation and application (U.S. Department of Defense, 1997a) (Appendix I). The directive establishes policy and assigns responsibility for "routine joint medical surveillance of all Military Service members during active Federal service, especially military deployments" (U.S. Department of Defense, 1997b, p. 1).

The directive notes the CDC definition of medical surveillance as "the regular or repeated collection, analysis, and dissemination of uniform health information for monitoring the health of a population, and intervening in a timely manner when necessary" (U.S. Department of Defense, 1997b, p. 2). It emphasizes the application of health information data to military activities to prepare and implement early intervention and control strategies. It states that "a surveillance system includes a functional capacity for data collection, analysis and dissemination of information linked to military preventive medicine support of operational commanders" (U.S. Department of Defense, 1997b, p. 2).

The directive states as policies that: medical and personnel information systems be designed, integrated, and used in a manner compatible with military medical surveillance; such systems be continuously in effect throughout military service and be *specifically configured to assess the effects of deployment on the health of service members*; and service members be made aware of significant health threats and corresponding protection before and during deployment. Medical surveillance will encompass the periods before, during, and after deployment to monitor threats and stressors, assess disease and non-battle injuries of all kinds, and reinforce the use of preventive countermeasures and the provision of optimal medical care during and after deployment. There shall be a serum repository to be used exclusively for the identification, prevention, and control of diseases associated with operational deployments of military personnel.

The directive designates the Secretary of the Army as the DoD Executive Agent for medical surveillance for deployment and for maintenance of the related Armed Forces Serum Repository. However, medical surveillance is the continuous responsibility of the DoD components (Army, Navy, and Air Force). During a deployment, this responsibility becomes shared with the joint task force (JTF) commander and the commander in chief of the appropriate combatant command (U.S. Department of Defense, 1997a). Policies for health surveillance of the Ready Reserve are to be consistent with the policies established for the active component.

DoD Joint Instruction

The instruction (U.S. Department of Defense, 1997a) (Appendix I) accompanying the directive details the specific actions necessary for medical surveillance before, during, and after deployments and outlines roles and responsibilities at these three stages. It anticipates that new systems will be developed to facilitate medical surveillance, such as automated medical record devices, and that a geographical information system will be used to conduct spatial analyses of the environmental and disease exposures of company-sized and larger units. The environmental exposure data will be capable of being linked to service members' individual medical records. It specifies that pre- and postdeployment health screening assessments be carried out, to include a mental health assessment. It also states that during a deployment, the Defense Manpower Data Center shall provide collective data such as daily strength by unit and grid coordinates for each unit, and inclusive dates of each individual service member's deployment. These data shall be linkable to collective medical surveillance data and to service members' individual medical records.

DoD Joint Memorandum on Deployment Health Surveillance and Readiness

In December 1998, the Chairman of the Joint Chiefs of Staff published a memorandum entitled Deployment Health Surveillance and Readiness to provide routine, standardized procedures for assessing readiness from a health perspective and conducting health surveillance in support of deployments (Joint Chiefs of Staff, 1998) (Appendix J). It states that health surveillance during a deployment includes identification of the population at risk, recognition of and assessment of hazardous exposures, use of specific countermeasures, and monitoring health outcomes. It details surveillance requirements before, during, and after deployments. It also includes, in its Enclosure D, a useful Tri-Service Reportable Medical Event List that should be updated on a regular basis.

Joint Publication 4-02 Doctrine for Joint Health Service Support

The policies described above still await incorporation into doctrine. Joint Publication 4-02 is under revision to reflect these policies.

National Science and Technology Council, Presidential Review Directive 5

In response to a recommendation from the Presidential Advisory Committee on Gulf War Veterans' Illnesses, a National Science and Technology Council Interagency Working Group developed an interagency plan to address health preparedness for and readjustment of veterans and families after future conflicts and peacekeeping missions. The resulting plan, released in November 1998, is called, *A National Obligation: Planning for Health Preparedness for and Readjustment of the Military, Veterans, and Their Families after Future Deployments* (National Science and Technology Council, 1998).

The plan addresses broad topics of deployment health, record keeping, research, and health risk communications. In the chapter on deployment health, the supporting narrative describes the Force Health Protection Strategy, including threat analysis, countermeasures, medical surveillance in the area of operations, and data analysis. Medical surveillance in the area of operations is explained as follows: "During the operation, monitoring the health status of the force and the health threats to determine short- and long-term risks to health and to take appropriate countermeasures" (National Science and Technology Council, 1998, p. 11).

Many of the policies and recommended strategies described in the documents above are evidence that DoD is taking the need for improvements in medical surveillance seriously. In sections that follow, a variety of tools are described that can contribute information to a medical surveillance system. Rather than being developed as part of a systematic plan for improved surveillance, however, each has been developed or planned to address other specific needs. Some coordination and examination of the "big picture" of health surveillance is needed to consider the tools available to make the process more effective and efficient for medical surveillance. The Joint Preventive Medicine Policy Group (or JPMPG) is a group of preventive medicine officers representing all of the services that has provided input to policy making. However, they do this work in addition to their full-time work, and have not been involved as early in the process as needed. Earlier involvement of such a group, providing them with adequate time and resources, could facilitate such coordination.

CURRENT SERVICE PRACTICES AND PLANS

Although the military's stated goal is for medical surveillance that is seamless over the career of the service member, present surveillance practices must necessarily differ in some aspects between garrison and deployed settings. This section reviews the current practices and plans for military surveillance in both settings in light of the policies noted above. For the purposes of this report, *deployment* is defined as it is in the memorandum Deployment Health Surveillance and Readiness, that is, "a troop movement resulting from a JCS [Joint Chiefs of Staff]/unified command deployment order for 30 continuous days or greater to a land-based location outside the United States that does not have a permanent U.S. military medical treatment facility (i.e., funded by the Defense Health Program)" (Joint Chiefs of Staff, 1998, Enclosure A, p. 1).

Garrison

Despite the radically increased operational tempo of U.S. military operations in recent years, at any given time, most military service members are not deployed but are in garrison or ashore. During this time routine medical care and preventive measures will take place, and these activities can also provide information that will serve as a baseline for assessment of changes resulting from or concurrent with deployments.

Recruit Assessment Program

The military is developing a survey instrument proposed to be given to new military recruits immediately upon reporting for basic training. Although baseline health information is already obtained from recruits during Military Entrance Processing, it is limited in scope, is not computerized, and often is not readily accessible (Hyams and Murphy, 1998). The Navy and Air Force have administered a psychological screening program to recruits since the 1970s; it is now called the Biographical Evaluation and Screening of Troops Program. The proposed new instrument, which is currently undergoing pilot testing, would collect preservice demographic, medical, psychological, occupational, and risk factor data on all U.S. military recruits and establish a computerized database of baseline health information. The Recruit Assessment Program (RAP) questionnaire would be administered to incoming personnel within their first week of training and would be given to active-duty, National Guard, and Reserve troops.

The Institute of Medicine (IOM) study team views the collection of uniform survey data from recruits upon accession into the military as an important contribution both to the individual medical record and to a population database for better understanding the development of disease in military populations generally. The data can help provide the foundation of the medical record maintained for the service member throughout his or her military career and potentially after it. It is thus critical that the instrument be developed in coordination with the continuing development of the Health Evaluation and Assessment Review (HEAR) (see below) and that it be compatible with the VA and DoD joint records system. It can provide baseline information about the health of recruits before their military service, as well as permit the testing of hypotheses about risk factors for disease development in military populations in the future. It is important that the instrument used be carefully developed with validated components and that it be pilot tested. The developers have undertaken or planned both of these. The Armed Forces Epidemiology Board favorably reviewed the RAP proposal in December 1997. Once implemented, the instrument should be periodically reassessed and refined with input from appropriate independent experts.

Periodic Health Assessments

In addition to planning the collection of health information from recruits as they enter the military, DoD is moving to implement an annual collection of health status and risk factor information from all service members. The HEAR was initially developed by the Air Force to "promote prevention and wellness, and evidence-based population health management" (Fonseca, 1998, Overheads, p. 2). Some features are similar to the Health Risk Appraisal used for many years by the Army. Its use has begun across the services, but data are not yet readily available to physicians.

The HEAR began as a scannable paper and pencil questionnaire that addressed topics of demographics, behavioral health risks, mental health, activity limitation and perceived health, medical care utilization, chronic conditions, and family history. It was envisioned to be useful both to the patient and to the health care provider, noting potential health concerns to the patient and to the provider in separate reports (Fonseca, 1998).

Later versions of the HEAR are designed for use as computer-assisted interviews. The later versions cover additional topics, such as nutrition, safety, reproductive health, and dental health, and include expanded sections on mental health and behavioral risk factors. Skip patterns are built into the questionnaire so that the interviewee does not face irrelevant questions. The computerized questionnaire is to be a component of the Preventive Health Care Application (PHCA). PHCA is a computer system for health maintenance to include the HEAR and an immunization tracking system. Through PHCA, HEAR results are provided to health care providers with certain responses flagged to facilitate intervention. Versions of the HEAR now in development will gather information about a service member's children and additional future versions are envisioned to be able to use information from previous surveys or other sources (DoD hospital records, for example) to determine which questions are necessary.

The IOM study team believes that the routine collection of health status and risk factor data through an instrument such as the HEAR can provide a useful component of an ongoing medical surveillance system. However, its goals should be clearly articulated, and the survey instrument should be focused with the use of survey questions validated in other settings or validated by comparison with personal interviews carried out by medical professionals. These longitudinal data may not themselves be useful for answering questions of causation of future clusters of illness, but they may help to provide a better understanding of predeployment factors. The fact that it is entirely self-reported information is a limitation, but routine capture of this information should make it a more reliable source of information about pre- and postdeployment health than data hastily gathered immediately before or after a deployment. Ultimately, the information is expected to be incorporated into the overall medical record which is likely to contain laboratory test results as well as physicians' notes. Incorporation of the baseline data gathered in RAP would help to shorten the questionnaire and eliminate unnecessary redundancy.

The HEAR is envisioned as both a clinical tool to facilitate individual preventive care and a tool to gather population-based data. The study team believes that it can serve a valuable function on both fronts with careful review, refinement, and incorporation of questions designed to note potential warning signs for the manifestations of medically unexplained symptoms, as discussed elsewhere in this report. It can also collect better information about reproductive health to facilitate surveillance for adverse reproductive outcomes addressed later in this chapter. In its current form the questionnaire focuses on diagnosed diseases, uses language that the service members may not understand, and uses categories different from those helpful to epidemiologists. The questionnaire will need modification so that it asks questions about symptoms and will require rigorous field testing and input from experts in survey development. Considerable work in health-tracking instruments has been carried out in the past several decades (Newhouse, 1993), and this information and expertise would be useful to apply to this situation.

Although the HEAR is being planned for use across the active duty services (Institute of Medicine, 1998), it is not yet planned for use with reserve-component troops. Discussions are still under way within the military about how this could take place. Given the increasing reliance on the reserve components, it is appropriate that they too be involved in health surveillance efforts to facilitate the maintenance of a healthy force. However, the fact that members of the reserve components receive most of their health care from civilian providers poses particular challenges. If the HEAR questionnaire flags a health problem in need of attention, the reservist may have to be referred for care to his or her civilian provider. Administration of the HEAR to members of the reserves would allow collection of ongoing baseline data and allow a better understanding of predeployment health than that provided by the hastily administered predeployment questionnaire.

In addition to periodic health assessments that include physical examination and laboratory testing when required, it is also important that both hospitalization and ambulatory visit databases be available and be linked to the remainder of an individual's medical record. Currently this linkage is possible only through the Defense Medical Surveillance System (DMSS), which will be described later, but with the development of a computer-based patient record it should become inherent to the medical record system. This is discussed more fully in Chapter 5.

Periodic Blood Draw

Part of the DoD plan for improved medical surveillance related to deployments incorporates the collection and storage of sera from each member of the military. Samples of sera that remain from the mandatory periodic (at least every 2 years) test for human immunodeficiency virus (HIV) infection are sent for stockpiling in Rockville, Maryland, and are under the care of the Armed Services Serum Repository. Samples from members of the National Guard and Reserves as well as from active-duty forces are collected and stored. The study team believes that collection of a serum sample within the 12 months preceding deployment, as specified in the DoD Joint Instruction on Medical Surveillance (U.S. Department of Defense, 1997a) provides an adequately recent predeployment sample should comparison with sera collected following a specific deployment be needed.

The Armed Services Serum Repository has proved to be useful in addressing questions about exposures to infectious agents by deployed forces. Sera obtained pre- and postdeployment from forces deployed to Bosnia were analyzed for antibodies to tick-borne encephalitis virus and hantavirus to assess the risks of infection with these agents. Similarly, sera from the Gulf War era were analyzed to assess seroconversion due to sandfly fever.

The study team finds the serum bank to be a valuable component of the health surveillance system, with uses beyond assessment of the hazards of specific deployments. These uses extend to assessment of broader health questions within the military and civilian populations. Recent applications of the serum bank include a large serological survey of military personnel for the prevalence of hepatitis C virus antibodies, and studies have examined potential serologic precursors of Hodgkin's disease and testicular cancer (Kelley, 1999b).

Although only the serum of blood samples is saved and stored, the cellular portion of blood could prove to be a future resource for assessment of exposures. DNA adducts of toxic compounds could be evaluated without intrusion into the privacy of the DNA code. However, at present the use of DNA information for anything but the identification of remains raises large ethical, legal, and social issues that the military must address even as society as a whole strives to evolve widely accepted policies. A series of special rules and procedures ensures the protection of privacy interests in the tissue specimen samples for identification of remains and any analysis of the DNA from these samples (U.S. Department of Defense, 1996c).

Surveillance for Drug- and Vaccine-Associated Adverse Events

Prevention of infectious diseases and protection of deployed forces from chemical and biological threats often require the use of vaccines, antiparasitic drugs, antibiotics, compounds that ameliorate the effects of nerve gas, and insect repellents. It is incumbent on the military to maintain accurate records of drug and vaccine use and to carry out effective surveillance for potential adverse events that may be related to a drug and or vaccine administration. Specific inquiries and definitive studies can be triggered when surveillance detects adverse events that may be linked to the use of drugs and biologicals.

Low-incidence events and possible combination effects are difficult to detect and relate to specific causes. Although difficult, precise evaluation of rates of adverse reactions to vaccines is essential. However, continued use of effective preventive measures will depend in part on how effectively and credibly such surveillance is carried out and how effectively the military responds to suspected adverse events. The first requirement for an effective program to monitor the effects of drugs and vaccines is maintenance of accurate records of vaccinations and drug use. This necessitates both computer-based patient records and a central database. A second requirement is mandatory reporting of medical conditions that may be related to drug and vaccine interventions singly or in combination. The IOM Committee on Interactions of Drugs, Biologics and Chemicals in U.S. Military Forces recommended in 1996 (Institute of Medicine, 1996b) that the services expand the Reportable Disease Surveillance System to include a larger list of conditions including neurological conditions, immune suppression and autoimmune conditions, and conditions related to liver and kidney toxicity. DoD has not acted on this recommendation.

Laboratory-Based Surveillance

Laboratory-based surveillance is the collection of diagnostic information on health events from central laboratories rather than from hospital discharge code databases or from clinicians. Implementation of a managed health care system within DoD over the last several years (with many fewer and shorter hospital stays and more outpatient treatment) has made the latter information sources insufficiently specific to be useful for epidemiology (Kelley, 1999a). The low sensitivity of provider-based reporting (Vogt et al., 1983; Hinds et al., 1985; Thacker et al., 1986; Standaert et al., 1995) and the low sensitivity and specificity of reporting based on the ninth revision of the *International Classification of Diseases* (ICD-9) for some conditions (Wenger et al., 1988; Guevara et al., 1996) are important reasons for the emphasis on laboratory-based surveillance (Harrison and Pinner, 1998).

At the same time, the managed health care system has taken a toll on the laboratory capability for public health surveillance. The new capitation systems reward the collection of information useful for treatment of individual patients but do not reward the collection of information useful for evaluation of the larger population. For example, a clinician does not need to know the precise strain of influenza virus with which a patient is infected to provide appropriate care for that patient. However, for public health reasons it is important to know the influenza virus strains causing current infections so that future vaccines will provide coverage against the prevalent strains and better protect the larger population (Harrison and Pinner, 1998).

Another relevant factor is the specificity level of diagnostic codes. Even for conditions diagnosed in the laboratory, surveillance in the military is carried out by using ICD-9-based reporting, with the single exception of the reporting of HIV infection. ICD codes are rarely useful for surveillance of infectious disease because the categories are generally too broad. Reliance on ICD-9-based reporting could produce a dichotomy in the quality of surveillance data between the civilian and military sectors (Harrison and Pinner, 1998). In one study, the ICD-9 code for pneumococcal pneumonia detected only 58 percent of cases of bacteremic pneumococcal pneumonia, and the positive predictive value was only 59 percent (Guevara et al., 1996). A study of *Haemophilus influenzae* infection indicated that the sensitivity of discharge diagnosis codes was 52 percent for meningitis and 24 percent for bacteremia (Wenger et al., 1988).

Recently, there has been a renewed effort to strengthen laboratory-based surveillance within DoD; this parallels a similar effort in the civilian community (McDonald et al., 1997; Centers for Disease Control and Prevention, 1997; Harrison and Pinner, 1998). One needed change for the military is in reporting requirements. Although military laboratories are required to report 21 different conditions to local civilian jurisdictions, they are not required to report any of these conditions directly to military health surveillance authorities. Central reporting of reportable conditions as well as information, on, for example, antibiotic resistance patterns within the military could provide information to support preventive measures for both deployed forces and their dependents. Laboratory-based reporting could also help with the timely recognition of bioterrorism (Kelley, 1999a).

Improvements to laboratory-based surveillance do not require a new infrastructure with new laboratory space and staff. Existing resources could be reinforced and reorganized to better address the public health questions. What is necessary is the ability to carry out unusual tests on unusual infections of public health importance, expertise to develop or implement special procedures, protocols to evaluate unknown agents, and capabilities for molecular epidemiologic studies. One of the critical needs is to better capture and use data that are already being generated but that do not make their way to a central location for analysis and dissemination (Kelley, 1999a).

The information systems in use by laboratories do not efficiently collect and report data (Bolton, 1999). The Composite Health Care System used by DoD medical treatment facilities can generate an infection control report for a particular location, but data cannot be aggregated across different sites. As a result, electronic mail is used to report data to relevant bodies, or sometimes these data are simply logged into notebooks by hand (Bolton, 1999). Tremendous improvements to information systems are possible and are needed for laboratory data collection and reporting.

In 1997 the VA Infectious Disease Program Office implemented a national laboratory-based automated electronic surveillance tool called the Emerging Pathogens Initiative. Software installed at 142 VA facilities nationwide searches Patient Treatment File and laboratory data each night to match criteria for 14 pathogens of interest. Data are transmitted monthly from each site to the VA Austin Automation Center for review and processing and are ultimately provided to VA headquarters for assessment and response. The program has provided number of cases, case rates, and demographic data for several diseases of particular surveillance interest and might be considered a model of interest to the military.

The study team finds that measures are needed to reinforce the laboratory capability for public health surveillance within the military. Adequate people and resources are needed to support an effective laboratory-based surveillance system and to improve the information technology systems for such a system. Diagnoses should be coded with as much specificity as is sought in the civilian sector.

Defense Medical Surveillance System

The Defense Medical Surveillance System (DMSS) is a system of databases managed by the Army's Center for Health Promotion and Preventive Medicine. Data from several military medical databases as well as personnel and deployment rosters are linkable through this passive system. The databases include those for military inpatient data (since 1990), ambulatory care data (since 1996), reportable diseases, acute respiratory diseases, health risk appraisals, and HIV infection status (Table 4-1). Analysts at DMSS are able to link personnel and medical databases to pose epidemiologic questions for a range of population levels, including the entire military or a particular service or for a range of deployment or demographic category-specific groups. The DMSS provides a valuable resource for military medical surveillance.

TABLE 4-1. Selected Data Tables Integrated Within the Defense Medical Surveillance System

Table	Source	Frequency	No. of Records	Service	Period of Time
Person[a]	DMDC	Monthly	6.4M	All	1990–1999
Demog[a]	DMDC	Monthly	53.9M	All	1990–1999
MEPS	MEPC OM	Monthly	6.4M	All	1985–1999
Deploy_PGW[b]	DMDC	Once	696K	All	1990–1991
Deploy[c]	DMDC	Monthly	282K	All	1993–1999
SIDR	CEIS	Monthly	1.6M	All	1990–1999
OJE_SIDR	PASBA	Weekly	6.5K	All	1996–1999
Deploy_Forms[d]	DST	Monthly	137K	All	1996–1999
SADR	CEIS	Monthly	22.5M	All	1996–1999
HIV_Tests[e]	Testing Labs	Weekly	20M	All	1985–1999
DoDSR	DoDSR	Weekly	23.2M	All	1985–1999
Casualty[f]	DIOR	Yearly	19.3K	All	1985–1998
HRA	CHPPM	Yearly	784K	Army	1990–1998
Reportable Events[g]	MTFs	Daily	48K	Army	1994–1999

[a] Person/Demog contain all persons on active-duty and in the reserve component.
[b] Deployment roster for the Gulf War.
[c] Deployment roster for major deployments since the Gulf War.
[d] Health assessment questionnaires administered before and after major deployments.
[e] Data from mandatory HIV tests performed on DoD personnel and applicants at Military Entrance Processing Stations.
[f] Casualty data on active-duty deaths.
[g] As outlined in the Tri-Service required list of reportable events.

NOTE: DMDC = Defense Manpower Data Center; MEPCOM = Military Entrance Processing Command; MEPS = Military Entrance Processing Stations; SIDR = Standard In-Patient Data Record; CEIS = Corporate Executive Information System; PASBA = Patient Administration Systems and Biostatistics Activity; SADR = Standard Ambulatory Data Record; DoDSR = U.S. Department of Defense Serum Repository; DIOR = Directorate for Information, Operations and Reports; HRA = Health Risk Appraisals; CHPPM = U.S. Army Center for Health Promotion and Preventive Medicine; MTF = Military Treatment Facility; K = thousand; and M = million.

SOURCE: U.S. Army Medical Surveillance Activity (1999).

A subset of data from DMSS without personal identifiers is available for analysis via remote access through an application called the Defense Medical Epidemiologic Database (DMED). With DMED, users can perform queries regarding disease and injury rates and relative disease burdens in active duty populations. Registration and access to DMED is available through the Army Medical Surveillance Activity web site, http://www.amsa.army.mil.

Global Surveillance for Infectious Disease Threats to Military Operations—Role of Overseas Medical Laboratories

Information on infectious diseases endemic in regions of high military and strategic interest to the United States is an important component of predeployment medical intelligence. It enables the armed services to implement preventive measures tailored to known threats that can severely hamper military operations. Appropriate vaccines, prophylactic drugs, insect repellents, and pesticides can be most effectively used if the disease threats are recognized and fully understood. Epidemiological studies of infectious diseases in local populations are the best sources of such information.

Since the turn of the century, military medical organizations conducting infectious disease research in regions of military interest have been a rich source of information used to guide military preventive medicine doctrine and policy. Seven different overseas medical research laboratories are in operation. Laboratories in Thailand, Brazil, Kenya, Indonesia, Egypt, and Peru focus on infectious diseases, whereas a laboratory in Germany conducts psychosocial research related to military personnel and their families (Gambel and Hibbs, 1996). These laboratories, operated by military medical research personnel augmented by local national scientists, conduct biomedical research and provide insight into regional epidemiological events. They are primarily involved with advanced product development, including efficacy testing in accordance with licensing requirements. They have proved to be a uniquely capable test bed for treatment and preventive medicine measures against a host of militarily important diseases such as malaria, leishmaniasis, hepatitis, bacterial diarrheas, Japanese encephalitis, scrub typhus, leptospirosis, and dengue (Gambel and Hibbs, 1996).

In addition to carrying out testing of diagnostic tests, vaccines, chemoprophylactic agents, and insect repellents to benefit both military and civilian populations, the overseas laboratories have provided sophisticated laboratory support during military deployments such as Operations Desert Shield and Desert Storm (the Gulf War) and Operation Restore Hope (Somalia), and during major field exercises. The laboratories are also an important training resource for the infectious disease and preventive medicine specialists, epidemiologists, microbiologists, entomologists, and research scientists needed by the military during deployments.

In addition to carrying out testing of diagnostic tests, vaccines, chemoprophylactic agents, and insect repellents to benefit both military and civilian populations, the overseas laboratories have provided sophisticated laboratory support during military deployments such as Operations Desert Shield and Desert Storm (the Gulf War) and Operation Restore Hope (Somalia), and during major field exercises. The laboratories are also an important training resource for the infectious disease and preventive medicine specialists, epidemiologists, microbiologists, entomologists, and research scientists needed by the military during deployments.

As infectious disease threats continue to change and emerge worldwide, the value of these laboratories to military preventive medicine increases. However, funds and personnel resources for these laboratories have been substantially reduced over the past several years, diminishing the ability of these units to carry out their missions (Institute of Medicine, 1999a).

While it cannot remedy the personnel problems at the overseas laboratories, the new DoD Global Emerging Infectious Disease Surveillance and Response System will provide for some improvements in global surveillance. The program began with a presidential directive in June 1996 to carry out four surveillance goals: systems research, development, and integration; response; training; and capacity building (Walter Reed Army Institute of Research, 1998). The improved funding planned for these laboratories will help to improve their eroded capability. However, the professional personnel issues remain a concern, in that limited personnel slots are budgeted to provide support to these laboratories—qualified personnel can be recruited but not retained. Thus, the service medical departments have insufficient professional personnel quotas to fully staff the overseas laboratories (Institute of Medicine, 1999a).

Deployment

Pre- and Postdeployment Questionnaires

Beginning with the deployment to Bosnia, DoD has instituted an effort to carry out brief health screens on personnel before and immediately after specified deployments. The screens include questions on physical and mental status and are meant to help determine the medical readiness of individuals for the deployment and any change in health status upon their return.

The data collected from these questionnaires are not very useful for providing a thorough baseline measure of health status for personnel or assessment of the health of personnel upon their return. Before deployment, the questionnaires are given at a time when the service member is harried and anxious. After a deployment, the service member is in a tremendous hurry to complete paperwork hurdles to return home. Thus, although these questionnaires might in some cases be useful for pinpointing the start of a service member's concerns about his or her health or documenting some unexpected or unusual exposure, they are not critical for routine medical surveillance. At present there are concerns that the postdeployment questionnaires are not carefully reviewed, so that any red flags that they might raise about exposures during deployments are not being noted (Green, 1999). In addition, predeployment questionnaires are apparently not being completed for many of the troops deployed to Kosovo (Bailey, 1999b). The study team believes that the information potentially gathered from these pre-and postdeployment questionnaires could be better gathered from a regularly administered survey such as the HEAR, when the information is more likely to be valid and the responses can be more readily addressed.

Capture of Ambulatory Care and Inpatient Data During Deployments

During a deployment, the most important component of medical surveillance is the capture of ambulatory care and inpatient data. These data can provide information to allow implementation of preventive interventions and can also help with the recognition of patterns suggestive of chemical or biological warfare agent use (Institute of Medicine, 1998). They also provide records of reported health problems that could prove useful after a deployment.

Weekly reports of disease and non-battle injury rates (DNBI) within each unit are reported up the medical chain of command. Visits to sick call are logged into one of the DNBI categories, which include combat/operational stress reaction; dermatological; gastrointestinal, infectious; gynecological; several different categories of injuries; ophthalmologic; psychiatric, mental disorders; respiratory; sexually transmitted diseases; unexplained fever; all other medical/ surgical; and dental (Joint Chiefs of Staff, 1998). DNBI reports can provide a useful source of data on these conditions.

No consistent automated means of carrying out this information capture and dissemination is yet available; the different services use different systems. Although these systems are similar and accomplish similar ends, they are all fairly new and could benefit from an exchange of lessons learned for considering a system that could be applicable in a variety of situations with data shared across services. The proposed Theater Medical Information Program (TMIP) is planned to incorporate this capability, but the program it would use to carry out this function has not yet been designated.

There are several challenges to a DoD-wide approach, however. The information management community is responsible for the development of automated medical surveillance systems, and the preventive medicine community is only peripherally involved (Institute of Medicine, 1998). Systems already in use by some services would not be readily applicable across the services because most Army battalion aid stations still do not have computers and are using "stubby pencil" technology (Institute of Medicine, 1998, 1999b).

Another important aspect of the ambulatory and inpatient data collected during deployments is the quality of the data collected. While it is understandable that during the heat of battle attention to record keeping might be decreased, the system should work well in non-battle conditions. The study team learned that the commitment to collecting and reporting ambulatory data at the unit level is variable and frequently low. Furthermore, those assigned to such work are often not adequately trained for the task (Institute of Medicine, 1999b). Further problems arise when the DNBI tracking systems are perceived as workload reports, leading to the reporting of administrative events or encounters that are not relevant to disease or injury (Institute of Medicine, 1999b). Each time that a new rotation of service members is deployed, training must be repeated. Additional challenges arise in joint-operations settings, in which the three different cultures of data collection and three sets of case definitions come into play. Mental health visits during deployments are not being captured in any electronic system and only infrequently in medical records (Institute of Medicine, 1999b).

The data referred to above are aggregate data. Individual-level data are only beginning to be collected by one of the services (Institute of Medicine, 1999b) and require active entry by providers after hours because of limitations in the numbers of terminals available. The availability of health care data on individuals is clearly critical to understanding the health outcomes of individual service members after a deployment.

Inpatient data are derived from administrative systems not designed for epidemiologic surveillance. The data can therefore be difficult to interpret without understanding, for example, that pregnancies in a theater of operation require medical evacuation. Therefore, for administrative reasons, those who are pregnant require hospitalization. Data from health care provided by host nation facilities and individuals, which are important in the Southwest Asia theater of operations, are not captured (Institute of Medicine, 1999b). As the medical infrastructure deployed ("medical footprint") in future deployments is very likely to decrease, the problem of capturing data from care provided by host nations will continue or grow.

Theater Medical Information Program

TMIP is being planned as a system integration program that will coordinate functioning health information systems. Although it holds promise for the future, when health information systems such as the Composite Health Care System II are further developed, it does not provide additional capability at present. Ultimately, it is planned to be integrated into the line communications, to "organize medical functions into logical, manageable business areas," and to "implement seamless, interoperable systems based on standards based infrastructure" (U.S. Department of Defense, 1998c). Although it is planned to be deployed in 1999, no training, implementation, or infrastructure is yet available to support it (Institute of Medicine, 1999b).

Identifying Deployed Populations

In a system that has not improved since the Gulf War, information about which units are deployed to a theater and who is present in the units is gathered separately by each service and is transmitted to the Deputy Chief of Staff for

Personnel and then to the Defense Manpower Data Center. The information is often inaccurate or out of date with respect to the movement of individuals within and in and out of the theater of deployment. Health concerns raised after the Gulf War highlighted the difficulties of finding out where units had been on given days and at given times and, beyond that, the near impossibility of knowing the locations of individuals. The same problems had been brought out by efforts to estimate exposure to Agent Orange during the Vietnam War.

A series of committees and panels considering the health problems of Gulf War veterans have noted the need for an improved ability to track the movements of deployed individuals, particularly to be able to better know about exposures that they might experience (Institute of Medicine, 1996a; Presidential Advisory Committee on Gulf War Veterans' Illnesses, 1996b).

Despite an apparent consensus that such information is necessary, it is not clear that current deployments involve any improved capabilities. Slowly, plans are being made for a new system called the Defense Integrated Military Human Resources System to provide improved personnel data for all uses, but these plans are still in early stages (St. Claire, 1998) and are thus difficult to evaluate. It is important that representatives of the preventive medicine community such as the Joint Preventive Medicine Policy Group as well as other users of the system be involved as the system requirements for the system are developed.

For the purposes of medical surveillance during a deployment, personnel information including the numbers of service members in a given unit are needed to provide denominators for the calculation of rates of reportable diseases and injuries. An improved system of collection and dissemination of these data will be helpful to the preventive medicine community as well.

Deployment Exposure Data

A clear lesson learned from the Gulf War was the need for the collection of better exposure data during deployments. Exposures of interest include both environmental exposures and exposures to vaccines and other protective agents. The report from a study carried out concurrently (National Research Council, 1999b) addresses exposure assessment from environmental agents, and Chapter 5 in this report discusses DoD efforts to better document immunizations in the individual medical record. Documentation of environmental exposures in individual medical records is a tremendously challenging task, but one that will be necessary to better address questions of long-term health risks from deployment exposures.

Postdeployment Medical Surveillance

Immediate Postdeployment Surveillance

The new surveillance policies described earlier have brought changes in procedures for medical surveillance immediately after a deployment. One component is the completion of a postdeployment questionnaire as described earlier. The questionnaire includes questions pertaining to both physical and mental health symptoms and provides service members the opportunity to express concerns that they may have about their health and that could be followed up with further examinations when they return from a deployment. Service members are to complete the screening before departure from the area of operation or, failing that, within 30 days of their return. Postdeployment assessments of reserve component personnel must be completed before release from active duty.

In conjunction with the postdeployment screening, however, is the collection of an additional blood sample from troops who participate in a designated deployment. Serum from 10 milliliters of blood from each redeploying service member is sent to the Armed Forces Serum Repository. The sample is intended to be collected while service members are still in the theater of operation, but failing that, it is to be collected within 30 days of the return home.

As noted earlier, the study team believes that a regularly administered survey, such as an improved version of the HEAR, should obviate any benefit from pre- and postdeployment surveillance questionnaires. The postdeployment serum samples have proved to be useful and should be collected as deemed necessary for pre- and postdeployment comparisons.

Routine Postdeployment Surveillance

Aside from the completion of a brief self-reported health questionnaire and the collection of a blood sample from returning service members, no plans for additional special efforts for medical surveillance of returning troops have been articulated by the DoD or VA. Those who remain on active duty in the military would resume care under their unit's regular garrison or shore provider. This would include an annual HEAR survey and physicals at periodic intervals. Any hospitalizations or visits to the clinic that they experience would ultimately be included in databases linked by DMSS, although with some lag time.

It is far more difficult to monitor the health of the population of service members who separate from the military after a deployment or members of the National Guard and Reserves who return and are then deactivated. No longer eligible for care from the DoD after past deployments, they have been on their own for medical care unless they suffer from health problems that are determined to be service connected, which entitles them to care through the VA medical system. They thus receive care from an array of civilian providers or if they are medically uninsured, may be hindered from seeking medical care at all. Since their medical care is provided by many different sources, there is no way to easily track their health care and be alerted by unusual rates of illnesses or health care use. In fact, without additional information gathering and analysis there is no way to determine the "usual" or expected rates of illnesses or health care for this group.

New legislation improves upon this situation. Language in the Veterans Benefits Improvement Act of 1998 (P.L. 105-368) provides that service members who serve on active duty in a theater of combat operations during a period of war or hostilities be eligible for medical care for a period of 2 years following their return. The care would include hospital care, medical services, and nursing home care.

It is crucial that this medical care be provided by caregivers familiar with features of the deployment and the particular concerns of returning veterans. As a result of the health concerns of veterans after the Gulf War, VA has put a tremendous effort into informing its caregivers about the concerns of veterans, with mixed success. After future major deployments, similar efforts are needed to familiarize caregivers with the experiences and concerns of veterans so that they can provide care appropriate to needs of veterans.

The 2 years following a deployment are a critical time in the development or precipitation of medically unexplained symptoms. It is important that deployed service members (active and reserve components) be monitored so that health care providers can respond to health problems and unexplained physical symptoms that will become apparent over time. One possibility is to administer the HEAR to a sample of all veterans after a deployment. Those still on active duty will complete it periodically as part of their routine care, but it would need to be mailed to those veterans who have separated from the military, requiring expense and concerted effort. A sample of recently separated service members who had not deployed could be included for comparison. The HEAR would be a questionnaire with which service members are familiar, and their predeployment responses to the same questions would be available for comparison. Responses that suggest that the veteran has many physical symptoms could be responded to with care and counseling as needed to try to prevent the further progression of the problem and the development of chronicity (this is described in more detail in Chapter 6).

A survey instrument such as the HEAR must be used with consideration and acknowledgment of the characteristics of self-reported data. Several studies have indicated that health information provided through self-reporting is not necessarily concordant with data from more objective sources such as medical records (Gordon et al., 1993; Kriegsman et al., 1996; Fowles et al., 1997; Bergmann et al., 1998). However, an individual's perception of his or her health status is a critical aspect of health. If people perceive themselves to be in poor health, then they are likely to have some need for care and support, even if the needs and problems are as yet medically unexplained. It is important to address these individuals' health concerns to prevent further progression or disability.

Deployment-Related Registries

Medical care was not readily available for many veterans who were concerned about symptoms that they experienced after deployment to the Gulf War.

In time, both VA and DoD established programs to provide medical evaluations and referrals for these veterans. The VA Persian Gulf Registry Health Examination Program (established in 1992) offers a free, complete physical examination with basic laboratory studies to every Gulf War veteran, whereas DoD's Comprehensive Clinical Evaluation Program (established in 1994) provides similar evaluations to Gulf War veterans still on active duty. Together, these two programs have provided health evaluations to more than 100,000 veterans with health concerns related to their Gulf War service.

Such registries were developed to meet a clear need in the veteran community for health care and for information about the deployment and the illnesses reported by Gulf War veterans. Indeed, the programs have developed to the point where they provide such information far better than civilian caregivers would be able to. The registries do not, however, fill the role of providing medical surveillance in a way that would be desirable after future deployments. Although they do capture health information from veterans who are concerned about their health, they are not based on a case definition of an illness.

After future deployments, the fact that medical care will be covered for 2 years after a designated conflict should permit changes in the way that health information is gathered from veterans who are concerned about their health. Rather than naming a special deployment-specific registry with a protocol unique to the deployment, veterans can simply receive health care as needed from the designated sources. The information should be captured and can be used to the extent to which it is used now to provide data on the symptoms and diagnoses experienced in this population. According to the National Science and Technology Council's Presidential Review Directive 5, DoD and VA plan to institute deployment-specific registries again as needed after future deployments (National Science and Technology Council, 1998). The study team discourages this approach, preferring that quality care be provided to service members after a deployment without a need for attribution to the deployment.

Long-Term Surveillance

Monitoring the health of a cohort of veterans over a long period grows increasingly difficult as, over time, veterans separate from the military and receive their medical care in the civilian sector. Although the ascertainment of mortality for such a group remains relatively straightforward, the collection of any information about morbidity requires far greater resources. DoD and VA plan to work toward the use of a medical record that is seamless between the two organizations (this is discussed in Chapter 5). Such a record would be of help, but it could not address the large numbers of veterans who seek health care outside the VA system. Health data for these veterans would have to be gleaned through surveys or very expensive reviews of medical records where they could be obtained. The available data should be used to try to assess the health of deployed forces over the long term, with an effort to note the limitations of the data and with research to better understand the biases in the data.

Reproductive Outcomes

A number of adverse reproductive outcomes have been reported by recent veterans, and it remains plausible that current and future military personnel will continue to express such concerns. This is due in part to the increasing percentage of females in the military, greater societal awareness about reproductive health issues in general, and increasing scientific recognition of the reproductive and developmental toxicities of various environmental or occupational exposures (as well as several lifestyle factors).

Increasing concern about adverse reproductive effects may reflect, in part, the clustering of some outcomes in select subpopulations. Clusters of miscarriages, birth defects, and childhood cancers have been reported in civilian populations. Although the cause of most clusters is often not known despite concerted study, there is a growing (albeit limited) literature to support the reproductive and developmental toxicities of many chemicals and other exposures including those that are voluntary (e.g., cigarette smoking).

Surveillance for reproductive outcomes should be considered a part of overall health surveillance. The reason for such an approach is simple. Reproductive processes are broad in scope and have an impact on human health throughout life. For example, nulliparous women are at increased risk of several gynecologic cancers, and men with impaired fecundity may be at increased risk of testicular cancer (Depue et al., 1983; Brinton et al., 1989; Meirow and Schenker, 1996; Moller and Skakkebaek, 1999). Hence, adverse reproductive outcomes have the additional potential to affect morbidity (and, indirectly, mortality) over one's lifetime. Consideration of reproductive health is in keeping with the mission to deploy healthy, fit, and physically and mentally ready military forces.

Surprisingly, much of the attention given to so-called adverse reproductive effects focuses on perinatal outcomes such as birth defects; less attention is given to the spectrum of potential reproductive and developmental outcomes. Surveillance for birth defects alone will not provide the military with a complete picture of reproductive health in deployed forces. To achieve this, information must be collected on a spectrum of endpoints that reflect the processes underlying human reproduction. It should be noted that a complete and updated reproductive and urologic history is critical for assessing adverse effects after deployment-related exposures. It is imperative to have a baseline reproductive history for both men and women, given the tendency for adverse pregnancy outcomes to be repeated in successive pregnancies (Bakketeig et al., 1979; Khoury et al., 1989; Lie et al., 1994; Raine et al., 1994).

There is little surveillance for reproductive outcomes in the general U.S. population, which makes it exceedingly difficult to obtain baseline estimates for military purposes. One notable exception is the live birth registries maintained by all states. Since 1985, all states submit birth certificate data by tape to the National Center for Health Statistics (NCHS). Although birth certificates may vary across states in terms of the type of data recorded, NCHS offers the U.S. Standard Certificate of Live Birth as a model for use by individual states. Thus, a minimal data set is available for all states.

The literature focusing on the accuracy and reliability of birth certificate data suggests that both vary by type of data item listed on the certificate (Carucci, 1979; Buescher et al., 1993; Piper et al., 1993; Emery et al., 1997; Costakos et al., 1998; Green et al., 1998) as well as by type of hospital reporting information (Parrish, 1993). Typically, agreement is highest for statistical and demographic data (>92 percent) and is lowest for medically relevant data about the pregnancy (Carucci, 1979; Buescher et al., 1993; Schoendorf et al., 1993). For key perinatal outcomes such as preterm delivery, live birth registries may be subject to misclassification bias on gestational age (Emery et al., 1997). The lowest rate of accuracy is found for birth defects (Snell et al., 1992). Tremendous underreporting of birth defects on birth certificates has been reported, stemming in part from delays in diagnosis or clinical variations in the recognition of defects.

Live birth registries can be linked with death registries to assess perinatal and infant mortality outcomes. Live birth registries also can be linked to other state registries such as birth defect or fetal death registries, if such registries are available. However, few states have such registries, and if they do they tend to use passive and not active surveillance mechanisms. Live birth registries may provide useful information on vital status and other outcomes such as multiple births, reductions in birth size and gestational age, and secondary sex ratios. Another important aspect of live birth registries is that they maintain a minimal data set on other potential confounders of adverse pregnancy outcomes (e.g., prior history of adverse outcome or lifestyle factors such as smoking or weight gain). Use of vital registry data for military populations must take into account whether the military component (active-duty or reserve status) or deployment status affects reporting of live births (or fetal deaths) or the accuracy of the recorded information.

It is important to note that surveillance for rates of live births or standardized fertility ratios alone will provide only crude data on the reproductive health of deployed forces. Essentially, live births reflect successful reproduction but do not necessarily provide insight into adverse outcomes that do not manifest in a live birth. Indeed, only 25 percent of all pregnancies result in a live birth (Kline et al., 1989). Accurate and reliable information on live births serves as denominator data when estimating rates of other adverse perinatal outcomes such as the prevalence of birth defects, low birth weight, or pre- or postterm delivery.

Surveillance for birth defects may be of particular concern for ensuring the reproductive health of deployed forces given growing evidence about the developmental toxicities of many chemicals and related environmental exposures, reported clustering of defects in select subpopulations, and the emphasis on birth defects in the media. Ascertainment of birth defects is not a straightforward process and is often hindered by a lack of available data or mechanisms for identifying defects for any given population. In the United States, 31 states have congenital malformation registries, 4 are in the process of implementing registries, and 3 are considering them. States that use passive surveillance mechanisms rely largely on hospital discharge records and may underascertain birth defects. Surveillance for birth defects requires considerable effort if reliable estimates are to be ascertained. Discussion of methodologic issues and a minimal data set are beyond the scope of this report and are provided elsewhere (Eskenazi, 1984; Holtzman and Khoury, 1986; Kallen, 1988).

Further problems associated with monitoring of birth defects include how defects should be defined and counted. For example, should both major and minor defects be counted? Should multiple or single defects be counted? Should genetic defects be counted or excluded? Recognition of birth defects varies across practitioners, and requirements mandated by states also vary (if reporting is required at all). Also, it is important to note that the majority of fetuses with birth defects are spontaneously aborted before birth, hence the need to refer to the prevalence of defects among live births. Recently, upon completion of a feasibility study, the Emerging Illness Division of the Naval Health Research Center concluded that the construction of a DoD-wide birth defects registry is feasible using a hybrid of active and passive surveillance mechanisms (Bush et al., 1999). Although such a registry might prove to be helpful in addressing concerns about birth defects following future deployments, a more sensitive indicator of reproductive health effects might be gathered through the collection and monitoring of reproductive health histories. A modified or refined version of a regularly administered survey such as the HEAR might accommodate this function.

Given that partners can change over time, it is imperative for any surveillance system to use unique identifiers so that individuals (parents and children) can be followed over time and linked with other health databases. As discussed earlier, baseline reproductive histories should be periodically updated, especially before and after deployment, and they should query personnel about subtle outcomes. Prevention of exposure to known and potential reproductive and developmental toxicants by deployed forces will help to ensure the reproductive and overall health of deployed forces (Palmer et al., 1992; Leon et al., 1998), including that of their dependent children. In sum, reproductive processes are broad in scope and have the potential to affect health status throughout life. The military cannot afford to ignore such human health endpoints.

At this time, the evaluation and analysis of data necessary for surveillance take place in a variety of settings in the different services, with special resources involved for specific deployments. While key databases are included in the DMSS and this unit has progressed toward capability for DoD-wide analysis, services also carry out their own surveillance activities. The study team acknowledges that some surveillance resources may necessarily be service-specific or deployment-specific, but urges DoD-wide coordination and oversight from a central authority and encourages the ongoing efforts in this direction through DMSS. Surveillance needs of the reserves must be included. The need for leadership and coordination in data analysis is related to the need described elsewhere in this chapter for leadership authority and accountability for coordination for preventive medicine and environmental and health surveillance across the U.S. Department of Defense and the individual services.

Confidentiality of Health Information

Several of the military's current and proposed instruments (both proposed by the military and recommended by this report) collect sensitive health-related data (e.g., mental health status, reproductive health issues, HIV infection status, childhood sexual abuse, and alcohol abuse). As these instruments are developed and used, questions should arise, such as how will the data be used, who will use them, and what protections are available to prevent abuses of the data and to protect the interests of those who complete the questionnaire?

It is anticipated that the data will be used for subsequent clinical decision making and management and for research. Both types of uses may be analogous to some uses of ordinary civilian medical records. For instance, it is unremarkable for a civilian medical record to include information about alcohol abuse or mental illness when that information is of potential utility in managing a variety of maladies. Similarly, health services research makes use of civilian records to study resource utilization, institution and provider performance, and other processes and outcomes.

Challenges arise when personal health information is used for purposes other than the provision of health care. For instance, will such data be used to determine assignments, postings, promotions, or other service-related matters? Given that the record may be maintained throughout a recruit's military career and perhaps after the military career, might the data be used to determine eligibility for future health benefits?

Because DoD is the employer, the issues here parallel those that arise in the context of occupational health. Although it is sometimes argued that employers should be able to use health data to make employment decisions, a noteworthy counterargument is that health records are inferior to on-the-job performance as tools for evaluating an individual's success.

Because reservists get care from civilian providers, and some active-duty service members may also seek private care, questions regarding the confidentiality of civilian records may arise. Military physicians or others currently cannot have access to civilian provider medical records without the consent of the patient. Therefore this consent and information about the intended uses would be needed to establish any links with civilian providers.

Currently, military medical records include a sheet entitled "Privacy Act Statement—Health Care Records" signed by the patient as the record is begun. It notes the following routine uses of the data:

> The primary use of this information is to provide, plan and coordinate health care. As prior to enactment of the Privacy Act, other possible uses are to: Aid

> in preventive health and communicable disease control programs and report medical conditions required by law to federal, state and local agencies; compile statistical data; conduct research, teach; determine suitability of persons for service or assignments; adjudicate claims and determine benefits, other lawful purposes, including law enforcement and litigation; conduct authorized investigations; evaluate care rendered; determine professional certification and hospital accreditation; provide physical qualifications of patients to agencies of federal, state, or local government upon request in the pursuit of their official duties. (DD Form 2005, February 1976)

As described in Chapter 5, the data from these instruments will be stored electronically. This will have the positive effect of making it comparatively easy for appropriate health professionals to access the data. It also means that it might be comparatively easy for inappropriate persons to access the data. As the instruments continue to be developed, it is important that clear statements of the intended uses of the data be provided and that guidelines and policies for considering subsequent modifications to that list be developed and made available. In addition, identification of the kinds of personnel who will have access to the data should be noted. (Note that such an effort will be complicated to the extent that the medical record is planned to be made available to nonmilitary entities, including the VA medical system, after an individual's discharge.) Finally, confidentiality and electronic security policies, referred to in Chapter 5, as well as the extent to which surveillance constitutes human subjects research, should be clarified.

FINDINGS AND RECOMMENDATIONS

Finding 4-1: The collection of uniform survey data from all recruits upon entrance into the military can provide valuable baseline health data from individuals and provide population data useful for understanding the development of disease and injury.

Recommendation 4-1: The Recruit Assessment Program should be implemented to collect baseline health data from all recruits (active-duty, National Guard, and Reserve) and should be periodically reassessed and revised in light of its goals. Its data should be used prospectively to test hypotheses about predisposing factors for the development of disease, injury, and medically unexplained symptoms.

Finding 4-2: Annual collection of health risk information through a survey should facilitate the implementation of preventive measures within the entire military population and provide valuable baseline health information. The instrument should be carefully designed for maximum benefit of health assessments and preventive medicine efforts, including those for medically unexplained physical symptoms and reproductive health.

Recommendation 4-2a: Annually administer an improved Health Evaluation and Assessment Review to reserve as well as to active-duty personnel to obtain baseline health information. When it suggests that an intervention is warranted, alert the individual and encourage him or her to seek care in the civilian sector.

Recommendation 4-2b: Refine the Health Evaluation and Assessment Review by drawing on additional survey instrument and subject matter experts. Make the categories more clinically relevant, and modify or add questions relevant to signs of medically unexplained physical symptoms (sleep disturbances or general symptoms without apparent medical explanation). Modify or add questions relevant to fertility to provide more sensitive indicators of adverse reproductive effects. Validate the questionnaire with comparison of results to those obtained through individual interviews.

Finding 4-3: The potential uses of and protections for sensitive health information are not necessarily known to service members.

Recommendation 4-3:

- **When sensitive information is collected from service members, make clear statements of its intended uses including the types of personnel who will have access to it.**
- **Develop and make available guidelines and policies for the drafting of such statements and the identification of such personnel.**
- **Establish a process to review ethical issues related to data collection and use.**

Finding 4-4: The Armed Forces Serum Repository is important and necessary.

Recommendation 4-4: Continue the Armed Forces Serum Repository by ensuring that the policies regarding timing and frequency of the serum collections in the Joint Medical Surveillance Directive and Instruction are adhered to.

Finding 4-5: The current disease reporting and surveillance system has not been expanded to increase the likelihood of detecting potential adverse effects of drugs and vaccines.

Recommendation 4-5: The U.S. Department of Defense should follow the recommendation of the 1996 Institute of Medicine study, *Interactions of Drugs, Biologics, and Chemicals in U.S. Military Forces* (Institute of Medicine, 1996b) and include potential adverse medical effects of drugs and biologics in the list of reportable conditions.

Finding 4-6: Improved laboratory surveillance is possible through better capture and use of data that are already being generated but that do not make their way to a central location for analysis and dissemination. Current information technology systems for the reporting of laboratory information to central locations are not user-friendly and provide barriers to the effective collection and dissemination of information.

Recommendation 4-6: Reinforce the laboratory capability for public health surveillance within the military. Mandate central reporting of laboratory findings of reportable conditions. Commit adequate personnel and resources to support an effective laboratory-based surveillance system with the information technology systems needed for efficient collection and reporting of data. Code diagnoses with levels of specificity comparable to those used for civilian health surveillance practices. Continue to provide increased resources to overseas laboratories for surveillance in regions of military interest.

Finding 4-7: The pre- and postdeployment health questionnaires do not provide useful baseline or postdeployment health status information because of the circumstances under which they are administered. The predeployment questionnaire is compromised by the mental state of the deploying soldier and the implicit influence from commanders not to flag any problems, and similarly the postdeployment questionnaire is completed in a rushed manner when other interests (getting home or getting compensation) may dominate.

Recommendation 4-7: Discontinue pre- and postdeployment questionnaires unless they are warranted for military reasons other than gathering baseline and postdeployment health status information (as readiness indicators, for example, or to flag topics in areas in which improved risk communication is needed). In their stead, annual administration of an improved Health Evaluation and Assessment Review should provide better information on the health of the service member to provide baseline and postdeployment assessments.

Finding 4-8: Reporting of aggregate disease and non-battle injury (DNBI) data during deployments has improved, although the quality of the data probably has not. Data on the health of *individuals* is still not adequately recorded in a manner that can be used later. Data from host nation and referral care, which are important contributions to care in some deployment theaters, are not captured. The U.S. Department of Defense needs to select a single data collection and reporting system for deployments workable in different settings. This is planned to occur through the Theater Medical Information Plan development process.

Recommendation 4-8: As quickly as possible, implement a deployment disease and non-battle injury (DNBI) surveillance system that is integrated with the patient care information system and that automatically reports information to a central medical command. Continue efforts to capture data at the individual as well as the aggregate levels during deployments. Provide adequate training to those who report the data at the small-unit level and assign accountability for the quality of the data provided. Provide more preventive medicine support in the field during deployments both to improve the quality of the data reported and to provide sufficient support for disease outbreaks. Develop means of capturing inpatient data from all providers who serve U.S. service members during deployments.

Finding 4-9: It is crucial that exposures that occur during deployments be recorded in individual medical records. Some progress has been made in developing means of recording the receipt of medical prophylactics such as immunizations, but it remains unclear how environmental surveillance data will be documented in individual medical records. A necessary step will be improvement in the collection and documentation of information about the locations of troops on a daily basis, as discussed by a sister NRC report (National Research Council, 1999b).

Recommendation 4-9: Integrate the efforts of environmental surveillance, preventive medicine, clinical, and information technology personnel to ensure the inclusion of medically relevant environmental and other exposures in the individual medical record.

Finding 4-10: Formerly, people who separated from the military following a deployment were eligible for government (U.S. Department of Veterans Affairs) medical care only when they were determined to have a service-connected condition. The Veterans Benefits Improvement Act of 1998 (P.L. 105-368) provides that service members who serve on active duty in a theater of combat operations during a period of war or hostilities be eligible for medical care for a period of 2 years after their return. The provision of this care without need for establishment of a service connection provides a valuable opportunity to ascertain the health needs of this population, including medically unexplained symptoms. It will be important to determine who uses this care and how well data surrounding this care can be captured from the U.S. Department of Defense and U.S. Department of Veterans Affairs providers and their contractors.

Recommendation 4-10: Carry out studies to evaluate the data captured from the 2 years of care provided after a deployment. Try to determine the extent to which the data are representative of the population of service members who deployed and whether they could be used to indicate the health of service members after a deployment.

Finding 4-11: Despite the limitations of self-reported data, the Health Evaluation and Assessment Review is another means by which the health of the forces can be monitored after a deployment. Service members who remain on active duty will continue to complete it, but special effort would be required for its administration to a sample of service members who separate from the military.

Recommendation 4-11: In addition to continuing to provide the Health Evaluation and Assessment Review (HEAR) to active-duty troops, annually administer the HEAR to a representative sample of service members who have separated from the service for 2 to 5 years after a major deployment to track health status and identify concerns including medically unexplained symptoms. Also administer the HEAR to those separated service members who seek health care during the 2 years after a deployment. Evaluate the validity and usefulness of the information collected.

Finding 4-12: Deployment-specific registries such as those established for Gulf War veterans do not fill the role of providing medical surveillance in a way that would be desirable after future deployments. Although they do capture health information from veterans who are concerned about their health, they are not based on a case definition of an illness. After future deployments, the fact that medical care will be provided for 2 years after a designated conflict would permit changes in the way that health information is gathered from veterans who are concerned about their health.

Recommendation 4-12: Avoid whenever possible the creation of deployment-specific registries. Depend, instead, on the data provided by routine medical care under the Veterans Benefits Improvement Act of 1998 (P.L. 105-368) and the annual Health Evaluation and Assessment Review.

Finding 4-13: Concerns over long-term health effects of deployments have increased. Data are needed to answer questions about the long-term effects of deployments and a variety of deployment-specific exposures.

Recommendation 4-13: Carry out surveillance to look for differences in mortality and morbidity between deployed veterans and comparison populations over the long term after major deployments. Include inpatient and ambulatory care data for service members who remain on active duty; data from the Health Evaluation and Assessment Review administered to active-duty service members, members of the reserves, and a sample of separated veterans; and inpatient and outpatient data from U.S. Department of Veterans Affairs facilities. Follow up with additional studies as indicated.

Finding 4-14: No systematic collection of standardized data on the reproductive histories of service members exists. Basic endpoints (i.e., gynecologic and urologic disorders, menstruation, sexual dysfunction, and impaired fecundity and fertility) are not consistently available as part of the medical record. Although the Health Evaluation and Assessment Review asks for some reproductive information, it is not designed to elicit the breadth of information needed.

Recommendation 4-14: The U.S. Department of Defense should develop, test, and field a questionnaire to capture reproductive endpoints. The questionnaire should be used to obtain reproductive histories upon joining the military and should be updated periodically as part of the Health Evaluation and Assessment Review or some other regularly administered instrument. Reproductive histories should inquire about a spectrum of fecundity- and fertility-related outcomes to ensure that reproductive health (and not just childbearing) has not been compromised.

Finding 4-15: A military birth defects registry would provide an insensitive measure of developmental toxicity stemming from maternal or paternal exposure(s) but would be an improvement over currently available information. This approach would be more complete and timely than record linkage studies with state-based birth defects registries. However, the conceptualization and establishment of such a registry require concerted effort and expertise to ensure the utility of the collected data, including consideration and planning for the methodologic nuances of birth defects and barriers to case ascertainment beyond that carried out in the recent Naval Health Research Center feasibility study.

Recommendation 4-15: The U.S. Department of Defense should proceed to establish a birth defects registry, although it should clearly acknowledge the critical limitations of such a registry. As described earlier in the chapter, birth defects are a very insensitive measure of developmental toxicity. Outside expert input should continue to be used to make decisions about the registry's surveillance strategy, case ascertainment process, classification scheme, inclusion or exclusion of genetic defects, unit of analysis, and choice of denominator.

Finding 4-16: The military health system has evolved and is developing several different tools (such as the Recruit Assessment Program, the Health Evaluation and Assessment Review, the Defense Medical Surveillance System, and deployment surveillance systems) that play or that could play a role in providing health surveillance information for military populations. These tools have not been planned to be part of a coordinated system of health surveillance and preventive medicine, and thus are not maximally efficient. A central authority is needed for environmental and health surveillance analysis and dissemination.

Recommendation 4-16: Clarify the leadership authority and accountability for coordination of preventive medicine and environmental and health surveillance across the U.S. Department of Defense and the individual services.

5

Medical Record Keeping

An Institute of Medicine committee studying the health consequences of the Persian Gulf War noted that "the single most troublesome problem encountered in attempts to conduct epidemiologic studies of illnesses among Persian Gulf war veterans has been the inability to retrieve information on medical care events such as hospitalizations, outpatient visits, and diagnosis and treatment from DoD and VA medical records in a uniform and systematic manner" (Institute of Medicine, 1996a, p. 128). The committee went on to state that "current systems are fragmented, disorganized, incomplete, and therefore poorly suited to support epidemiologic and health outcomes studies" (p. 128). As a result, the number one recommendation from the committee was to have the U.S. Department of Defense (DoD) and the U.S. Department of Veterans Affairs (VA) work together to develop a "single, uniform, continuous, and retrievable electronic medical record for each service person" (p. 10). They envisioned that the record should include all relevant health items, allow linkage to exposure and other data sets, and have the capability to incorporate relevant medical data from other institutions with appropriate confidentiality protections.

The Presidential Advisory Committee on Gulf War Veterans' Illnesses (1996b) directed the National Science and Technology Council (NSTC) to develop an interagency plan to address health preparedness for and readjustment of veterans and families after future conflicts and peacekeeping missions. NSTC recommended that DoD "implement a fully integrated computer-based patient record available across the entire spectrum of health care delivery over the lifetime of the patient" (National Science and Technology Council, 1998, p. 23). The goal was to "ensure the accuracy, timeliness, security, and retrievability of information that must be entered into records or automated systems that document personnel history for active, National Guard, and reserve service members and veterans" (p. 23).

In accordance with its charge, the study team reviewed DoD's approach to medical record keeping and provides recommendations to enhance the capability of information systems to support the health of deployed U.S. troops. As part of the review process, the study team held three workshops that covered various aspects of DoD's approach to medical record keeping. The study team also solicited advice from additional experts on medical information systems, Edward Hammond and Clement McDonald, who participated in DoD briefings and the review. The study team and other experts consider the computer-based patient record (CPR) essential for DoD to meet the health care needs of service members before, during, and after deployments (Institute of Medicine, 1997). Additional information systems are necessary to support population-based surveillance beyond medical record surveillance, such as for laboratory-based surveillance, reportable conditions, and disease non-battle injury (DNBI) reporting (Chapter 4). This chapter summarizes the study team's observations, findings, and recommendations.

While this study and report focused on the global needs for effective automation of military medical records, information is available elsewhere providing more detail about the current medical record keeping practices of the military services. A recent report provides information about specific medical record keeping practices during the Gulf War, how policies and practices have been modified to respond to identified problems, and plans for the future (Office of the Special Assistant to the Deputy Secretary of Defense for Gulf War Illnesses, 1999).

INFORMATION NEEDS OF THE MILITARY HEALTH SYSTEM

As the largest health care system in the world, the military health system has an extraordinary need to acquire, manage, analyze, and retain health information on recruits, active-duty personnel, reservists, and veterans. While care of the individual service member should be its first priority, the record-keeping system in the military health system must meet several needs simultaneously to fulfill the needs of Force Health Protection:

1. provide access to an individual's health data anytime and anywhere that care is required,
2. support record keeping for the administration of preventive health services,
3. facilitate real-time medical surveillance of deployed forces and timely medical surveillance of the total force,
4. provide comprehensive databases that support outcomes studies and epidemiological studies, and
5. maintain longitudinal health records of service members beginning with recruitment and extending past the time of discharge from the military.

Each of these requirements is briefly elaborated upon below.

Individual Care

Informed decision making requires access to comprehensive data on patients at the time that care is delivered. The mobile nature of military personnel, including deployments abroad, makes use of CPRs the only practical option. Because service members may be deployed to locations where access to the CPR may be problematic, other methods of providing necessary health information at the point of care must also be considered. It is unlikely, however, that large amounts of data are required outside of a medical treatment facility. For specific situations, such as medical evacuation, portable storage devices may be useful.

Preventive Care

Although preventive care is part of care to individuals, its universal application to members of the force (e.g., mass immunizations) and the need to track compliance with guidelines warrant special attention. Service members need immunizations to protect them from hazards associated with special deployments. These include immunizations against respiratory diseases prevalent in training camps, against natural disease hazards during deployments, and against biological warfare agents. CPR systems perform well when used to identify service members who are eligible for a specific preventive medicine service, remind health professionals to perform the service, and track members' health statuses (McDonald, 1976; McDonald et al., 1984, 1992; Shea et al., 1996; Tang et al., 1999). Reminder and tracking functions should be incorporated into the CPR to ensure the greatest possible integration of preventive medicine practices with routine care.

Another part of prevention is to "do no harm." Adverse drug reactions cause significant morbidity in hospitals (Bates et al., 1995; Leape et al., 1995; Classen et al., 1991; Lazarou et al., 1998). Adverse events also occur in the ambulatory care setting, including the military ambulatory care setting. Computer-based decision support associated with physician order entry can effectively reduce the incidence and costs of adverse drug interactions (Classen et al., 1991; Evans et al., 1993; Lee et al., 1996; Shiffman et al., 1999). Military CPR systems should include automated decision support to detect potential drug allergies and drug-drug interactions as well as other decision support functions (Johnston et al., 1994).

Medical Surveillance

In addition to providing data to support immediate care of individuals, the military health system must support ongoing medical surveillance of the military force to ensure maximal preparedness for the military mission and to detect health threats promptly. Useful information for surveillance will come not only from individual medical records, but also from sources such as mandatory reportable conditions, aggregate DNBI data, and laboratory databases. Consequently, the ability to consolidate data from all regions in the world must exist and must be available in a timely manner. To analyze aggregate data, common representation of data is required. At a minimum, common data definitions and common data models must exist for all relevant health items to be consolidated. Also, since the interpretation of data depends on how data are gathered, the use of common applications to acquire data increases the consistency of data collected at different locations.

The operational utility of surveillance data to commanders (particularly in theaters of operation where the risk of chemical or biological agents is high) depends on both the accuracy of the data and the timeliness with which commanders can access and interpret aggregate data. Real-time linkages between medical units and upper echelons of command are needed so that surveillance data can be used to detect and immediately respond to health threats.

Correct interpretation of real-time surveillance data during an engagement and epidemiological studies of war-related illnesses after a deployment also depend on accurate documentation of exposures. Data systems containing detailed records of duty locations and environmental exposures, such as those discussed by one of the companion reports to this one, *Strategies to Protect the Health of Deployed U.S. Forces: Detecting, Characterizing, and Documenting Exposures* (National Research Council 1999b), must be interfaced with the CPR so that links between exposures and illnesses can be studied and adverse health effects can be treated or prevented.

Databases for Epidemiologic Studies

It is crucial that health information collected from individuals be gathered in a manner that permits asking epidemiologic questions about deployed populations. Two unmet requirements after past deployments have been the need to conduct good epidemiologic studies of the effects of putative deployment exposures and the need for information to assess the long-term health status of deployed individuals. Meeting these needs requires record-keeping systems that can link personnel information, location information, individual exposure information, and health outcome information.

Longitudinal Record Keeping

Manifestations of the health effects of war are often delayed and are sometimes prolonged. Consequently, information-gathering activities should continue for years, perhaps indefinitely, after discharge from the military, as discussed in Chapter 4. For discharged service members who later receive their health care from VA, ongoing follow-up requires interfaces between VA and DoD health information systems. For service members and reservists who receive care from civilian health care providers, mechanisms for the capture of essential health data from the Recruit Assessment Program (RAP) and Health Evaluation and Assessment Review (HEAR) instruments are necessary.

Defining, understanding, treating, and preventing illnesses that follow deployment of U.S. troops require diligent and comprehensive record keeping. The following section examines some of the major information systems activities under way and planned in DoD.

MAJOR INFORMATION SYSTEMS ACTIVITIES

To gain an understanding of the ongoing information systems activities in support of Force Health Protection, the study team heard briefings on several projects including the Composite Health Care System (CHCS), the Government CPR (GCPR) project, the Preventive Health Care Application (PHCA), the Personal Information Carrier (PIC), and various survey instruments. Observations for each project area are summarized below.

Composite Health Care System

The CHCS is a clinical information system project that began in the early 1980s. The scope of clinical information stored in CHCS is currently limited to ancillary data such as laboratory results and pharmacy data. CHCS is deployed at 86 medical treatment facilities worldwide, and each CHCS stores data in a local database. Unfortunately, data from the local databases cannot be linked to construct a consolidated database. The lack of data integration also makes it difficult to provide a continuous record for service members. The study team heard several examples of the difficulties in accessing information from disparate CHCSs. For example, when a service member changes duty stations or is deployed, data stored in one CHCS cannot be transferred to the CHCS at another location. Laboratory data critical to effective medical surveillance can be transferred to another facility only by electronic mail because laboratory results are stored in local CHCS databases. The CHCS hardware and software were described as "difficult and expensive to operate and maintain, and the system has an architecture that does not readily provide expansion of capabilities to meet current and future military health system mission needs" (U.S. Department of Defense, 1998a). Because of the limitations of CHCS, a second phase of CHCS (CHCS II) was initiated in 1997, and the original program was named CHCS I.

The CHCS II program includes development of a CPR, immunization tracking, health risk assessment, pre- and postdeployment health status tracking, and security services. CHCS II has been planned as a "system of systems" (U.S. Department of Defense, 1999c). A "best-of-breed" approach (an approach that identifies applications that serve specific tasks and interfaces them to a central system) has been adopted as the strategy for information systems in the military health system. Although this strategy takes advantage of multiple niche products, it presents a significant challenge to data integration because the different products do not share a common data model or database (Hammond, 1999; McDonald, 1999). The best-of-breed approach tends to favor growth of independent, task-specific applications without sufficient consideration of the overall integration strategy. The need for data integration must be proactively interjected into the process of defining, specifying, and prioritizing information requirements. To the extent possible, the needs of all three services should be considered concurrently to maximize reuse of data and software programs. Attempts to combine data gathered from different applications into a single database are fraught with difficulty and often are not possible. Development and maintenance of interfaces to multiple systems requires substantial effort and must be updated every time any one program is updated. To work at all, there must be a well-articulated and precisely defined technical architecture that spans all branches of the military. Similarly, a common approach to data standards by all who need data (e.g., caregivers, epidemiologists, and preventive medicine professionals) should be adopted. Otherwise, the same or similar data will be collected multiple times instead of being collected once and reused (Hammond, 1999; McDonald, 1999).

A consistent theme observed throughout the briefings was a mutual lack of awareness and coordination among the various project participants involved with information-gathering activities and systems. In general, each need for data has been addressed by a separate data-gathering activity at the individual service level. It was common to find that each branch of the military had its own processes and programs for the gathering of data. Effective central oversight authority common to all three services to ensure that independent efforts are coordinated or, better yet, consolidated into a single activity that serves the needs of all three services was not apparent. The study team received very few details about the implementation plans and milestones for many of the important medical record-keeping projects including CHCS II, the final common pathway for information systems projects. Although the intent is that all applications be integrated into CHCS II, the study team heard no concrete technical plans for the integration. In addition, it is not clear that CHCS II data from different regions will be consolidated. According to one briefing, CHCS I data will not be integrated with CHCS II data (L. Ray, 1998). Compromising the ability to share data among applications would undermine the vision of creating a uniform CPR for all service members and would prolong the state of data fragmentation described in previous studies.

In addition to developing technical plans for data integration, organizational plans need to be developed to standardize policies and practices relating to medical record keeping. The study team heard of differences in policies between the services regarding whether certain information should be recorded and of differences in the forms used to record information. In short, whether and how medical information was recorded varied on the basis of the type of data involved (e.g., outpatient care, inpatient care, immunizations, or investigational drug use), the location of the service member (e.g., garrison, deployed, and location of deployment), and the branch of service. Policies, procedures, and practices should be standardized so that consistent and comprehensive data can be stored in the CPR throughout the military enterprise.

A new program, the Theater Medical Information Program, is planned to be a field-deployable system that will link information databases. It is planned to "support mission-critical information and data from across the areas of medical command and control, patient movement, medical logistics, health care delivery, and manpower, personnel, training, and resources" (U.S. Department of Defense, 1998b, p. 4). CHCS II is anticipated to be only one of many systems or modules that it links and integrates (U.S. Department of Defense, 1998c). Although CHCS II is scheduled to begin worldwide deployment in 2000 (U.S. Department of Defense, 1999f), many of its features and characteristics are still under development, and it is likely to be several years before it is ready to provide the functions described above. The Theater Medical Information Program is fully funded through 2004.

Since CHCS II will be a key component used by the Theater Medical Information Program for the care of the service member during a deployment, it is vital that the two systems work together well to meet the needs of deployment. CHCS II must be developed and implemented with a priority for the readiness mission.

A separate area of concern for the study team was the medical record-keeping needs of the reserve component. As described in Chapter 8, members of the reserves do not receive their health care from the military health system but from civilian providers through their employers' insurance or paid for by themselves. Thus medical records for reserve forces are not readily available to the military system. Because reservists increasingly constitute a significant portion of deployed forces, ensuring that health care providers have adequate information to care for reservists during deployments and that epidemiologists have sufficient population data for this group should be a high priority. The reserves are at increased risk of adverse health consequences (Iowa Persian Gulf Study Group, 1997), perhaps because of the episodic nature of their participation in the military. Consequently, the health information management needs of the reserve component should be explicitly addressed in the information systems strategy. Currently, they are not.

One means to acquire health status information from reserve members would be through annually administering the HEAR survey to members of the reserves, as recommended in Chapter 4, and through administering the RAP instrument to all recruits as currently planned by DoD and recommended in Chapter 4. It is important that data be captured electronically and be retrievable as part of a computerized patient record for reserve members. While such a CPR for reservists would not be as complete as that for those who are active-duty service members, it should provide information useful during deployments and for surveillance.

Government Computer-Based Patient Record Project

As part of his commitment to resolving the health information management issues that impeded study of Gulf War illnesses, the President directed DoD and VA to work together to ensure that service members' health information can be passed seamlessly from the military health system to VA (White House, 1997). In 1998, the GCPR project was established to accomplish this goal. The GCPR project is a cooperative venture involving the DoD, the Veterans Health Administration, and the Indian Health Service to facilitate seamless exchange of patient data among government health information systems. The effort is to be standards based and is to include input from and cooperation with private-sector standards-setting organizations. The study team applauds and supports the goals of the GCPR project. Their intention to work with and build on existing work of health care standards organizations (e.g., HL-7) is excellent. The early focus on building and refining reference models is well placed. However, the GCPR project team may be underestimating the level of effort and time required to make substantive progress in this area. For example, the Institute of Electrical and Electronic Engineers' MEDIX standards group and HL-7 have been working on the Reference Information Model (RIM) for over 12 years. It may be unrealistic to expect that the GCPR project team can complete an information model, even of a limited domain, in a matter of a year. The model of any one domain is interrelated with the global, or overall model. Furthermore, their plan to draw on available bodies of work, extend them to meet GCPR needs, and make those extensions available to the international community (GCPR Framework Project, 1999c) is not part of the standards-development process. Such "extensions" performed outside the context of the consensus-based standards process tend to cause divergence from standardization, rather than to strengthen it.

Due to a delay in finalizing the contract with the prime contractor, the study team did not receive any details of the proposed architecture, project plans, and implementation approach during the workshop briefings. While the draft report was being reviewed, the study team received two documents providing an overview of the technical architecture proposed by Litton/PRC for the GCPR Framework, the basis for developing a "virtual" longitudinal patient record (GCPR Framework Project, 1999b,c). The overview document (GCPR Framework Project, 1999b) describes an architecture that relies on a proposed standard for distributed object services (CORBA—Common Object Request Broker Architecture) to identify the patient, locate the various repositories of patient information, translate the meanings of data in heritage systems (existing systems of DoD, VA, and HIS) into a common information model, and ensure system security. The project plans to integrate heritage systems, commercial off-the-shelf systems, and government off-the-shelf systems in a "best-of-breed" approach.

The GCPR team is committed to demonstrating the ability of their Framework to: "(1) share patient data with no loss of meaning or usefulness, and (2) be able to cooperate in the joint execution of tasks" (GCPR Framework Project, 1999b, p. 3). It is important that the proof of concept prototype demonstrate the

Framework's ability to meet these objectives. For example, using their chosen domain of laboratory data, it would be useful to evaluate the Framework's ability to mediate the application of decision support rules stored in one system to laboratory data that are combined from other heterogeneous data sources.

The study team and external advisors find the architecture described to be reasonable conceptually, but are concerned about the feasibility, practicality, cost, and maintainability of the approach. Within a limited domain (e.g., exchanging lab test results), it should be possible to develop a proof-of-concept prototype as proposed by the GCPR project team. The challenge will be to assess the scalability of both technical and non-technical aspects of the prototype to a large health system the size of the DoD, VA, and IHS.

A key element of the proposed GCPR Framework is the virtual database, "a single interface to a variety of distributed, heterogeneous data sources" (GCPR Framework Project, 1999b, p. 8). While it is technically possible to wrap (that is, translate a proprietary interface into a standard interface) heritage systems in a CORBA environment, the ability to maintain the "meaning and usefulness" of the data will prove quite challenging. Although a CORBA-wrapped object may be able to communicate with other CORBA components and services, limitations in the heritage system will persist. For example, if some context of data (e.g., date/time stamp, authentication of the person entering data, medications being taken by patient) were not stored in the heritage system, it will be impossible to answer a query requiring such information. Another example where wrapping heritage systems will not necessarily satisfy critical system requirements involves security. The documents mention encryption and digital certificates—techniques to secure communication of data, but do not address the administrative security features needed in each repository to protect identifiable patient information. If a heritage system does not support role-based access or does not record audit trails of all accesses and updates, applying a CORBA wrapper will not raise the functional capabilities of the system to meet Health Insurance Portability and Accountability Act (P.L. 104-191) requirements.

The GCPR documents do not describe how deficits in data collection will be handled to achieve the goals of medical record keeping and medical surveillance. For example, if some important information (e.g., exposure data) is not captured in the heritage system, the feasibility of conducting recommended medical surveillance activities will be limited. If the goal of the GCPR project is merely to access existing data in legacy systems, a simpler Web-based approach could be entertained. A key motivation for creating a computer-based patient record is to efficiently capture comprehensive information about all service members and to make relevant views of that information available to decision makers. Consequently, accommodating the need for entering new data and reconciling data elements among the various heritage systems should be addressed in the architectural plans.

The information management component of the GCPR Framework acts to synthesize "a virtual patient record . . . out of disparate records stored on different systems in different locations" (GCPR Framework Project, 1999b, p. 11).

The GCPR project team proposes to accomplish this "by unifying the information in these records in a common representation, by using a clinical lexicon to standardize terminology and a Common Information Model to provide a shared semantic base of understanding" (p. 11). The study team has significant concerns about the feasibility of this goal, since none of the needed standards currently exists or is likely to be developed in the next few years. No acknowledgment is made of the costs of developing or maintaining such standards. It is also not clear how changes made to the heritage systems will be incorporated into the information model and how these would propagate to other systems that may rely on the data from the source system.

The original time line presented to the study team called for operation of a proof-of-concept laboratory version of a virtual patient database (linking data from heritage systems) by September 1999, and for operation of a full pilot system by February 2000, followed by testing at a live site. More recent time lines call for the prototype phase to finish by February 2000, the pilot tests to finish by March 2001, and enterprisewide implementation by August 2002 (GCPR Framework Project, 1999d). Given the people and organizational challenges associated with standards development and the technical complexity of the project, the study team is concerned that the project will not meet its goals according to the proposed time lines.

Health Assessment Instruments

To gather health information from all service members, a number of survey instruments have been or are being developed. The study team was briefed about plans to automate several of the health assessment instruments that were described in Chapter 4. The study team's summarized observations are below.

Preventive Health Care Application

PHCA includes two modules: software to capture data from the Health Evaluation and Assessment Review (HEAR) survey and an immunization tracking module (ITM) (U.S. Department of Defense, 1999e). Deployment of PHCA with HEAR began in the spring of 1999; ITM entered beta testing in February 1999. Both applications draw on data stored in the local, stand-alone PHCA database. PHCA receives demographic data from CHCS I through a one-way interface. Data stored in the local PHCA database cannot be uploaded to CHCS I.

The study team attended separate demonstrations (different vendors were involved) of HEAR and ITM. The computer-based implementation of the HEAR survey was a verbatim translation of the paper-based survey form. Although there are many opportunities to streamline the data-collection process when the paper-based survey is converted to a computer-based format, the program did not take substantial advantage of that capability beyond incorporating skips to appropriate questions.

The second component of PHCA is ITM. The ITM software is divided into several modules, most of which communicate with each other through batch processes. Multiple vendors are involved. The ITM program downloads demographic information (which originates from CHCS) from the local PHCA. It downloads vaccine supply data from a separate vaccine inventory program through a batch interface. During mass immunizations, a stand-alone program called Mass Immunization (MI) is used on a laptop computer to track immunizations. MI downloads demographic data from ITM. Once immunization data are entered into MI, they are uploaded to ITM and are subsequently uploaded to the Defense Eligibility Enrollment Reporting System (DEERS). The study team was struck by the use of several different software programs, many written by different vendors, to document the administration of a vaccine. PHCA has not been used during the ongoing mass anthrax immunization program because it was not yet fully developed at the start of the immunizations. Instead, each service adapted a different service-specific system to track anthrax immunizations before uploading the information into DEERS. DEERS itself is primarily an administrative system; its use for medical records was an expedient made necessary because the medical records systems were not adequate.

The study team was particularly concerned that PHCA data from HEAR and ITM were stored in a local database at the medical treatment facility. Consequently, medical surveillance data gathered through the HEAR survey resides locally. If an individual transfers to another duty station, HEAR data would have to be transferred by filling out a paper form (DD Form 2766) and hand entered into the PHCA system at the new station. The stand-alone nature of PHCA substantially limits its utility as a repository of patient information and as a medical surveillance tool. It is planned that PHCA will be able to upload data for transfer when CHCS II is implemented, although concrete plans have not yet been defined (ACS Government Solutions Group, 1999).

Pre- and Postdeployment Questionnaires

The current pre- and postdeployment health assessment questionnaires (which can be found in Appendix J) are intended to be administered immediately before and after a deployment, respectively. The questionnaires consist of scannable forms, and the data are stored at the U.S. Army Center for Health Promotion and Preventive Medicine. These data are not yet linked to HEAR data or to other health data. It was not clear that the data have been used in any decision making to date.

Recruit Assessment Program

A new questionnaire that is planned to be administered as the Recruit Assessment Program is being developed to collect baseline data on all U.S. military recruits. The intent is to collect data on a scannable form. Since the program is still entering a pilot stage, no decision has yet been made regarding the computer program into which the data will be entered or how much of the data-collection activity will be coordinated with the HEAR survey program or the pre- and postdeployment questionnaire activities.

Overall, the study team was concerned about the lack of coordination among the various data-gathering projects in the different services. Although most of the survey developers expected data from their surveys to be entered into a computer, each survey typically uses its own dedicated software program. Epidemiology researchers and preventive medicine professionals were not adequately consulted in the development of many of the survey instruments. Understanding the requirements of both the primary and the secondary users of data at the outset would improve the chances of designing a common survey instrument that serves multiple purposes. Minimizing the number of surveys administered and their frequency of administration is highly desirable, considering the logistical challenges associated with the collection of accurate data from troops being deployed. The ability to analyze aggregate data from multiple sites is critically dependent on the compatibility of the applications used to gather data and the database definitions used to store the data. One approach to ensuring comparable data is to use a common software application to gather the data. Another approach is to ensure that the multiple applications used comply with data standards so that the data can be integrated easily. Without establishing shared data standards ahead of time, data obtained through different software programs cannot be combined easily.

Deployment Medical Surveillance System

In the absence of CPRs, medical surveillance is fragmented and not available in real time. The study team heard of some special efforts to improve central reporting and surveillance during deployments. For example, the study team was briefed on the collection of disease and non-battle injury (DNBI) medical surveillance data from Bosnia and from Southwest Asia. In both theaters, diagnoses assigned to outpatient encounters are recorded in the sick-call log by using the 10th revision of the International Classification of Diseases. Twenty-five codes are used. These data are reported weekly to the Joint Task Force under the Joint Task Force surgeon.

The data have several limitations. One of the biggest challenges is ensuring that the encounter diagnoses are accurately abstracted from the progress notes. In general, the task of filling out the classification sheets is assigned to a nonclinician with no training in abstracting. Furthermore, the frequency with which reports are submitted may not be sufficient to detect important outbreaks or sentinel diseases. In addition, multiple diagnoses for individual subjects are coded as separate events, which may distort the percentage calculations. These surveillance data are stored on local servers and thus are not combined with other data. Without a central strategy for collection, consolidation, and analysis of field data, medical surveillance will continue to be fragmented and incomplete.

Another problem with incomplete data collection during deployments involves inpatient data. Both policies and practices differ significantly among different deployments and among the different services in the military. For example, inpatient data from Bosnia are sent to the Patient Accounting and Reporting Real-Time Tracking System (PARRTS), a central patient reporting and tracking database, whereas inpatient data from Southwest Asia are not because PARRTS is not expected to be part of the planned Theater Medical Information Program now under development. Furthermore, when a service member is treated in a host nation facility or at a military health system-sponsored facility, data are not captured in the medical surveillance system. Although more deployment surveillance data are being reported to central facilities now than during the Gulf War, collection, consolidation, and timely analysis of health data about U.S. troops are far from complete and systematic efforts to correct this situation are lacking.

Although the Theater Medical Information Program is planned to carry out the function of facilitating medical surveillance during deployments, it is likely to use modifications of existing programs. Developers should take into account the different demands of different deployment settings. Many of the problems identified above are not problems related to technology alone but are problems related to the training and equipment available to those carrying out necessarily active data-collection roles. An important change will be the implementation of systems that permit less active and time-intensive collection of data. If this change is implemented, medical surveillance will then involve the active scrutiny and analysis of data collected passively.

Personal Information Carrier

The study team was briefed about the PIC, which is being developed to store medical data in a form that service members could carry with them at all times. The PIC, which was conceptualized as a "smart card" (a computer processing unit and memory embedded in a small device), would store an individual's medical status and history, including medical documents, x-rays, and vaccination records (National Science and Technology Council, 1998). The study team heard a number of different purposes described for the PIC. At times it was described as the official complete medical record for each service member (U.S. Department of Defense, 1997c). At other times it was described as an information carrier to communicate information from the field to the central CPR (Page, 1999). Most recently, it is planned to "serve as the abridged Electronic Theater

Medical Record in settings where computer network connectivity is not available, providing in-theater health care providers with immediate access to accurate clinical information" (U.S. Department of Defense, 1999d, p. 1). The information on the PIC is to be read by a proprietary access device. Data would be transferred to a portable computer that would upload the PIC information to the central CPR periodically whenever a network connection was available.

The descriptions of the PIC did not justify clearly the use of high-capacity smart-card technology or adequately assess the feasibility of its use under adverse conditions such as the battlefield. Smart-card technology such as that proposed for the PIC has been proposed since the 1980s for possible application in civilian health care. To date, there have been no significant uses of the technology in any sizable installation. There are several reasons for the lack of success so far: (1) data on the card are frequently out of date (e.g., laboratory test results); (2) each card technology requires proprietary card readers, which are not widely available; (3) there is no predominant card technology; (4) there are no data content or format standards for the storage of data on the card; (5) the costs of the cards and the readers are significant; and (6) damage or loss of the card may result in lost information. Most of these issues apply to use by the military health system as well. Some additional requirements are unique to the military (e.g., durability, readability, and size). Earlier feasibility studies of PIC devices raised concerns about their tolerance of muddy conditions (U.S. Army Medical Department, 1997). Despite these limitations, however, there may be niche applications for PIC use in the military. One possible use would be to capture and communicate medical histories and interventions about a service member undergoing medical evacuation. For this use scenario, however, a PIC is needed only for cases of medical evacuation, not as a personal medical record for all service members. The logistical and financial implications of these two scenarios are drastically different. Although testing of candidate PICs is under way, a clear justification and use scenario is needed.

INFORMATION SYSTEMS ACQUISITION AND DEVELOPMENT PROCESS

Recognizing the need to consolidate 80 to 90 legacy information technology projects into a more manageable structure, in 1996 the military health system designated each military service to be responsible as executive agent for a subset of systems focused on a particular area of interest. The five areas of interest are clinical, logistics, resources, executive information, and theater medical systems. In February 1999, the five business areas, as well as information technology infrastructure and customer support, were consolidated under a single Program Executive Officer (PEO), who is responsible for all acquisition tasks necessary to support approved functional requirements (Tibbets, 1999a).

Functional requirements are developed by the Functional Integration Workgroup, consisting of clinicians, resource managers, logisticians, and health care administrators who are senior officers below the general or flag rank. The information requirements are reviewed by the military health system Program Review Board, consisting of the medical chief information officers of the Army, Navy, Air Force, and the military health system, as well as representatives of the medical comptrollers of the Army, Navy, and Air Force. The information requirements are sent to the Theater Functional Steering Committee for approval, and then are approved and funded by the Information Management Proponent Committee (Tibbets, 1999b).

Once the information technology projects are prioritized and funded, the approved projects are sent to the PEO for implementation (U.S. Department of Defense, 1999b). The PEO has full life-cycle responsibility for the approved projects, including development or procurement, worldwide deployment, and operation of the systems. Work is outsourced to industry through competitively awarded contracts. In time, the PEO plans to migrate the military health system to an information technology architecture that consists of multiple software applications running in a single worldwide network computing environment, providing for progressively greater degrees of information interoperability, data center consolidation, and remote management of information technology assets from data center to desktop (Tibbets, 1999a).

While the study team notes that the previous process for prioritizing, funding, and procuring information technology seemed to encourage selection of individual systems to address individual needs, it is not yet clear how well the new system will work to encourage development of an architecture to accommodate the diverse needs. The study team urges continued emphasis on broad-based input to the development of functional requirements, and external input as feasible throughout the process.

CONFIDENTIALITY OF HEALTH INFORMATION

Given the mandatory nature of health data collection in the military, including the collection of sensitive information (e.g., human immunodeficiency virus infection status and mental health status), stringent regulations, policies, and procedures are necessary to maintain system security and to protect the confidential health information of all service members and their dependents. Included in the legislative mandates of the Health Insurance Portability and Accountability Act of 1996 (P.L. 104-191) are provisions governing system security and the confidentiality of patient data (Health Insurance Portability and Accountability Act of 1996, 1996). When they become law, the military will have to comply with them in the same manner that civilian providers do. The Secretary of Health and Human Services released the Notice of Proposed Rule Making for security regulations in August 1998, drawing heavily on the recommendations of the Institute of Medicine study of current security practices (National Research Council, 1997). Final regulations are expected by the end of 1999.

SUMMARY

There are many challenges to the development, implementation, and maintenance of a health information system to serve the diverse needs of the military. It is not surprising that there are separate activities in each of the services. In some cases these are driven by immediate needs, and in other cases they arise out of a lack of awareness of existing solutions or projects under way elsewhere in the military. To meet the health needs of U.S. forces deployed abroad, however, a unified CPR system that supports the readiness mission is essential. At the core of a unified record is a common data model and common data content definitions that facilitate integration of data from distributed sites and systems. Interfacing of the data from heritage systems will continue to pose substantial barriers to conducting medical surveillance and epidemiological studies of the health of and illnesses suffered by deployed troops. Data integration should be the goal from the beginning. Acquisition and development plans should begin with a clearly articulated technical architecture, a common data model, and common data standards.

The process of developing an integrated CPR for the military health care system is complex, yet it is essential to ensure military readiness and a healthy force. It involves tremendous expenditures of money and resources and requires extensive expertise. With so much at stake, the study team recommends that an external advisory board participate in the effort by providing ongoing review and advice regarding the military health information systems strategy. Composed of members of academia, industry, and other governmental organizations such as the National Library of Medicine, this group would provide synergy and potential leverage between the military and civilian health information system sectors. The study team believes that this partnership will increase the likelihood of success for the overall endeavor.

The study team recommends that a comprehensive review of the military health information systems strategy be undertaken to enumerate the information needs; define an expedient process for the development of an enterprisewide technical architecture, common data model, and common data standards; identify critical dependencies; establish realistic time lines; assess the adequacy of resources; and perform a realistic risk assessment with contingency plans. A truly integrated CPR accessible for medical care, medical surveillance, and epidemiological research is absolutely essential to the health and readiness of U.S. troops deployed abroad. A thoughtful review of the current strategy will increase the chance of success.

FINDINGS AND RECOMMENDATIONS

Finding 5-1: Medical information system development and acquisition within the U.S. Department of Defense have been piecemeal. There is no clear effective central authority to ensure that data from all software systems can be consolidated to serve the needs of those involved with individual care and medical surveillance.

Recommendation 5-1: Clarify leadership authority and accountability for establishment of an integrated approach to the development, implementation, and evaluation of information system applications across the military services. Establish a top-level technical oversight committee responsible for approving all architectural decisions and ensuring that all application component selections meet architecture and data standards requirements.

Finding 5-2: Several current and proposed information systems address task-specific information needs at a local level without sufficient consideration of the overall integration strategy and the need for a common architecture. Thus, multiple overlapping projects address similar information requirements.

Recommendation 5-2: Coordinate the evaluation of information needs for maximum reuse of data elements, data-gathering instruments (e.g., surveys), and software systems across the military health system.

- Assess information requirements across the military enterprise in the context of a global data model and a common architecture for the computer-based patient record.
- Include primary and secondary data users (e.g., preventive medicine professionals and epidemiologists) in the process of specifying, selecting, and developing data-gathering instruments and information systems.
- Analyze the logistical and work flow effects of data-gathering activities as part of the specification and design process.

Finding 5-3: Medical record-keeping practices vary widely on the basis of the type of data involved (e.g., outpatient care, inpatient care, and immunizations), the location where medical service is provided (e.g., a garrison or a deployment location), and the branch of service.

Recommendation 5-3: Develop standard enterprisewide policies and procedures for comprehensive medical record keeping that support the information needs of those involved with individual care, medical surveillance, and epidemiological studies.

Finding 5-4: There are many challenges to the development, implementation, and maintenance of a health information system to serve the diverse needs of the military. An assessment of the readiness of the information technology organization to meet the challenges according to the necessary time lines would alert the leadership to areas that require additional resources, management attention, or contingency planning. Ongoing external input could help to take into account benefits, costs, reliability, feasibility, cross-military ease of use, and the ability to use such systems for subsequent individual and population health studies.

Recommendation 5-4: Conduct an independent risk assessment of the military health information system strategy and implementation plan. Establish an external advisory board that reports to the Secretary of Defense and that is composed of members of academia, industry, and government organizations other than the Department of Defense and the Department of Veterans Affairs to provide ongoing review and advice regarding the military health information system's strategy and implementation.

Finding 5-5: The conceptual architecture proposed for the GCPR Framework Project provides an open-systems architecture to interface heritage applications with new applications. However, limitations of the heritage systems will impede development of fully integrated records and functional decision support. The study team is concerned about the feasibility, practicality, cost, and maintainability of the approach when scaled beyond the limited proof-of-concept prototype that is planned. The GCPR team acknowledges that "the technical solution being pursued in the GCPR Framework project has a moderate to high probability of failure . . . " (GCPR Framework Project, 1999a, p. 21).

Recommendation 5-5: To reduce the risks of the entire GCPR Framework Project, the GCPR project team should ensure that the Phase I prototype is sufficiently representative of the complexity expected for the total project. The prototype should include evaluation of the following:

- **Integration of data from heterogeneous sources while preserving the meaning of the original data**
- **Implementation of decision rules stored in one system acting on data from another system**
- **Entry of data in a new system and its reconciliation with data in heritage systems**
- **Incorporation of existing standards in the prototype and identification of gaps in available standards**
- **Measurement of performance characteristics of the virtual database and estimation of the performance of a comprehensive system with all the data components and middleware services in operation**
- **Estimation of the level of effort and costs of maintaining the middleware services**

Finding 5-6: The health information needs of reserve service members are not being adequately addressed. Although there are challenges to gathering data on reservists, no substantive initiative to acquire or link health data for this group exists.

Recommendation 5-6: Develop methods to gather and analyze retrievable, electronically stored health data on reservists. For example, ensure that data from the Recruit Assessment Program and the Health Evaluation and Assessment Review collected from reserves (as recommended in Chapter 4) are captured as part of a computerized record permitting retrievability and population-level analysis as well as the addition of new data from periods of deployment or activation.

Finding 5-7: The need for high-capacity smart-card technology for a universal personal information carrier is not clearly justified, and its fit with the remainder of the information infrastructure for the military system is not clearly articulated.

Recommendation 5-7: Reexamine the information requirements for the personal information carrier (PIC) and develop a justification for applying the appropriate technology to satisfy the information requirements.

- Identify specific scenarios for the use of the PIC and the relevant military population affected.
- Define the minimum data needed for the provision of care in the battlefield setting.
- Explore practical alternatives for the provision of access to necessary emergency information at the point of care and estimate the infrastructural costs associated with each option.

Finding 5-8: The military mission requires collection, storage, and communication of sensitive, individually identifiable health information for each service member.

Recommendation 5-8: Make available to service members the regulations, policies, and procedures regarding system security and protection of individually identifiable health information for each service member.

- Comply with all system security regulations adopted by the Secretary of Health and Human Services to the extent practical in the military.
- Develop confidentiality policies to comply with federal privacy legislation and regulations in accordance with the Health Insurance Portability and Accountability Act of 1996 (PL 104-191).

Finding 5-9: Funding of major projects is uneven. The Government Computer-Based Patient Record project operates year by year, the Theater Medical Information Program project is fully funded, and the second version of the Composite Health Care System project is funded for deployment but not additional development.

Recommendation 5-9: Treat the development of a lifetime computer-based patient record for service members as a major acquisition, with a commensurate level of high-level responsibility and accountability. Clear goals, strategies, implementation plans, milestones, and costs must be defined and approved.

6

Prevention Measures for Deployed Forces

Measures to protect the health of deployed forces take place throughout the life cycle of the service member. Although some of them are continuous activities, for the sake of discussion they can be categorized into measures that take place before, during, and after a deployment (the deployment cycle). Some activities, like risk communication, must take place in different forms throughout the deployment cycle. After a general discussion of risk communication, this chapter considers preventive measures for different stages of the deployment cycle.

RISK COMMUNICATION

Risk communication is a critical process in public health and is a critical process in military health as well. In the civilian community, tremendous interest and effort have led to the development of an understanding of risk perception and risk communication over the last few decades, particularly in the area of risks from environmental hazards and other public health challenges such as smoking and AIDS. The processes of risk perception and risk communication are complex and have generated a substantial and growing body of literature (Slovic, 1987; McCallum et al., 1991; Fischhoff, 1995; Gustafson, 1998).

Risk communication raises a number of interesting and important ethical issues (see, e.g., Cothern, 1996). They are shaped by the following considerations:

1. If a risk is disclosed too early or is based on inadequate evidence, the communicator may be faulted for unnecessarily alarming or even causing panic in potentially affected people, or for underestimating the risk.

2. If a risk is disclosed too late or is based on too high a standard for evidence, the communicator might be faulted for withholding information that would have allowed for informed decisions by (potentially) affected people.

Risk is a probabilistic concept. Some risks are likely to lead to harm, some are unlikely to lead to harm, and some fall between these extremes. Should a very low risk be communicated if the communication itself can have bad consequences? In some cases, risk communication can be riskier than the risk being communicated.

Moreover, the science of risk analysis is imprecise: any particular risk calculation is uncertain and open to revision (Graham and Rhomberg, 1996). Accuracy is achieved not with a precise value that is placed on a particular risk but with a range of values. It is also important to distinguish between the likelihood of a risk being realized, the severity of the risk if it is realized, and the time of onset and duration of the harm if it is realized. Furthermore, those exposed to a risk will vary in the importance that they attach to likelihood, severity, and timing.

What is *risk communication*? The field evolved from the growing need to explain controversial decisions about environmental and occupational hazards, and through social scientists' efforts to understand how people reacted to information about hazards. The decisions often involved technical content and uncertainties difficult to convey in messages for the general public. Initially the term *risk communication* was commonly used to describe one-way messages from experts to nonexperts, but in the last decade there has been a shift of focus from merely the messages themselves to the entire process (National Research Council, 1989). The National Research Council report, *Improving Risk Communication*, described risk communication "as an interactive process of exchange of information and opinion among individuals, groups, and institutions" (p. 21). It construed risk communication to be successful "to the extent that it raises the level of understanding of relevant issues or actions for those involved and satisfies them that they are adequately informed within the limits of available knowledge" (p. 21).

Although in specific situations two-way exchange is vital, it is neither feasible nor appropriate that all communications about risks in the military be dialogues. Different situations warrant different degrees of exchange, falling on a continuum between none and extensive. In many situations a simple one-way brief on the hazards to be faced must be sufficient. In some instances the adequacy of a simple briefing cannot be assumed and feedback is needed to verify that the intended message has been understood. Most challenging perhaps, are those situations that require full discussions that aspire toward meeting the definition of risk communication given above to include active dialogue among all the groups involved. The challenge for the military will be to identify which situations require which levels of interaction between the concerned parties and to plan for these situations. Clearly, a prerequisite for such planning is identification of the various situations in which risk communication does and should occur.

In the statement of task, the study team is charged with addressing "improvements in risk communication with military personnel in order to minimize stress casualties among exposed or potentially exposed personnel" (Appendix B). It is the opinion of the study team that successful risk communication, as defined above, can provide an important contribution not just in minimizing stress casualties but also in improving trust and credibility and in ultimately improving the morale and effectiveness of the fighting force.

Many factors other than the findings of scientific research enter into individuals' perceptions of risk. The extent to which the risk is voluntary or imposed by others, involves a familiar or an unfamiliar risk or is associated with dreaded consequences as well as other factors are all involved in the perceived magnitude and acceptability of a risk. Personal factors are also important: education, cultural background, values, psychological outlook, health, and trust level. Although the provision of a primer on risk communication is beyond the scope of this report, a large body of literature is available (Slovic, 1987; National Research Council, 1989; McCallum et al., 1991; Fischhoff, 1995; Gustafson, 1998). The substance of this literature indicates that when it is carried out well, risk communication can contribute to improvements in mutual respect and trust. It can also help people to make better decisions leading to actions that better reflect objective risks and that consequently reduce morbidity.

A critical site for risk communication in the military is at the level of the service member in his or her unit. Over years of dealing with stress-related casualties during combat, military psychiatry has developed an approach that emphasizes leadership and unit cohesion as critical components in mission accomplishment and prevention of psychological symptoms, physical symptoms, and stress casualties (Stokes, 1998). The nature of the communication between a commander and his or her unit and between members of the unit is clearly both an indicator of and a contributor to the cohesion of the unit.

Another critical juncture for dialogue about risks and health is between health care providers and service members after deployments. The extent to which health care providers listen to their patients' concerns and show understanding and responsiveness while sharing relevant information with them is important. As described for medically unexplained symptoms in Chapter 3, it is helpful for the care provider to acknowledge both the incompleteness of medical and scientific understanding and the areas in which evidence and knowledge are more complete. Because of the complexity of the topic and the possibility of wide variability among providers, specific guidelines are needed concerning what providers say to patients about medically unexplained symptoms, and training is needed to ensure that they follow these guidelines.

In the years since the Gulf War, portions of both the U.S. Department of Defense (DoD) and the U.S. Department of Veterans Affairs (VA) have been forced to consider risk communication issues with more care than in the past. In responding to the concerns of veterans regarding illnesses following their Gulf War deployment, DoD has faced repeated risk communication challenges. The incomplete information and changing messages provided in the summer of 1996 about the destruction of chemical munitions at Khamisiyah, Iraq, in March 1991, were particularly damaging to DoD's credibility. It is universally agreed that losing credibility is much easier than restoring credibility, emphasizing the need for a proactive orientation toward risk communication. In its report on the government's activities in response to Gulf War illnesses, the Presidential Advisory Committee on Gulf War Veterans' Illnesses (1996b) made several recommendations related to the topic of risk communication. Among them was the recommendation that DoD and VA immediately develop and implement a comprehensive risk communication plan "in close cooperation with agencies that have a high degree of public trust and experience with risk communication" (p. 51), such as the Agency for Toxic Substances and Disease Registry and the National Institute for Occupational Safety and Health.

In response, the Clinical Working Group of the Persian Gulf Veterans Coordinating Board developed the Comprehensive Risk Communication Plan. This plan provides many suggestions that can be used by different groups as they undertake risk communication efforts. The guide was included as an appendix in the report, *A National Obligation: Planning for Health Preparedness for and Readjustment of the Military, Veterans, and Their Families after Future Deployments* (National Science and Technology Council, 1998). In the body of the same report, DoD, VA, and the U.S. Department of Health and Human Services (DHHS) endorse the following goal regarding risk communication:

> Goal 5. Establish an effective health risk communication program that educates and informs active military personnel, veterans, and their families throughout the deployment lifecycle and beyond on issues related to health risks and available services. (p. 15)

The study team was encouraged to learn that the goal of an effective health risk communication program was endorsed by the Interagency Working Group from DoD, VA, and DHHS in the National Science and Technology Council document. In the information-gathering workshop of January 1999, the principal investigators and advisors for the present study sought to clarify the extent to which the responsibility of pursuing this goal within DoD had been assigned (Institute of Medicine, 1999a). It appears that although the military services have some limited programs in risk communication, risk communication has not yet been made a priority at the department level.

The Clinical Working Group of the Persian Gulf Veterans Coordinating Board has also recently released a revised version of their risk communication plan. The Comprehensive Risk Communication Plan for Gulf War Veterans "is designed to improve federal efforts to provide a clear and accurate dialog on the health consequences of Gulf War service" (Persian Gulf Veterans Coordinating Board, 1999, p. 3). It provides good advice and sensible suggestions for improving communications with Gulf War veterans. Much of the advice is relevant to communications for deploying forces as well. With a goal of rebuilding and earning veterans' trust in DoD and VA and regaining credibility that has been lost since the Gulf War, the plan outlines objectives including engaging in ongoing dialogue on health risks, increasing veterans' abilities to cope with symptoms, improving communication, and keeping veterans informed about the health effects of service in the military. The plan notes the critical need for clear goals and evaluation of efforts, and it outlines several research needs for communication with military personnel. The present study team believes all of these points are important for deployed forces generally.

The study team believes that a clear commitment to improvements in risk communication is needed from DoD. Responsibility should be designated to attempt a cultural change within DoD and the military services so that dialogue and exchange about risks are facilitated at all levels. Aspects of risk communication need to be incorporated into the training of line commanders and health care providers. However, the process is an ongoing one that is not conveniently complete with a 1-day or 1-week course. Instead, it requires ongoing reevaluation and effort. The questions whether, when, and how to communicate risk involve a number of nuanced and difficult judgment calls. There is no algorithm for making these calls. It is not sufficient to suggest that a communicator simply "tell the truth" when the truth in a given situation cannot be determined. As well, failing to disclose even very small risks will be regarded by some as a form of deception.

In addition, DoD and the services need to have a discussion about what problems the tool of risk communication may be used to try to solve. Such a discussion can lead to goals for reducing these problems. Evaluation of the extent to which these goals are met can point out both successes and needs for changes.

A recent encouraging example of the use of some of the principles of risk communication within DoD is in the ongoing effort to vaccinate all service members against anthrax. The Anthrax Vaccination Program took proactive steps to inform commanders, service members, their families, and the wider community about the vaccine and the need for it through a variety of messages tailored to target audiences. This effort also illustrates the fact that risk communication is a process that does not end with the first batch of brochures but requires ongoing dialogue in response to the concerns of those involved.

What other risks should be discussed with the service members? It would be impossible as a practical matter to itemize and rank all risks faced by military personnel. There are a number of reasons for this: there are too many, some are minor or trivial, some are or should be assumed (e.g., telling a combat-bound soldier he or she might be wounded by gunfire), and so forth. Since there are almost an infinite number of risks associated with any deployment, these need to be prioritized. However, the priorities suggested by casualty numbers and historical data will not necessarily coincide with the concerns of the service members, who may have other criteria for assigning risk. In general, the risk communication should include battle-related risks, environmental health risks, and psychological hazards. Risk communication should include an introduction to medically unexplained symptoms. To better address the specific concerns of the troops, information about the nature of these concerns in specific situations is needed, and the collection of this information must be an ongoing process.

An advisory group would fill an important function in this process. The use of a panel to advise communicators has a precedent and analog in the practice of including members of affected groups in biomedical research design and evaluation and on ethics review boards (institutional review boards). This improves acceptance from members of affected groups, as well as providing advice from the perspective of those to whom risk communicators are communicating. Since the task of risk communication is inherently fallible—that is, one can plan on having to manage errors—the existence of such groups can be quite helpful in justifying various risk communication strategies both before and after the fact. Service members from a range of levels and their family members could provide input on their information needs and health concerns. Experts from outside the military could provide ongoing access to the body of knowledge on risk communication developed from civilian experience. Indeed, experts from VA and DHHS were important to developing the Guide to Health Risk Communications found in the National Science and Technology Council (1998) document.

Risk communications do not have to be emotional. Indeed, carefully crafted information about risk is seldom frightening, paralyzing, or counterproductive. Whenever possible, risk communications should be combined with information about how to minimize the risks and deal with the negative outcomes should they occur. They should attempt to increase instead of decrease feelings of control.

In addition to the hazards of deployment that are acknowledged in advance of a particular deployment, health issues that require attention and risk communication are certain to arise during and after deployments. DoD needs to plan for these situations, even though it cannot know in advance what the specific risks or concerns will be. DoD's plan should include plans for the early identification of problems and concerns and the criteria to be used to determine when and how risk communications should take place. An especially important decision is who will serve as the spokesperson during the period when answers to questions raised are unavailable or only provisional.

Data from studies of patients and others encountering difficult or threatening situations suggest that providing a framework or context for interpreting the situation and their likely responses to it can reduce both stress and physical symptoms, even when people cannot change the situation. The study team commissioned Jean Johnson, R.N., Ph.D, to write a paper that addresses the question, "What does the research on informational interventions to reduce the stress of medical procedures tell us about communicating to troops the risks of deployment?" Her review of the evidence suggested that the provision of sensory and procedural information to patients before medical ordeals is often beneficial in reducing outcomes such as pain, emotional distress, poor psychological well-being, medical complications, and length of hospital stay (Johnson, 1998). Preparatory information influences perceptions and interpretations in a manner that enhances peoples' ability to cope with stressful experiences (Johnson, 1998). Suls and Wan (1989) concluded from their review of the research that descriptions of peoples' typical experiences were most effective for facilitating coping. Studies with other populations also support the concept that preparatory information can help reduce stressful reactions (Inzana et al., 1996). This body of research suggests that alerting troops to the stresses and emotions that they are likely to feel during combat may improve their ability to cope and decrease the negative consequences that sometimes follow from these stressful situations.

Risk communication is not a panacea, and many may have unrealistic expectations about what it can accomplish. To quote the 1989 National Research Council report on risk communication:

> it is mistaken to expect improved risk communication to always reduce conflict and smooth risk management. Risk management decisions that benefit some citizens can harm others. In addition, people do not all share common interests and values, so better understanding may not lead to consensus about controversial issues or to uniform personal behavior. But even though good risk communication cannot always be expected to improve a situation, poor risk communication will nearly always make it worse. (p. 3)

The reasoned creation of policies that acknowledge that risk communication is probabilistic, uncertain, and (sometimes) error prone can serve to reduce error and ethically optimize the practice of risk communication.

Further discussions about risk communications specific to the periods before, during, and after deployment follow. Findings and recommendations about risk communication are provided at the end of the chapter.

PREVENTIVE MEASURES BEFORE DEPLOYMENT

Preventive measures that take place before a deployment include those that occur upon entrance into the service, during training and routine garrison life, and immediately before a deployment.

Preventive Measures on Entrance into the Service

Risk Communication

The first opportunity for risk communication between DoD, the services, and service members occurs as service members are recruited and begin their military service. During this time there may be a tendency to downplay the risks inherent in military service, but the risks of death or injury should be raised and discussed frankly.

Accession Standards

DoD has developed accession medical standards with the purpose of bringing in recruits who are healthy and who can be deployed worldwide. The standards are uniform across the services and are described in DoD Directive 6130.3 (U.S. Department of Defense, 1994a). According to the directive, new applicants must join the services (1) free of contagious diseases that will endanger the health of other personnel, (2) free of medical conditions or physical defects that cause excessive loss of time from military duty for necessary treatment or hospitalizations or would likely result in separation from the military for medical unfitness, (3) medically capable of satisfactorily completing required training, (4) medically adaptable to the military environment without the necessity of geographical area limitations, and (5) medically capable of performing duties without aggravation of existing physical defects or medical conditions (U.S. Department of Defense, 1994a).

Roughly 355,000 physical examinations are conducted on potential new recruits each year, with about 250,000 new recruits entering the services annually. Approximately 15 percent of new applicants are turned away for disqualifying medical conditions. Waivers of the standards for certain medical conditions can be granted with approval of the service's Surgeon General (Ostroski, 1999).

Accession medical standards have improved and have become more stringent with improvements in medicine and technology. The Accession Medical Standards Working Group and Accession Medical Standards Committee were begun in 1995 to bring some systematic tracking and evaluation to the standards. The Steering Committee is co-chaired by the Deputy Assistant Secretary of Defense (Military Personnel Policy) and the Deputy Assistant Secretary of Defense (Clinical and Program Review), with members including representatives from the Office of the Assistant Secretary of Defense (Force Management Policy), Office of the Assistant Secretary of Defense (Health Affairs), Office of the Assistant Secretary of Defense (Reserve Affairs), Offices of the Service Surgeons General, Offices of the Service Deputy Chiefs of Staff for Personnel and Chief of Personnel and Training, and Headquarters U.S. Coast Guard. The working group consists of action officers from these offices (Clark et al., 1999). They review and revise the physical standards for enlistment, induction, and appointment described in the directive. The committee's main objectives are to make sure that military personnel are fit both medically and physically, to make sure that existing medical problems are not compromised further because of training and deployment, and to ensure a cost-effective, healthy force (Ostroski, 1999).

An important change in the system took place in 1998, when the Accession Medical Standards Directive was revised to use the 9th revision of the International Classification of Diseases to track disqualifying, waived, or medically discharged conditions. This system will provide a means of assessing the effectiveness of the standards and the medical experiences of people granted waivers for otherwise disqualifying medical conditions through research carried out by the Accession Medical Standards Analysis and Research Activity group at the Walter Reed Army Institute of Research (WRAIR).

Some of the medical issues that have been the focus of new approaches or reevaluation of the standards for new applicants are asthma, attention deficit hyperactivity syndrome, refractive eye surgery, knee surgery, and hepatitis B and C. The Surgeons General waive disqualification for certain conditions such as asthma and attention deficit hyperactivity syndrome on a case-by-case basis (Clark et al., 1999; Ostroski, 1999).

Although the accession medical standards are uniform across the services, they are not necessarily implemented identically across them. For example, in the area of psychiatric disorders, potential recruits are not necessarily screened for many of the disqualifying conditions. The Navy and Air Force use certain screens for psychiatric and psychological conditions that the Army does not use (Institute of Medicine, 1999a).

Retention Standards

Reports following the Gulf War suggested that some service members who were deployed to it were not medically fit to carry out their missions (Presidential Advisory Committee on Gulf War Veterans' Illnesses, 1996a). In response to its charge to review compliance with active duty retention standards, the study team was provided a workshop briefing on the topic. Although DoD provides general guidance on separation or retirement for physical disability (U.S. Department of Defense, 1996d), each service has its own medical fitness standards. It is DoD policy that "the sole standard to be used in making determinations of unfitness due to physical disability shall be unfitness to perform the duties of the member's office, grade, rank or rating because of disease or injury" (U.S. Department of Defense, 1996d, p. 2). Because the different services have different missions and working environments, implementation of these guidelines is not uniform across the services. The retention standards are a list of medical disabilities, described in Instruction 1332.38 (U.S. Department of Defense, 1996e). If an individual is identified as having one of these medical disabilities, he or she must undergo a review to determine whether the extent of the disability makes the person unable to perform his or her duties.

The review involves the work of two boards. The Medical Evaluation Board review consists of an evaluation by the individual's attending physician, perhaps a specialist, who writes a narrative summary of the service member's medical condition. This narrative is combined with statements from the member's commander as well as efficiency reports and medical records. The evaluation is then reviewed and signed by three physicians, at least one of whom is at least the second in command of a medical center or a hospital.

The second of the two review boards is the Physical Examination Board. This review board is primarily made up of nonmedical officers who have responsibility for evaluating whether the service member can perform the day-today duties of his or her particular military occupational specialty despite the medical condition. The Physical Examination Board then makes a determination of either fitness to remain in the service or the need for separation from the military (Wortzel, 1999). Retention standards are periodically reviewed by the services' medical specialty consultants for necessary updates.

With limited information gathering on this topic, the study team did not note any problems with the retention standards themselves—the challenge for the services is to implement them effectively. Similar to trends in civilian health care, the services are shifting their emphasis away from physical examinations toward a prevention-based approach to care. Physical examinations are generally required every 5 years except for pilots, who receive them more frequently. As described in Chapter 8, meeting the requirement for periodic physical examinations is difficult in some of the reserve components. Furthermore, physical exams do not tend to be the way most health problems in service members are identified; they are found instead when the service member reports it or reports to sick call (Wortzel, 1999). In contrast to the physical exams, the Health Evaluation and Assessment Review (HEAR) will be administered annually, and should thus provide a more current means of assessing service member health status. For this reason it is particularly important that the HEAR also be provided to reserve members, as recommended in Chapter 4.

Recruit Assessment Plan

As described in Chapter 4, the military plans to administer a survey to new recruits upon reporting for basic training to collect baseline health information. The information should be helpful for the implementation of preventive measures for the individual, and over time, as the database provides information on risk factors in the military population, it should be useful for prevention on a population basis.

Preventive Measures During Training and Routine Garrison Life

Doctrine

Doctrine for medical aspects of nuclear, biological, and chemical (NBC) defense is developed by the Army Medical Department Center and School in conjunction with the other services, and exists in several forms. Joint Publication 4-02, *Doctrine for Health Service Support in Joint Operations* (Joint Chiefs of Staff, 1995), is being revised. It will describe the requirements for health service support in an NBC environment. Additionally, there is the *Handbook on the Medical Aspects of NBC Defensive Operations* of the North Atlantic Treaty Organization (NATO) (U.S. Department of the Army, 1996) and Army document FM-8-285, *The Treatment of Chemical Casualties and Conventional Military*

Chemical Injuries (U.S. Department of Defense, 1995). The Army also provides document FM-8-10-7, *Health Service Support in a Nuclear, Biological, and Chemical Environment* (U.S. Department of the Army, 1993), which provides operational doctrine for combat health support in an NBC environment. This document is also under revision. Additional resources are under development on low-level radiation exposure, treatment of biological warfare agent casualties, and protection from potential long-term effects of exposures to an NBC-environment (Flowers, 1998). Doctrine will also be developed on the use of the FOX chemical reconnaissance vehicle, which is used in Bosnia to identify toxic industrial chemicals.

Doctrine on personal protective measures for insects exists in the form of DoD Instruction 4150.7, *DoD Pest Management Program* (U.S. Department of Defense, 1996a). Additional information more relevant to individual protection measures is available in Armed Forces Pest Management Board Technical Information Memorandum No. 36, "Personal Protective Techniques Against Insects and Other Arthropods of Military Significance" (Armed Forces Pest Management Board, 1996). This document notes the critical importance of command emphasis on ensuring compliance with personal protective strategies.

Army Regulation 40-5 provides "a comprehensive disease prevention and environmental enhancement plan of action for the U.S. Army at fixed installations and in support of field forces" (U.S. Department of the Army, 1990, section 1.1). The regulation describes a program that ranges from field sanitation procedures to environmental laboratory services to the epidemiology consultant service. Additional detail or focus is provided in various field manuals.

Training

Given the array of health threats during deployments (reviewed in Chapter 2), it is important that service members learn about typical health risks during deployments and the appropriate countermeasures during their training. Early attention to such issues conveys the message that they are taken seriously by the services, and is likely to increase the level of adherence to further risk reduction instructions offered during deployments

Medical training on treatment is introduced in basic courses when care providers enter the services, and additional training is provided over time. For treatment of chemical and biological agent casualties, training is provided by the Army. In the recent past, satellite broadcasts have been used to train both military and civilian care providers in recognizing and treating infectious diseases or chemical injuries as a result of biological or chemical warfare or terrorism. Courses for professional care providers are also offered periodically at the U.S. Army Medical Research Institute of Infectious Diseases and the U.S. Army Medical Research Institute of Chemical Defense.

It is a different matter for the line commanders, however. Because they are ultimately responsible for the well-being of the troops, their understanding of the importance and some of the fundamentals of preventive medicine concepts is important. However, they receive very little training in preventive medicine during their basic and advanced courses (Parker, 1999).

It is important that basic preventive medicine measures be emphasized during the training of service members and particularly the training of commanders. Simple measures such as personal protective measures (PPMs) for arthropod bites can be crucial to the health of the forces. There is evidence that even though a highly effective system of PPMs has been available since 1991 (Armed Forces Pest Management Board, 1996), many soldiers are not aware of them (Gambel et al., 1998). Recent deployments have been affected by disease as a result of lack of awareness and lack of enforcement of existing preventive medicine doctrine by commanders in the field (Calow, 1999; Gambel et al., 1999).

Similarly, basic field sanitation may not be receiving the needed command emphasis. Alhough a system of field sanitation exists in Army regulations, the Field Sanitation Teams of deployed units frequently are not properly trained or equipped for their roles (Gambel, 1999).

Vaccines

Policy

Vaccines make up a critical component of the existing countermeasures against infectious diseases and other biological hazards, so service members receive many vaccines as routine aspects of their service. These immunizations protect them from (1) the everyday hazards of garrison life (e.g. cramped quarters with people from throughout the country), (2) infectious diseases endemic to the places to which they deploy, and (3) biological weapons that are determined to be threats in particular areas of deployment. Table 6-1 lists the vaccinations prescribed for military personnel as of 1995 (does not include anthrax). Differences in practices among the services are the result of different training cycles, different missions, and different exposures.

For immunizations not unique to the military, it is DoD policy to follow the U.S. Public Health Service general recommendations, which are developed by the Centers for Disease Control and Prevention's Advisory Committee on Immunization Practices and published in the CDC's *Morbidity and Mortality Weekly Report*. For immunizations unique to the military, the departments develop appropriate procedures in consultation with the Armed Forces Epidemiological Board, the Armed Forces Medical Intelligence Center, and the Armed Forces Pest Management Board, as needed (U.S. Department of Defense, 1986).

Principles, procedures, policies, and responsibilities for the immunizations program are detailed in a publication entitled *Immunizations and Chemoprophylaxis* which is issued jointly by the Army, Navy, Air Force, and Coast Guard (U.S. Department of the Air Force, 1995).

TABLE 6-1. Vaccinations Prescribed for Military Personnel

Disease or Agent	Army	Navy	Air Force	Marine Corps	Coast Guard
Adenovirus types 4 and 7	B	B	G	B	G
Vibrio cholerae	E	E	E	E	E
Hepatitis A	G	G	C,D	G	G
Hepatitis B	F,G	F,G	F,G	F,G	F,G
Influenza	A,B,X	A,B,R	A,B,R	A,B,R	B,C,G
Japanese Encephalitis	D	D	D	D	G
Measles	B,F	B,F	B,F	B,F	B,G
Meningococcus (types A, C, Y, W135)	B,D	B,D	B,D	B,D	B,G
Mumps	F,G	B,F,G	F,G	B,F,G	G
Polio	B,D,R	B,R	B,R	B,R	A
Plague	D,F	F	F	F	F
Rabies	F	F	F	F	G
Rubella	B,F	B,F	B,F	B,F	B
Tetanus-diphtheria	A,B,R	A,B,R	A,B,R	A,B,R	A,B
Typhoid	C,D	C,D	C,D	C,D	D
Varicella	F,G	F,G	F,G	G	F,G
Yellow fever	C,D	A,R	C,D	A,R	B,C,E

NOTE: A = All active-duty personnel; B = recruits; C = alert forces; D = when deploying or traveling to high-risk areas; E = only when required by host country for entry; F = high risk occupational groups; G = as directed by applicable surgeon general or Commandant, Coast Guard; R = reserve components; X = reserve component personnel on active duty for 30 days or more during the influenza season.

SOURCE: U.S. Department of the Air Force, 1995.

A special policy exists for immunizations against biological warfare threats and is detailed in DoD Directive 6205.3, *Immunizations Program for Biological Warfare Defense* (U.S. Department of Defense, 1993). The Secretary of the Army serves as the DoD executive agent for this activity. The policy states that personnel assigned to high-threat areas or predesignated for immediate contingency deployment (crisis response) or those identified and scheduled for deployment on an imminent or ongoing contingency operation to a high-threat area "should be immunized against validated biological warfare threat agents, for which suitable vaccines are available, in sufficient time to develop immunity before deployment to high-threat areas" (U.S. Department of Defense, 1993, p. 2). The policy further states that DoD shall develop a capability to acquire and stockpile adequate quantities of vaccines to protect service members against all validated biological warfare threats and that the research, development, testing, evaluation, acquisition, and stockpiling efforts for the improvement of existing vaccines and the development of new vaccines shall be integrated and prioritized. A description of the availability, safety, and efficacy of vaccines and therapies for chemical and biological agents is available in a recent report from the Institute of Medicine (1999c).

Vaccine Acquisition and Supply

DoD requires several vaccines that have limited or no market outside of the military. Licensed vaccines in this category include adenovirus type 4 and type 7 vaccines, plague vaccine, and anthrax vaccine. Research and development efforts will likely add several vaccines to this list in the future. Because of their limited market, maintaining a reliable manufacturing base for and supply of these vaccines for military use has proven to be very difficult. Large commercial vaccine companies have shown little or no interest in supplying DoD with small amounts of special vaccines if there is no other market. Reliance on smaller companies with less manufacturing capability and expertise has resulted in an unreliable supply of vaccines.

At present DoD has no manufacturer for the live oral adenovirus type 4 and type 7 vaccines, which are needed to prevent epidemics of acute febrile respiratory disease in recruit training camps (Gray et al., 1999). Previously manufactured vaccines were highly effective (Gaydos and Gaydos, 1995) and very cost-effective, but the sole manufacturer ceased production and neither vaccine is available. Efforts to find a new manufacturer, create and validate the manufacturing capacity, and obtain licensure for new products are under way but may take 2 to 3 years. Meanwhile, acute respiratory disease due to adenoviruses goes unchecked in Army and Navy recruit training facilities (Gaydos and Gaydos, 1995; Gray et al., 1999). Recently, two recruit centers where the vaccines were not available had large acute respiratory disease epidemics (Gray et al., 1999).

The vaccine against plague (which is caused by *Yersinia pestis*) proved to be very effective (Cavanaugh et al., 1974) at protecting troops in Vietnam, where plague is endemic. Previous manufacturers have ceased production of the vaccine against plague and have relinquished the license, leaving DoD without a supply of this vaccine for the foreseeable future.

The manufacturer of the current anthrax vaccine, BioPort, has had problems meeting regulatory requirements and standards, resulting in a costly program to upgrade the manufacturing process and facility so that it meets U.S. Food and Drug Administration (FDA) standards. Since this vaccine is made by a process devised more than 40 years ago, it is far from the optimal product possible today using modern biotechnology production and purification methods. The current vaccine requires multiple doses and contains many extraneous proteins. A much more efficient vaccine that has a uniform content and that requires fewer doses can be developed. The Committee on R&D Needs for Improving Civilian Medical Response to Chemical and Biological Terrorism Incidents recommended that a second-generation anthrax vaccine be developed for civilian use (Institute of

Medicine, 1999c). Developing a second-generation anthrax vaccine would be an appropriate action for DoD as well.

Responsibility for the vaccine supply is divided among several organizations within DoD and the individual services. Procurement of licensed vaccines is done by the services and by Defense Supply Center Philadelphia. The Assistant Secretary of Defense for Health Affairs has both policy and procurement decision-making roles. Research and development responsibility for vaccines for biological defense resides with the Joint Program Office and is carried out through the Joint Vaccine Acquisition Program (JVAP) by a prime contractor. The U.S. Army Medical Research and Materiel Command has responsibility for developing vaccines against diseases other than those caused by biological weapons. JVAP has not yet developed any vaccines, and no manufacturers have yet been identified to supply the products under development (Institute of Medicine, 1998).

Vaccine procurement has been a challenging problem for DoD for many years, and recent events indicate that optimal solutions have not yet been found. A proposal to build a government facility to manufacture vaccines was rejected in 1991 because it was considered too expensive. Current efforts on vaccines against adenovirus, *Y. pestis*, vaccinia virus, and several other agents have a high risk of failure on the basis of previous experience. Multiple problems have arisen from isolated attempts to procure vaccines of no commercial interest from small manufacturers. The current fragmentation of responsibility for vaccine acquisition within DoD may contribute to the problem by failing to consolidate the medical, technical, and program management expertise needed to address these complex problems under a single authority. The Institute of Medicine report *Emerging Infections: Microbial Threats to Health in the United States* (Institute of Medicine, 1992) recommended both an integrated management structure and government production facilities as a means of addressing the growing need for a reliable vaccine supply. Since that time the availability of commercial products has declined and the level and locations of military deployments have increased. The study team urges DoD to reconsider the concept of government production facilities for vaccines.

Identification of Biological Warfare Threats

Annually and as required, the Chairman of the Joint Chiefs of Staff in consultation with the Commanders of the Unified Commands, the Chiefs of the Military Services, and the Director of the Defense Intelligence Agency must validate and prioritize the biological warfare threats to DoD personnel. The Armed Forces Epidemiology Board annually identifies vaccines available to protect against validated biological warfare agents identified as threats and recommends appropriate immunization protocols (U.S. Department of Defense, 1993).

Vaccine Coverage

A survey carried out for the Armed Forces Epidemiological Board in the spring of 1998 found substantial variation in the rates of vaccination against influenza, tetanus-diphtheria, yellow fever, and typhoid among the convenience sample of units included in the survey (Birch and Davis, 1998). Unit coverage rates ranged from 43 percent to 100 percent for single required vaccines, with most units' rates being 90 percent or greater. Units considered likely to be deployed had higher coverage rates than other units, and active-duty units had higher coverage rates than reserve units.

Immunization Record Keeping

The Joint Instruction *Immunization and Chemoprophylaxis* (U.S. Department of the Air Force, 1995) requires a written medical form and PHS-731 card (also known as the "yellow shot card") for each service member. Service policies and practices vary, however, reflecting the status of service record automation, and no one data source yet provides complete data for units or services. In some cases data reside in a number of independent readiness systems used within the services (Birch and Davis, 1998).

The study on immunization coverage by Birch and Davis also found that important data were missing from many records. More than 90 percent of the data sources on typhoid vaccine did not include the name of the vaccine or the route of administration, so it was impossible to determine those who were up to date for the vaccine (Birch and Davis, 1998). Such data are also important, for example, if certain lots were found to be ineffective.

DoD plans to provide immunization tracking through the Preventive Health Care Application, a computerized health information system that is still under development (described further in Chapter 5). In the meantime, the different services are using their own interim systems to collect and report immunization data.

Anthrax Vaccine

As described above, the U.S. military routinely immunizes service members against many infectious disease threats. However, the Secretary of Defense announced plans in December 1997 to ultimately vaccinate all U.S. military personnel against anthrax, a biological warfare agent. Such a mass immunization was unprecedented. The decision reflected the increasing recognition of a valid threat of the use of anthrax as a biological weapon against U.S. forces.

Because of its logistical and public relations ramifications, the decision was a major one. The logistical challenge of immunizing the entire force is tremendous. The current anthrax vaccine, licensed by FDA in 1970, involves a series of six inoculations per service member over an 18-month period (at 0, 2, and 4 weeks and then at 6, 12, and 18 months), followed by an annual booster. Immunization of the estimated 2.4 million service personnel over a 7- to 8-year period requires tremendous planning and ongoing administrative effort.

The public relations challenge is also considerable. The anthrax vaccine is among the many agents to which service members in the Gulf War were exposed and that veterans have considered to be a possible contributor to or cause of illnesses among Gulf War veterans. Although no evidence supports the hypothesis that the anthrax vaccine was a causal factor, concerns continue in the veteran and service member communities and are sustained through the media and the Internet.

The vaccination program is being carried out in three phases that began in May 1998. In Phase I, the forces assigned or rotating to high-threat areas of Southwest Asia and Korea are being immunized. Forces that deploy early into high-threat areas are being immunized in Phase II, and the remainder of the total force and accessions will receive immunizations in Phase III beginning in fiscal year 2003 (Randolph, 1998). After Phase III, the program will be sustained with annual boosters.

The Army is the executive agent for immunizations for Biological Warfare Agents (U.S. Department of Defense, 1993) and for the Anthrax Vaccine Immunization Program (AVIP). As executive agent, the Army monitors the services' implementation of AVIP, oversees the vaccine acquisition and stockpile effort carried out by the Joint Program Office for Biological Defense (JPO-BD), and is the focal point for the submission of information from the services.

Anthrax immunization is a command responsibility that is part of force protection. Commanders are responsible for implementation, education of their personnel, and tracking the anthrax immunization series. The Surgeons General of the services have logistical oversight. JPO-BD centrally funds and maintains the stockpile of vaccines and defined production capabilities (U.S. Department of the Navy, 1998).

Preventive Measures Immediately Before Deployment

Frequently, little time is available between notification that a service member will be deployed and departure, and there are many competing demands for this limited time. Service members have myriad nonmedical activities that need to be done, such as paperwork to update their wills. Medical necessities include acquiring adequate supplies of medications and prescription glasses and last-minute requisite immunizations. The predeployment health questionnaire must also be completed. The service members also have many personal matters to attend to in preparation for departure. Among these competing demands, preventive medicine measures may not always be fully implemented.

The predeployment preventive medicine briefing is an example. Before a deployment, the troops are given briefings about the health threats they will encounter in the theater of operations and the countermeasures that they will need to use. It is important that these briefings take place. The discussions of potential risks and their countermeasures should emphasize those risks considered of greatest importance on the basis of such criteria as prevalence, potential harm, and preventability and should include discussion of some of the service members' chief concerns.

Starting with Operations Desert Shield and Desert Storm (the Gulf War), an additional tool used to provide information to troops and commanders during a deployment has been available: booklets with environmental and preventive medicine information for different areas of deployment. These are produced by both the Division of Preventive Medicine at WRAIR and the U.S. Army Research Institute of Environmental Medicine (USARIEM) and are intended to be taken along during the deployment. The USARIEM guides are designed for small-unit leaders, whereas the WRAIR booklets are designed for all military personnel, for small-unit leaders, medical planners, and health care providers (Huycke et al., 1997).

Such information booklets provide valuable reinforcement of the information provided to the service member through training and briefings. They cannot be considered replacements for training and briefing, however, because the information is sufficiently important that the service member should receive a briefing. The booklets should be distributed in a timely manner and written at the reading levels of the target audiences. Their effectiveness, however, should be evaluated (Huycke et al., 1997) because there is no evidence that they are read, understood, remembered, or used by service members. Since 1996, the U.S. Army Center for Health Promotion and Preventive Medicine has coordinated the publication of these reports. Additional products have been developed, including decks of playing cards with prevention tips on them, and one-page pamphlets and laminated cards with information on particular hazards, such as ticks and rodents for soldiers deployed to Bosnia.

PREVENTIVE MEASURES DURING DEPLOYMENT

Risk Communication

As exposures or health concerns arise during deployments, commanders at all levels must be prepared to provide service members with the best information available to them. Procedures are needed to ensure that concerns about emerging problems are shared across levels, facilitating their recognition and investigation and aiding in the development of well-considered communications.

Combat Stress Reactions and Control

As noted in Chapter 2, the importance of unit cohesion in affecting the rates of psychiatric breakdown in combat came to be recognized in World War II.

Today, unit morale and leadership are acknowledged across the services to be among the most important factors for preventing combat stress reactions (Manning, 1994; D. R. Jones, 1995; Mateczun, 1995; Rock et al., 1995).

Once an acute stress reaction ("battle fatigue") has occurred, several aspects of response are considered crucial to returning the service member to duty without long-term sequelae. The principles of battle fatigue management, first described by Salmon (1929) in World War I, are proximity, immediacy, and expectancy, as described in Chapter 2. The U.S. Army has used the mnemonic PIES to capture these principles and that of simplicity of treatment, whereas the U.S. Navy and Air Force have taught the same principles with the acronym BICEPS, where B and C are for brevity (treatment will be brief [hours or days]) and centrality (treatment is at a central location and there is no evacuation until the individual has been evaluated by skilled professionals), respectively (Hazen and Llewellyn, 1991; Stokes, 1998). Hazen and Llewellyn (1991) cited sources that assert that with appropriate application of these fundamental principles, a recovery rate of 70 to 90 percent can be expected from prehospital treatment elements (Hazen and Llewellyn, 1991). During the Gulf War, evacuation policies and resources made it difficult to carry out a rapid return to duty in the service member's original unit, despite the potential harm of evacuation (removing needed proximity, immediacy, and expectancy, as described in Chapter 2) to the battle-fatigued soldier (Martin and Cline, 1996).

Although different parts of the military have been using the combat stress control tools described above for years, DoD has recently established a policy on the topic. DoD Directive 6490.5, *Combat Stress Control (CSC) Programs*, requires that each of the services implements plans to "enhance readiness, contribute to combat effectiveness, enhance the physical and mental health of military personnel, and to prevent or minimize adverse effects of Combat Stress Reactions" (U.S. Department of Defense, 1999a, p. 2). The policy also indicates that "leadership aspects of combat stress prevention shall be addressed in senior enlisted, officer and flag-rank training programs. Protective factors against combat stress reactions, such as frequent communication (in person) with troops, unit morale and unit cohesion, shall be emphasized" (p. 2). Furthermore, "CSC units shall train with operations organizations or platforms on a regular basis" (p. 2) and combat stress casualty rates shall be collected as a discrete category from other disease and non-battle injury casualty rates.

The study team applauds this policy and hopes that it will be implemented effectively and with dispatch throughout the services. The study team encourages studies to evaluate the impacts of the new programs where feasible.

Postcombat debriefing has also become a part of the military response to combat trauma. Debriefing entails the involvement of everyone in the group in a verbal reconstruction of the event in precise detail. A group consensus is sought to resolve individual misperceptions and restore perspective about true responsibility. Feelings about the event are discussed and validated as normal, as are some of the stress symptoms that unit members experience (U.S. Department of the Army, 1994).

A debriefing process was incorporated into the Navy's Special Psychiatric Rapid Intervention Teams in 1978, and the Army used debriefing techniques in response to several terrorist attacks in the 1980s (Koshes et al., 1995). Although there was no formal doctrinal mandate or training program for unit debriefings in the Gulf War, U.S. Army mental health teams did conduct them (Koshes et al., 1995; Belenky et al., 1996b). Critical event debriefings after traumatic events became common practice after the deployment of Army division mental health teams and combat stress control detachment teams to Somalia in January 1994 (Koshes et al., 1995). A particular form of debriefing developed by Mitchell (1983), called "critical incident stress debriefing" is designed for traumatic incidents involving preexisting civilian teams. The military uses a modification termed "critical event debriefing" (Koshes et al., 1995). The new DoD policy on Combat Stress Control (CSC) programs includes Critical Event Debriefings (to take place "as indicated") among the responsibilities of the CSC unit personnel after exceptionally stressful events (U.S. Department of Defense, 1999a).

Debriefing has become a part of the response to traumatic events out of the expectation that it can help prevent posttraumatic stress disorder (PTSD). However, a recent systematic review of psychological debriefing for the prevention of PTSD did not indicate that single-session debriefing reduced psychological distress or prevented the onset of PTSD. There was no evidence that debriefing reduced general psychological morbidity, depression, or anxiety (Wessely et al., 1997). Since DoD is drawing upon critical-event debriefings as part of its policy on combat stress control, it should evaluate its impact to the extent feasible. A recent Institute of Medicine report (1999c) noted similar research needs for the civilian community.

Use of Investigational New Drugs by the Armed Forces

Among the several force protection issues highlighted by the experiences of the Gulf War have been the difficulties surrounding the use of drugs or biologics that have not been licensed by the FDA.

FDA grants licensure to drugs or biologics that have been shown to be both safe and efficacious for the use in question. Drugs developed to protect against chemical or biological warfare agents or other dangerous infectious diseases can be demonstrated to be safe in humans with the usual procedures. However, the human efficacy trials usually required by FDA as direct evidence of efficacy are not possible for products that cannot be tested in the field against the natural disease and for which challenge studies are too dangerous. As a result, a large and growing number of much-needed products currently under development in military research and development programs have not proceeded to licensure by FDA.

A product under development is termed "investigational" when it is being tested in volunteer subjects under an Investigational New Drug Application (IND) and has not been licensed by FDA for the intended use. FDA controls the use of an investigational new drug and studies must be conducted under approved protocols.

This ordinarily necessitates review by an institutional review board and obtaining informed consent from the recipient of the product. It also requires the maintenance of detailed records of the drug administration and the results.

In the Gulf War, DoD faced the threat that Iraq might use chemical and biological warfare agents. Two medical products available to potentially protect against these agents were pyridostigmine bromide (PB) and botulinum toxoid (BT) vaccine. PB had been licensed and in use for many years as a treatment for myasthenia gravis, and data from studies with animals supported its effectiveness as a pretreatment against certain nerve agents. BT had been used routinely for more than 25 years as a vaccine for industry and laboratory workers with potential occupational exposure to botulinum toxins. Both were investigational products being administered and tested for military purposes under INDs.

Because DoD was concerned before the Gulf War that it could not follow the rules for administering products under IND status in battlefield circumstances, it requested that FDA waive the informed consent and other IND requirements. After several months of discussion, FDA did so in the form of an Interim Rule establishing the authority of the Commissioner of FDA to waive IND requirements in certain military exigencies (Federal Register, 1990). The Interim Rule had several requirements, including that the FDA decision must be based on a finding that obtaining informed consent is not feasible, that withholding treatment would be contrary to the best interests of military personnel, and that no satisfactory alternative product is available.

The use of PB and BT in the Gulf War was characterized by poor record keeping, inadequate data collection, and other violations of the terms agreed to in the FDA waivers (Rettig, 1999). In the years after the war, progress toward completion of the rule making for the Interim Rule was complicated and slow (Presidential Advisory Committee on Gulf War Veterans' Illnesses, 1996b; Rettig, 1999). In October 1998, the progress was overtaken by events when the U.S. Congress passed legislation providing that only the President can waive the requirement for informed consent when an investigational new drug is administered (P.L. 105-261, Section 731). The legislation requires that for informed consent to be waived it must be determined that it is not feasible, is contrary to the best interests of the member, or is not in the best interests of national security.

The new legal setting will place markedly increased responsibility on both FDA and DoD to work toward ways to provide service members with appropriate medical protection against battlefield hazards. FDA has indicated that it will propose to amend its new drug and biological product regulations

> to identify the kind of evidence needed to demonstrate the efficacy of drug and biological products used to treat or prevent the toxicity of potentially devastating chemical or biological substances when efficacy studies in humans ethically cannot be conducted because they would involve administering a lethal or permanently disabling toxic substance to healthy human volunteers without a proven treatment. (*Federal Register*, 1998, p. 21957)

No amended regulations have been proposed as of this writing.*

The new regulations will make it difficult to obtain an exemption from the informed consent requirement. They will make it possible to advance products to licensure provided that research is done to generate the data needed to meet the new FDA requirement. These events place an increased responsibility on DoD to begin, in communication with FDA, to accelerate the research needed to meet the new criteria. Both agencies must do much work to ensure that necessary research and development efforts proceed rapidly and that appropriate standards for proof of efficacy are established.

PREVENTIVE MEASURES AFTER DEPLOYMENT

Risk Communication

Risk communication after a deployment is a crucial component of the appropriate care and support for the service member upon his or her return. Health concerns and health problems are almost certain given the experiences of previous major deployments, and deployed forces will need information to understand them. As discussed in the *Comprehensive Risk Communication Plan for Gulf War Veterans* (Persian Gulf Veterans Coordinating Board, 1999), risk communication will be successful only to the extent that trust and credibility are present. Thus, efforts at risk communication must be part of an overall effort to see that returning service members are treated with gratitude and provided with medical care and support services to ease their readjustment.

Reintegration

The challenges of a major deployment do not end upon the service member's return. Service members must readjust to home life and perhaps civilian life (for those separating from the service or returning to inactive reserve status). A discussion of the challenges of reintegration and the programs provided for service members is found in Chapter 7.

Medical Management and Symptomatic Treatment of Medically Unexplained Symptoms

Clinicians and other persons working in medical surveillance must recognize that medically unexplained symptoms are just that, namely, they have no

---

*On October 5, 1999, FDA proposed regulations describing the evidence needed to demonstrate efficacy of new drugs for use against lethal or permanently disabling toxic substances when efficacy studies in humans cannot ethically be conducted.

current explanations. Therefore, conveying the limits of modern medicine coupled with a compassionate approach to patients with medically unexplained symptoms is essential to the management strategy for such patients. Until clear etiological factors are identified, the health care professional relies upon a body of knowledge about the management of medically unexplained symptoms (described below), and this approach has proven to be effective in many cases.

Because medically unexplained symptoms are a prevalent and persistent problem that is associated with high levels of subjective distress and functional impairment and with extensive use of medical care, the study team believes that it is important to institute an aggressive program of early diagnosis and symptomatic treatment. Although a program of primary prevention is not feasible given the current state of knowledge, the study team does believe that enough is known to recommend the implementation of a secondary prevention strategy. This would encompass the early detection of medically unexplained symptoms by primary care physicians and a graduated series of palliative, symptomatic treatment interventions.

There is good clinical evidence that medically unexplained symptoms are much harder to treat and ameliorate once they have become chronic and the individual has accommodated to the sick role and family roles are reconfigured (Kellner, 1986; Kroenke and Mangelsdorff, 1989; Kellner, 1991; Craig et al., 1993; Barsky, 1998). It is therefore important to identify patients with medically unexplained symptoms early, when there is a greater opportunity to restore the patient to his or her previous level of function and avoiding invalidism and assumption of the sick role. Two methods could be used to detect medically unexplained symptoms early. The first method is through the incorporation of a self-report questionnaire into the routine, comprehensive health assessments that all personnel periodically undergo. The HEAR (which is described in Chapter 4) will be administered annually to all active-duty service members, and the RAP (see Chapter 4) is planned to be administered to all personnel at the time of induction. Both assessments should include a self-report screening questionnaire to identify individuals with a high likelihood of having persistent medically unexplained symptoms. Questionnaires (such as the PRIME-MD, the Somatic Symptom Inventory, and the Somatoform Disorders Schedule) already exist to measure this that have adequate reliability and validity (Barsky et al., 1986, 1991; Swartz et al., 1986; Weinstein et al., 1989; Spitzer et al., 1994; Janca et al., 1995; Kroenke et al., 1998b).

The second method of early identification is through a heightened awareness of medically unexplained symptoms on the part of primary care providers. This is necessary throughout the military medical care system and should not be restricted only to the health care of deployed personnel. These providers need to know more about medically unexplained symptoms, to understand the problem in depth, and to acquire the clinical skills and strategies needed for optimal medical management of patients with these symptoms.

Having learned to recognize and identify the problem earlier in its course, the physician must then be able to bring specific knowledge and skills to bear to help the patient. These include the following: validating the patient's distress and then negotiating a mutually agreed upon set of therapeutic goals; shifting the focus of the medical care interaction from definitive diagnosis and outright cure to coping with residual symptoms and rehabilitation; providing the patient with an explanatory model of symptom amplification to account for the patient's symptoms; cautious and limited reassurance; and a search for a comorbid psychiatric disorder that may be contributing to suffering and functional impairment (Smith et al., 1986b; Barsky, 1997; Barsky and Borus, 1999). Primary care providers will require in-service training and workshops to become more knowledgeable about, comfortable with, and proficient in this clinical approach. The study team believes that a program of continuing education should be undertaken for all military primary care providers to improve their clinical ability to diagnose and treat medically unexplained symptoms. Although this educational effort would be extensive and expensive, the study team believes that it would be cost-effective in light of the high prevalence of medically unexplained symptoms, the high level of disability and functional impairment that it entails, and the enormous medical care costs that ensue when the condition is not optimally treated.

The primary care setting is the best locus for the treatment of medically unexplained symptoms. However, some patients' symptoms will prove to be refractory to the primary care provider's efforts. Such patients should be referred to more intensive, multimodal programs developed on a rehabilitative model. One such program has been established for some of the Gulf War veterans with medically unexplained symptoms (Engel et al., 1998). Modeled after the University of Washington's Multidisciplinary Pain Center (Loeser and Egan, 1989), this is a 3-week, intensive outpatient program with a highly structured physical activation plan and intensive psychosocial elements to address the chronic nature of reduced functioning and the many factors that reinforce it. Specific components of the multimodal approaches have been in use for many years, with the best studied of these involving a combination of cognitive-behavioral therapy (CBT) and physical reactivation. This approach has much in common with cognitive-behaviorally based programs now emerging for the treatment of a variety of functional somatic syndromes, including irritable bowel syndrome, fibromyalgia, chronic fatigue syndrome, headache, and atypical chest pain (Buckelew, 1989; Martin et al., 1989; Salkovskis, 1989; Blanchard et al., 1990; Skinner et al., 1990; DeGuire et al., 1992; Keefe et al., 1992; Sharpe, 1995; Speckens et al., 1995; Van Dulmen et al., 1996; Deale et al., 1997; Mayou et al., 1997; Clark et al., 1998). Controlled intervention trials with long-term follow-up have begun to demonstrate the effectiveness of CBT in reducing somatic symptoms, generalized distress, and disability (Buckelew, 1989; Martin et al., 1989; Peck et al., 1989; Salkovskis, 1989; Blanchard et al., 1990; Hellman et al., 1990; Skinner et al., 1990; DeGuire et al., 1992; Keefe et al., 1992; Sharpe et al., 1992, 1995, 1996; Payne and Blanchard, 1995; Speckens et al., 1995; Van Dulmen et al., 1996; Deale et al., 1997; Fulcher and White, 1997; Clark et al., 1998). These interventions help patients cope with symptoms by reexamining their health beliefs and expectations and by exploring the impact of the sick role and of stress and distress on their symptoms. Patients are assisted to find alternative explanations for their symptoms, restructure faulty disease beliefs, alter expectations, and learn techniques of focused attention and distraction. The cognitive-behavioral approach stimulates patients to assume a more active role in coping and rehabilitation, and it counters their belief that cure can result only from the application of a technological intervention to a passive patient. Behavioral strategies, such as response prevention, systematic desensitization, graduated exercise regimens, and progressive muscle relaxation, help patients resume normal activities, minimize role impairment, and curtail sick behaviors.

The implementation of these programs of secondary prevention will require careful and rigorous evaluation. The yield of screening questionnaires for detection of the early stages of medically unexplained symptoms (if incorporated into the HEAR or the RAP) must be assessed. Longitudinal studies are necessary to determine how well such instruments perform in terms of specificity, sensitivity, and positive predictive value. The highly specialized, multimodal, intensive treatment programs that the study team recommends need to be subjected to carefully controlled, randomized evaluation. It is difficult to design suitable control groups and to randomize patients in such studies, but these obstacles are not insurmountable. Finally, the effects of educational programs for primary care physicians also need evaluation. It is difficult to demonstrate changes in physician behavior and practice resulting from educational interventions, but medical care outcomes can also be assessed.

In addition to implementing and evaluating a comprehensive program of secondary prevention and treatment, the study team believes that a thorough program of research is also necessary. Current knowledge and understanding of medically unexplained symptoms are inadequate, particularly in light of their high prevalence and costs in personal distress and suffering, functional disability and impaired productivity, and ineffective and inefficient medical care. Prospective studies are necessary to assess the role of predisposing causes (such as a prior history of medically unexplained symptoms, psychiatric disorder, and trauma or abuse), precipitating factors (including deployment and other stressful events), and perpetuating and maintaining factors. Phenomenological and descriptive studies are needed to investigate the complex and poorly delineated relationships between medically unexplained symptoms and PTSD. Epidemiological surveys are needed to document the incidence, prevalence, and course of medically unexplained symptoms and to distinguish and delineate chronic, severe, and disabling medically unexplained symptoms from transient and less severe medically unexplained symptoms. Finally, as mentioned above, careful outcomes studies are needed to assess the outcomes after various treatment interventions.

In February 1999, DoD published a request for proposals on several research topics related to Gulf War illnesses (Commerce Business Daily, 1999). Among them was a solicitation for research on several symptom-based conditions, as well as a solicitation for studies of any of a variety of aspects of deployment health including development of physical symptoms following deployments. The study team encourages DoD to continue to try to involve academic institutions in education and research efforts related to medically unexplained symptoms.

FINDINGS AND RECOMMENDATIONS

Finding 6-1: Although there are encouraging signs that the importance of risk communication has been acknowledged within some quarters of the U.S. Department of Defense, additional indications of commitment to a cultural change throughout the entire system are needed from the top. Effective risk communication cannot be reduced to a list of do's and don't's. Constant reevaluation and change are needed as well as training, with the participation and input of service members from many levels.

Recommendation 6-1: Although responsibility for risk communication must permeate all levels of command, the U.S. Department of Defense (DoD) should designate and provide resources to a group within DoD that is given primary responsibility for developing and implementing a plan to achieve the risk communication goal articulated in the National Science and Technology Council's Presidential Review Directive. Such a plan should

- **Involve service members, their families, and outside experts in developing an explicit set of risk communication topics and goals. In other words, decide what information people need to know and when they need to know it.**
- **Consider how to deliver the information, including the intensity of communication needed for different types of risks. Some topics will necessitate full, ongoing dialogue between the involved parties, whereas others will require less extensive efforts. Incorporate procedures to evaluate the success of risk communication efforts and use these evaluations to revise the communication plan as needed.**
- **Include a response plan to anticipate the inevitable appearance of new risks or health concerns among deployed forces. The plan should include a process for gathering and disseminating information (both about the risks themselves and about the concerns of the troops) and for evaluating how communications about these issues are received and understood by service members and their families.**
- **Educate communicators, including line officers and physicians, in relevant aspects of risk communication.**
- **Carry out the interagency applied research program described in the National Science and Technology Council's Presidential Review Directive (Strategy 5.1.2).**

Finding 6-2: Recent efforts to make accession standards evidence based are laudable. The means appear to be in place to evaluate and improve accessions standards (no recommendation).

Finding 6-3: Each service member should be provided the essential skills, supplies, and equipment to stay healthy while he or she is deployed. Lack of effective preventive medicine training can compromise the health of deployed forces and missions.

Recommendation 6-3: Provide the time for field preventive medicine training for service members including members of the reserves and particularly for line commanders during basic and advanced training.

Finding 6-4: Vaccine procurement has been a challenging problem for the U.S. Department of Defense for many years and recent events indicate that optimal solutions have not yet been found. The IOM report on *Emerging Infections: Microbial Threats to Health in the United States* (Institute of Medicine, 1992) recommended both an integrated management structure and government production facilities as a means of addressing the growing need for a reliable vaccine supply.

Recommendation 6-4: The U.S. Department of Defense should reevaluate the concept of government facilities for vaccine production and stockpiling.

Finding 6-5: Advances in biotechnology make possible the development of a second-generation vaccine that would require fewer doses. An Institute of Medicine committee recently recommended operations research on the development of improved vaccines against anthrax.

Recommendation 6-5: The U.S. Department of Defense should begin development of a second-generation vaccine against anthrax.

Finding 6-6: The small booklets on environmental and preventive medicine information relevant to the area of deployment given to some deploying service members provide useful information, but they are not a substitute for personal protective measures training and there is no evidence that they are read and understood.

Recommendation 6-6: Evaluate the extent to which the preventive measures booklets relevant to the area of deployment are read and understood by service members including members of the reserves.

Finding 6-7: The U.S. Department of Defense's new policy on combat stress control programs should bring some consistency and needed visibility to the prevention and management of combat stress reactions. The emphasis on training for leaders and the collection of surveillance data on combat stress reactions are important. Since the impacts of some interventions are in question, additional research on them is warranted.

Recommendation 6-7: Seek ways to evaluate scientifically the combat stress interventions that are used.

Finding 6-8: The legislative requirement that the President grant waivers of the requirement of informed consent for products with investigational status is an appropriate policy solution to a difficult and complex issue. It will make such waivers much more difficult to obtain and place added responsibility on the U.S. Department of Defense and the Food and Drug Administration to conduct research and to license the products needed for protection of the health of forces and preservation of national security. Both agencies must recognize and act on this increased responsibility for the health of service members.

Recommendation 6-8: The U.S. Department of Defense in consultation with the Food and Drug Administration should review the status of all products with investigational status and ensure that research and development efforts that will lead to the licensure of essential products are implemented.

Finding 6-9: Medically unexplained physical symptoms have been a prevalent and persistent problem in military populations after major deployments. Information from the civilian literature indicates that early recognition and symptomatic treatment of the problem may help to avoid the development of more serious chronic problems.

Recommendation 6-9: The study team recommends that the U.S. Department of Defense develop an improved strategy for addressing medically unexplained symptoms involving education, detection, mitigation, evaluation, and research.

- **Undertake a program of continuing education for military primary care providers to improve their clinical ability to diagnose, treat, and communicate with patients with medically unexplained symptoms.** Incorporate the topic into the curricula of military graduate medical education programs such as the Uniformed Services University of the Health Sciences and the service schools for medical personnel. To the extent possible, make information about medically unexplained symptoms available and accessible to service members and to civilian health care providers for members of the reserves.
- **Carry out a pilot program to identify service members in the early stages of development of medically unexplained physical symptoms through the use of routinely administered self-report questionnaires and through informed primary care providers.**

- **Evaluate the efficacy of the pilot secondary prevention and treatment program, including the ability of screening questionnaires to detect early stages of medically unexplained symptoms.**
- **Treat medically unexplained symptoms in the primary care setting whenever possible, with referral to more intensive programs as necessary.**
- **Carry out a research program with prospective studies to assess the role of predisposing, precipitating, and perpetuating factors for medically unexplained symptoms. As feasible, involve academic health centers in the research efforts.**

7

Postdeployment Reintegration

INTRODUCTION

Family- and Work-Related Problems of Deployment

Although it has come to be well understood that deployments to combat or operations other than war can be highly stressful experiences, the challenges of the return home for service members and their families are frequently given less attention. Nonetheless, aspects of readjustment to the home environment have proved to be significant sources of concern to returning veterans. Many returning Vietnam veterans struggled with relationships with their bosses, coworkers, wives, family, and sexual partners (Egendorf, 1982). Egendorf and colleagues' interview of veterans for their *Legacies of Vietnam* study found that about 50 percent of the veterans interviewed showed signs of disturbing, unresolved war experiences that affected their everyday lives (Egendorf et al., 1981). The National Vietnam Veterans Readjustment Study found that 45 and 37 percent of men and women, respectively, serving in the Vietnam theater reported having at least one serious postwar readjustment problem and that roughly one in four Vietnam theater veterans continued to experience at least one such problem when they were surveyed in 1990 (Kulka et al., 1990). Veterans who were exposed to war-zone stress displayed poorer levels of adjustment in family roles and marital relationships than civilians or veterans from the same era who were not deployed to Vietnam (Kulka et al., 1990).

After the Gulf War, veterans reported concern about family-related matters, money, and employment. In one group, although 12 percent suffered moderate or severe war-zone stress reactions, 19 percent experienced moderate or severe family adjustment problems (Figley, 1993b).

Although no two deployments are alike, some of the experiences of recent deployments may be helpful when considering future needs and possible preventive interventions. Separation from family has always been an important stressor during deployments, but the changing makeup of the deployed force has led to some new challenges. During the Gulf War, the percentages of deployed women and reserve-component service members were larger than they have ever been. About 7.2 percent, or roughly 50,000 of the 670,000 service members deployed were women, 9.8 percent were members of the Reserves, and 6.2 percent were members of the National Guard (Gray et al., 1998). More single parents and military career couples were also among the deployed than in the past (Figley, 1993b). For example, 16 percent of Vietnam veterans were married with children during their service in Vietnam (U.S. Department of Defense, 1991), whereas 60 percent of Gulf War service members were married with children during their service in the Gulf (Dove et al., 1994a,b).

The first major deployment of women in a war was during the Gulf War, which also took a different type of toll on some families, in that significant numbers of men or extended family members were left in unaccustomed roles of caring for young children or infants. For financial reasons, many of these families chose to leave military bases to join relatives, but this placed them some distance from the support services available at the bases (Scurfield and Tice, 1992). Upon the return of service members from deployment, families needed to readjust both to changed roles and often to changed locations. For the more than 20,000 single parents or almost 6,000 couples deployed to the Gulf (U.S. Department of Defense, 1991), finding appropriate long-term child care was an additional source of stress before, during, and, perhaps, after deployment.

The health and well-being of the family members left behind is often a chief concern of deploying service members. Some have mentally or physically disabled dependents (elderly parents, special-needs children) whose medical care is a particular worry. The availability of adequate support services for these families during the deployment and into the reintegration period is crucial (Holloway, 1999).

The unprecedented call-up of National Guard and Reserve units for the Gulf War had a strong effect on service members and their families. Even after the fall of the Berlin Wall, many reserve personnel were under the impression that they were a reserve to the active component, to be called only in case of another world war. Following notification that they would be deployed, their unit mobilization plans included 30 to 90 days of training before deployment. Therefore, they had never planned to deploy in just a few days' time (Meyer, 1999). Others had not anticipated that they would ever be called to a regional conflict and felt inadequately prepared, either emotionally or in terms of training, for participation in warfare (Scurfield and Tice, 1992). Extremely rapid deployment of troops (some within 36 hours) allowed little preparation for departure. Reserve component members thus frequently left behind disrupted families and careers. This rapid deployment also affected thousands of service members and their families who served in European theaters away from combat during the Gulf War (Ford et al., 1998). After the deployment, many who were self-employed returned to find their businesses in trouble (Yerkes and Holloway, 1996). A recent literature review considering stress and the Gulf War postulates reservists and reserve units to be at greater risk for stress reactions for the several reasons cited above (Marshall et al., 1999).

Effects of Downsizing and Increased Operational Tempo

The National Guard and Reserves were not the only service members to return home to financial uncertainty. As the Gulf War deployment came to an end, the services were carrying out a substantial downsizing that meant many who might have liked to continue on active duty did not have that option (Johnson and Broder, 1991; Lancaster, 1992; Leavitt, 1996; McCormick, 1996; Landay, 1997). In 1992, when the U.S. Congress contemplated cuts of up to $15 billion in the defense budget, Defense Secretary Richard Cheney announced that 300,000 active-duty personnel would be let go to allow savings of that magnitude (Lancaster, 1992). The Army active-duty force was reduced from 800,000 people at the height of the Gulf War to about 500,000 by the end of 1995. In April 1995, Defense Secretary William Perry notified the Army that it must prepare for further personnel cuts to 475,000 people, the smallest number of Army personnel since 1939 (McCormick, 1996). The numbers of Selected Reserve personnel were at their largest (1.2 million) in 1989 (Leavitt, 1996). However, by 1998, the total had fallen to roughly 890,000 (Kohner, 1999a).

Decreases in support services frequently accompany decreases in numbers of personnel. Thus, at the same time people are downsized or encouraged to leave active duty, there are decreases in resources and support to make their transitions easier or mitigate their effects (Holloway, 1999). Often the people who provide such support services are members of the reserve component, and they are deactivated just as they are needed for the reintegration process.

At the same time that the sizes of the services have been decreasing, the operational tempo of the military has increased to an historic high. Between 1960 and 1991, the Army engaged in only 10 operational events, excluding training and alliance-related events. Since 1991, however, the Army has conducted 28 operational events. The Marines had 15 contingency operations during the years 1982 to 1989; however, since the fall of the Berlin Wall the Marines have had 62 contingency operations (Bateman, 1999). The Air Force is undergoing long-term deployments such as Operations Southern Watch and Northern Watch in Southwest Asia. The likely length of the deployment of U.S. forces as part of the North Atlantic Treaty Organization deployment to Kosovo is unknown as of this writing.

The added deployments and contingency operations have come at a time when the number of Army divisions has been reduced from 18 to 10, the number of Navy ships has been cut from 546 in 1992 to 333 today, and the number of Air Force fighter wings has been slashed from 25 to 13. The quality of life of members of the military is slowly eroding because of the increased operational tempo and the continued reduction in personnel and resources (Bateman, 1999).

The health of veterans themselves is another particular challenge of homecoming. After the return of the military from deployment to Panama, families reported concern and confusion over symptoms exhibited by some of the returned service members. Symptoms included isolation, moodiness, detachment, and sleep disturbances (Scurfield and Tice, 1992). The symptoms experienced by many Gulf War veterans also caused considerable concern to families, concern that was heightened following reports of "mystery illnesses" that began to appear in the media in the years following the return of service members from the Gulf War.

Given the array of challenges described above, the period of return and reintegration after a deployment is a time when service members face particular hardships. The section that follows reviews the literature for available evidence about steps that might be effective in assisting service members upon their return. A description of the programs that are currently in place in the military to help service members with reintegration follows.

MILITARY REUNION AND REINTEGRATION LITERATURE REVIEW

Information Gathering

Psychological, sociological, and medical literature databases were surveyed for information on reintegration and reunion topics for the period from World War II to the present. Databases were accessed through the National Library of Medicine's MedLine, the American Psychological Association's PsycFirst, PsycINFO, and PsycLit, and from Sociological Abstracts, Inc.'s Sociological Abstracts database.

Few studies on reintegration into the home environment for nonmilitary workers have been published in the searched literature. Similarly, few studies on the reintegration of military personnel of other countries were found. As a result, the literature review that follows primarily reflects findings from studies of U.S. military personnel and their families.

Coping with family separations and reunions is a frequent reality of military life. Although much has been written on the process of separation of family and the service member in terms of emotional outcomes and coping strategies, there is relatively little systematic research on the specific theme of reunion-reintegration and emotional behavior (Mateczun and Holmes, 1996). The following summarizes the current understanding of features of reunion and reintegration based on information found in the literature.

Family Factors

The nature of a service member's homecoming is related to the terms on which she or he left the family. The type and frequency as well as the interpersonal tone of communication during the period of separation also shapes expectations upon return. Leaving home at a time of unresolved conflict can result in hurtful discussions and angry feelings with family members while the service member is away. Leaving home on good terms enhances communication and, consequently, facilitates a pleasant homecoming (Yerkes and Holloway, 1996).

Families are encouraged to write letters, send electronic mail, telephone, and send audiotapes. Service members are encouraged to do the same, but it is suggested that they address the family members individually to personalize their communications (Black, 1993).

An easy transition back into the home environment also depends on how well a family has adapted to the long absence. Studies of prisoners of war (POWs) suggest that longer separations require more time for a family to reach equilibrium upon the POW's release and return (McCubbin et al., 1975; Nice et al., 1981). Wives of POWs who have children or wives of POWs who work or who are more active and socially oriented through community activities, family support groups, and church functions cope better than those who do not perform such activities (Black, 1993; Figley, 1993b; Wood et al., 1995). Work by Hunter (1984) indicated that those at great risk for poor adaptation to the separation were "immature, extremely dependent spouses, foreign-born spouses, and spouses who were isolated within a civilian community and expected veterans to make up for lost time by devoting more time to family matters" (Mateczun and Holmes, 1996, p. 376).

Factors in the marital relationships of POWs were also relevant for successful readjustment. Spousal agreement on the husband's future career plans was crucial, and agreement on relationship roles was more important than who actually performed the roles (Hunter, 1984; Mateczun and Holmes, 1996).

Reunion Period

The literature indicates that during the reunion period, the service member goes through three phases: return, readjustment, and reintegration (Mateczun and Holmes, 1996).

Return Phase

The return phase of reunion entails the anticipation of the reunion and the actual physical reunion of those who have been separated. This is a stressful period because changes in both the service member and his or her family have taken place during the separation, and there is apprehension about what these might be and how they will be responded to (Mateczun and Holmes, 1996).

Readjustment Phase

The readjustment phase is the time during which service members and their families tend to modify their behavior to fit back into a lifestyle together. As mentioned above, each family member will have changed over the course of the separation. The readjustment period involves reaching an understanding that these changes have occurred and allowing time to establish homeostasis (Figley, 1993a; Mateczun and Holmes, 1996). During the readjustment phase, the returning service members typically experience initial culture shock and emotional overload that may cause the spouses to be emotionally separate. Some couples may have some sexual difficulties during this time. These may be due to factors such as unresolved feelings about the separation, known and unknown marital infidelities, or unresolved, unchannelled aggression (Peebles-Kleiger and Kleiger, 1994). In some families, however, the opposite may occur during the readjustment phase. There may be feelings of physical closeness, euphoria, and excitement with children and spouses. Couples may go through a honeymoon phase during which talking and reestablishment of intimacy take place until the first argument sets in.

Reintegration Phase

The reintegration phase is a time when the service member eases his or her way back into a routine, and returns to the day-to-day civilian or garrison life. To avoid upsetting the balance established during the service member's absence, the veteran must slowly work his or her way back into the family. The married couple works to reestablish intimacy as children and parents also try to reestablish familiarity and connectedness (Peebles-Kleiger and Kleiger, 1994). Families may need to be reminded to give each other some time to get reacquainted and learn the new roles and perspectives that may have been acquired during the separation. Families who expect changes in each other may be better able to cope with those changes and renegotiate their new relationship (Blount et al., 1992).

Ordinarily, changes in the handling of financial matters, household chores, and other responsibilities among family members have been made while the service member has been away, and attempts to maintain a lifestyle like the one before the separation may no longer be welcomed. The spouse who is left at home as the head of the household often matures, develops greater independence and self-confidence, and provides a different lifestyle for his or her family in the absence of the spouse (Boss et al., 1979; Nice et al., 1981; Ford et al., 1993; Wood et al., 1995). A reliance on negotiation and compromise to work toward sharing the responsibilities can help during the reintegration phase.

Although the return home from a deployment and reintegration into the home and work environment are challenging enough for the typical active-duty service member, they pose particular challenges for those who retire or who are discharged from the military upon their return. These persons must not only readjust to the family and home routine but must also begin an entirely new work life, with the attendant stresses of the job search and a new set of expectations in a very different work culture (Wolfe, 1991; Figley, 1993b).

Return of the Wounded or Ill

Veterans who are wounded or ill also face special challenges. Family and coworkers expect a quick return to normal and wonder why, once the physical wounds are healed, the returned service member is not the same as before the deployment. Complete healing may come slowly for some, if at all. Approximately 479,000 (15.2 percent) of the estimated 3.14 million men who served in the Vietnam theater had posttraumatic stress disorder (PTSD) in 1990. An estimated 8.5 percent (610) of the 7,166 women who served in Vietnam had PTSD in 1990 (Kulka et al., 1990).

Role of Family in Readjustment

Families have an important role in promoting readjustment behaviors in the returned service member. This role can be manifested in four related ways: (1) detecting traumatic stress, (2) confronting the trauma, (3) urging the recapitulation of the tragedy, (4) facilitating resolution of the trauma-inducing conflicts (Figley, 1995).

Changed patterns of behavior can be detected because family members are aware of each others' habits and dispositions and can easily detect a behavior change or traumatic stress once the family member has returned from the deployment (Figley, 1995). Once the behaviors are recognized, family members are in a position to confront the traumatized person about them either by approaching him or her directly or in a more subtle and indirect manner (Figley, 1995). Families can promote readjustment behavior by encouraging the traumatized veteran to summarize what had happened before the return through answering five basic questions: (1) What happened to me that was so traumatic? (2) Why did it happen to me? (3) Why did I and others in the same situation act as we did? (4) Why have I acted as I have since then? (5) If something like this happens again, will I be able to cope more effectively? (Figley, 1988, 1995). Addressing these questions may be more difficult when the behavior change is a response to more subtle challenges than a particular traumatic event. For example, the veteran could be disappointed that the family he or she returned to differs from the one that he or she remembered and envisioned while on deployment.

Finally, families can help in facilitating resolution of the internal conflicts. For example, they can help with the healing by providing more positive or optimistic ways to view the stressful events and their consequences (reframing) (Figley, 1995). With supportive listening, they can help the traumatized person with clarifying insights and help with more appropriate assignment of blame and credit (Figley, 1995).

Family Roles in Readjustment in Non-Military Settings

Like families of military personnel, family members of corporate executives also must frequently reorganize the family system when a spouse is away on business. Although the absences are often not as prolonged as in military separations, a spouse is sometimes gone long enough to require a reorganization of family roles. Boss and colleagues used a coping inventory to study 66 corporate wives. A factor analysis indicated that wives coped with the stress of routine absence of a husband or father by fitting into the corporate lifestyle, developing maturity and interpersonal relationships, and establishing independence (Boss et al., 1979). Although several studies of coping behaviors for separations in the civilian community have been conducted, research is lacking concerning family coping upon reintegration (Boss et al., 1979; Mateczun and Holmes, 1996).

Prevention of War-Related Stress for Family Members

No studies have confirmed the effectiveness of specific programs for preventing war-related stress for families of service members (Figley, 1993b). However, Figley describes several factors associated with lower levels of family members' stress due to separation and reintegration: (1) preparation of the service member and his or her family for all aspects of deployment with briefings and educational materials; (2) frequent contacts with other families in similar situations to provide support groups for families and service members; (3) provision of educational programs for the community so that it can support and encourage the families of service members; (4) provision of accurate and timely information about the health, safety, and return schedule of the service member; and (5) provision of a contact point for returning service members to ensure provision by the military of adequate health and human services especially for those who do not live near military installations, for example, members of the reserves and their families (Hill, 1949; McCubbin et al., 1974; McCubbin et al., 1976; Hunter, 1982; Kaslow and Ridenour, 1984; Hobfoll et al., 1991; Wolfe, 1991).

PROGRAMS TO ASSIST FAMILIES AND SERVICE MEMBERS WITH REINTEGRATION

The armed services have developed various programs to assist service members and their families through their return and to ease the transition into the home environment. Because no studies have confirmed the effectiveness of specific programs to help families and service members, the military programs were developed on the basis of experience and anecdotal evidence. Few of the programs offered by the services are mandatory. Instead, it is generally up to service members to seek out the programs for themselves and their families.

Navy Support Services

Some of the earliest programs to assist service members with homecoming were developed by the Navy. The Navy's return and reunion programs are based on three assumptions: (1) separations due to deployments are normal, even though they are stressful events in Navy family life; (2) Navy families are not dysfunctional; they are basically healthy families; and (3) increasing a family's cohesion, adaptability, and communication supports the overall goal of the programs offered by the Navy (Tinney, 1998). Because they are a part of the Navy, Marines also have access to the Navy programs.

During deployment, several means are used to maintain communication between families and deployed personnel. For example, the Navy established services whereby families can make videotapes of themselves and send them to the service member. Aboard ships service members have opportunities to do the same. This service is rapidly being supplanted, however, by the increased use of electronic mail and sailor phones aboard ships (Stokoe, 1999).

This change has been evident at the world's largest naval base in Norfolk, Virginia, which contains 300,000 sailors, Marines, civilian employees, and family members. During the recent deployment Operation Desert Fox, the use of electronic mail was far greater than that during any other deployment and was a family's primary means of staying in contact with service members (Vogel, 1998). Some service members feel that electronic mail gives them a great boost in morale and allows them to help resolve problems at home faster because of the faster communication with family members (Della Cava 1998).

The Navy Family Ombudsman program is another way to keep families abreast of relevant news and information during the deployment and the return. The program was developed in 1970 and was standardized in 1994 to provide each command with an official representative to provide information and referrals to families, serve as a point of contact between the commands and families during deployment, and provide newsletters that contain family information (B. Ray, 1998).

The Navy established the first family service center in Norfolk, Virginia, and now has 68 centers throughout the world to provide assistance and counseling for families of service members (Tinney, 1998). In the early 1970s, Navy chaplains began providing informal support and help for sailors as they prepared for the return home. In 1980, an official return and reunion homecoming program was developed at the Norfolk Family Service Center (Stokoe, 1999). As part of this program, a team of two to six individuals, usually education and program specialists, meet with the sailors at sea and with family support groups at home before the service member's return. They find out what some of the apprehensions and common concerns are and then relay the information between groups to provide service members and families with better coping strategies (U.S. Army Combined Arms Command, 1991; Tinney, 1998). The time is spent facilitating group discussions and giving interactive presentations both in person and through closed-circuit television (Tinney, 1998). Programs for couples, single sailors, sailors reuniting with children, and others are also available (Tinney, 1998). Frequently, command leadership requires attendance for briefings covering financial concerns and reintegration with family (Stokoe, 1999).

Upon their return, Navy service members go through a redeployment process that includes checklists about their medical and dental status and any family problems that might exist (for example, family health problems). Since the service member is eager to return home, he or she may not necessarily bring up problems that might delay the return (Conner, 1999).

Lifelines is a new initiative introduced by the Secretary of the Navy. It uses the Internet (www.lifelines4qol.org), teleconferencing, satellite broadcasting, and cable television to respond to quality-of-life needs of active-duty members, reservists, U.S. Department of Defense (DoD) civilian employees, and their families. This system of care allows families and service members to access community information and services at their own pace in their homes or local libraries without traveling long distances (Stokoe, 1999).

Army Support Services

The other armed services have developed similar family center programs. The Army has provided increased support for service members and their families since the Gulf War. New guidelines, training curricula, briefings, workbooks, and videotapes have been developed to better educate soldiers and their families. These tools are a part of an Army-wide program called Operation READY (Resources Educating About Deployment and You) that was developed for both active duty and reserve component personnel including the National Guard (Barnard, 1999). Operation READY provides guidelines to facilitate helping soldiers and families with issues concerning reunion into the home environment. Using Operation READY, family centers assist families with financial matters and other needs while the service member is deployed. Family support groups formed at individual units, primarily at company levels, can receive help from the Family Assistance Center staff (U.S. Army Combined Arms Command, 1991; Barnard, 1999). Family Assistance Centers provide a contact that families can turn to for questions and concerns, provide referrals to agencies appropriate for their needs, and distribute monthly newsletters that provide accurate information about the troops during a deployment (U.S. Army Combined Arms Command, 1991).

Air Force Support Services

The Air Force family support centers provide a variety of programs for service members from all branches of the military. There are programs for relocation assistance, transition assistance, career focus, information and referral, personal financial management, volunteer services, resource networks for employment, family services, and family readiness (Coyle, 1999). An array of services provide support related to separation and reunion. Stress management classes are offered to couples and families during and after deployment to help in coping with the stresses of separation and reunion. At Bolling Air Force Base, the First Sergeant's Adopt an Airman program offers service members of all ranks an opportunity to talk about their deployments with a first sergeant and discuss fears and anxieties about returning home. The first sergeant acts as a liaison for higher-ranking officials and enlisted members (Coyle, 1999). The Hearts Apart program provides support groups to help families express their feelings and concerns during a deployment and prepare them for their reactions when their loved ones come home. The readiness program also provides video teleconferencing, video electronic mail, and international calling cards for frequent communication while the service members are away.

Programs to Help Support National Guard and Reserves

The three services have developed many programs to assist active-duty service members and their families in coping with the emotional and mental challenges of reintegration and reunion after a deployment. Although all components have addressed these issues to some degree since the Gulf War, the provision of support services in the National Guard and Reserve has been more inconsistent (Ogilvy-Lee, 1999). Individuals who join National Guard and Reserve units are civilians with regular jobs outside of military life. They frequently do not live close to military bases. When they are called to military duty they are given the assurance that their jobs will be waiting for them when they return. By law, their jobs are protected for 5 years, but even with this legal protection, some reserve members have reported subtle discrimination that is difficult to prove (Barnard, 1999). Members of the reserves who own their own businesses may return from service to find that their businesses have failed (Ogilvy-Lee, 1999).

The Army Reserve uses the Operation READY training program to prepare soldiers and their families for deployment and reintegration. The Army Reserve's Family Readiness Offices are located at its Regional Support Commands and 7th ARCOM (Army Reserve Command) in Germany. These Family Readiness Offices manage the mobilization assistance program (deployment assistance) for family members. They also manage the unit Family Support Group Programs that are essential in the Army reserve and receive strong program and command emphasis. Since units are geographically dispersed, the unit support groups are important in reaching out to help family members directly. Deployed soldiers maintain contact with family members by telephone and through informational mailings (e.g., newsletters). Operation READY reunion materials are used by family support group volunteers to help family members prepare for the soldiers' return. Soldiers are now provided reunion briefings at the demobilization station used for all Army Reserve soldiers returning to the United States after a deployment. Chaplains and Family Readiness Offices coordinate reunion workshops for both soldiers and family members about 6 weeks after redeployment (which is often the time of the end of the "honeymoon phase"), as requested by the units when problems begin to appear in families (Barnard, 1999).

During the Gulf War in 1990 and 1991, the deployment of many more Air Force reservists than in previous deployments raised concerns about providing support for their reintegration to the home environment. Although no official programs were in place for the Air Force Reserves immediately following the Gulf War, programs to provide help in separation and reintegration issues began in 1993 in response to a survey that showed a need for family support-type programs (Bassett, 1998). Rather than relying on volunteers, the Air Force Reserve Family Readiness Program employs professionals to provide help in separation and reintegration issues for Air Force reservists and their families. Counseling and educational workshops as well as relevant resource materials are available on installations. In contrast to the other service reserves and National Guard, Air Force Reserve personnel are located on active-duty installations and air reserve bases, thus enabling ready access to programs and support (Bassett, 1998).

The Navy and Marine Reserve forces are provided with the same family service centers, support groups, and programs provided to Navy active-duty forces if they have been deployed continuously for 2 weeks or more. As with the Army Reserves, however, there are problems of access for those reservists and their families who live far from a base. However, activities such as the Reserve Mobilization Exercises (drills and exercises that help reservists prepare for deployment) and the newly begun Lifelines have the potential to provide greater access to programs that help reservists and their families during deployment and reintegration.

The National Guard has a dual federal and state role and mission and is made up of the Army National Guard and the Air National Guard. During a period of 1 year from late August 1990 through August 1991, the National Guard set up 471 family assistance centers and served 257,731 military family members from all services throughout the 54 U.S. states and territories (Ogilvy-Lee, 1999). Each state and territory has a full-time State Family Program Coordinator, who oversees the unit family support programs. Support at the unit level for the Guard members and their families is provided to a significant degree by specially trained volunteers, who are assisted by a unit military member trained in family assistance. Training workshops, booklets, and referral within the state and the local community are used extensively to assist and support Guard members and their families. Guard units also have Operation READY program materials available to them. As noted by other directors of readiness programs within the reserve component, not enough family program funding and full-time employees are available to provide the support needed for the National Guard (Ogilvy-Lee, 1999).

VA Support Programs

The U.S. Department of Veterans Affairs (VA) also has programs to assist in the return and reintegration of service members into the home environment after deployments. The U.S. Congress authorized the establishment of Vet Centers in 1979 to provide readjustment counseling, particularly for needs surrounding war-related psychological trauma including PTSD (Flora, 1999). Vet Centers are administered by the VA's Readjustment Counseling Service (RCS), and are community-based, nonmedical facilities intended to provide maximum ease of access for local veteran populations and to emphasize postdeployment rehabilitation in an informal setting.

Currently, 206 Vet Centers in the United States and its territories provide services to veterans (both active-duty and reserve) of deployments to World War II, the Korean War, Vietnam, the Gulf War, Lebanon, Grenada, Panama, and Somalia (U.S. Department of Veterans Affairs, 1998a,b; Flora, 1999). The services include assessment for PTSD, counseling and psychotherapy, family counseling, educational and supportive counseling to help veterans with current civilian life, employment and educational counseling, and multiple referral services (Flora, 1999). Community outreach and local networking are important components of the services provided by the Vet Centers as are collaborations with local VA medical facilities. The Vet Centers serve as the community access point for VA health care for many veterans (Flora, 1999).

Vet Centers are typically staffed by a four-person team with a team leader, two counselors, and an office manager. Vet Center teams include psychologists, social workers, nurses, and other professional counselors and paraprofessionals. Roughly 80 percent of all Vet Center counselors and team leaders are veterans and about 60 percent have served in combat theaters (Flora, 1999).

Vet Centers serve approximately 130,000 veterans each year and interact with more than 700,000 veterans and family members. The Vet Centers also make over 100,000 referrals to VA medical facilities each year. More than 96,000 Gulf War veterans have been seen at Vet Centers since April 1991.

There are some indications that Vet Centers are helpful to veterans. According to a Vet Center Readjustment Counseling Service client satisfaction survey, more than 90 percent of veterans seen at Vet Centers said that they would recommend the Vet Center to other veterans. Also, the Gulf War veterans' prospective PTSD study, undertaken by RCS in collaboration with the VA's National Center for PTSD, found that the rate of PTSD decreased in a treatment-seeking veteran group (Litz et al., 1995). In addition, the final report of the Presidential Advisory Committee on Gulf War Veterans' Illnesses (1996b), praised the outreach services that the Vet Centers were providing to contact and inform Gulf War veterans.

After the Gulf War, the U.S. Congress established an additional readjustment counseling resource specifically for Gulf War veterans. The Persian Gulf Family Support Program operated from October 1992 to September 1994 to provide services such as those carried out at Vet Centers as well as Gulf War illness-related outreach from 36 VA medical centers. The outreach included briefings for National Guard and Reserve units, local veterans service organization chapters, and grassroots family support groups. At day-long Persian Gulf Health Days, educational seminars on illnesses, traumatic stress, and VA benefits were held for veterans and the general public. Veterans were able to enroll in the VA Registry at those seminars (Presidential Advisory Committee on Gulf War Veterans' Illnesses, 1996b).

Although evaluation of that program is beyond the scope of this report, the study team suggests that elements of the program found to be effective be implemented during rather than after future large deployments and given the flexibility to continue as long as the needs remain apparent. Special strengths of the Persian Gulf Family Support Program were its availability for both National Guard and Reserve components, its family-focused interventions, and its outreach. Screening tools were used to help identify problems of individuals and families and assess program effectiveness to some extent (Altheimer, 1999; Murphy, 1999; Rathbone-McCuan, 1999). Lessons learned from the program should be applied to similar programs in the future. However, since the final report of the program was presented to the U.S. Congress in 1994, no evaluations of the Persian Gulf Family Support Program have been conducted (Murphy, 1999; Rodell, 1999).

The plan recently released by an interagency working group in response to Presidential Review Directive 5 includes mention of the reintegration of service members after deployments. Among the goals articulated in the Deployment Health chapter is to "Preserve the health and well-being of those who have served and their families" (National Science and Technology Council, 1998, p. 12). Several related objectives with associated strategies are presented to address this goal:

> Strategy 3.1.1: Develop interagency solutions to provide access to the appropriate levels of financial support, health services, and readjustment counseling for military service members' transition to future military service or civilian life.
>
> Strategy 3.1.2. Establish a combined DoD [U.S. Department of Defense], VA, DHHS [U.S. Department of Health and Human Services] plan to respond promptly and in a coordinated manner to both the anticipated and unanticipated health needs and concerns of veterans returning from major deployments.
>
> Strategy 3.2.4. Prepare DoD and VA plans for providing individual and family counseling and mental health services for military members and members of their families, especially in preparation for and upon the return home of the deployed military member. (National Science and Technology Council, 1998, p. 13)

Although these strategies listed in the Presidential Review Directive 5 are indeed sound and reasonable, to the study team's knowledge no steps have yet been taken to carry them out.

FINDINGS AND RECOMMENDATIONS

Finding 7-1: The changing demographics of the deployed forces, increased operational tempo, and increased reliance upon the reserve component all bring heightened needs for support services for service members and their families both during and after deployments.

Recommendation 7-1: Planning and operational documents for military deployments should be required to include plans for supporting the return and reintegration of active-duty and reserve service members involved in the deployment. These plans should specify

- **anticipated problems and preventive and support strategies to deal with anticipated and unanticipated problems;**
- **the resources required to carry out the strategies; and**
- **proposals for how the required resources will be funded and made available.**

The funding consequences of the resulting requirements should be reflected in the regular funding cycle and in requests for supplemental funding associated with deployments.

Finding 7-2: Since the Gulf War, the services, including the reserve components, appear to have made progress in responding to the support needs of service members and their families during reintegration. The resources and personnel to provide support to the reserve components appear to be less robust and perhaps lacking, however, given the increasing operational tempo and reliance upon these reserve forces.

Recommendation 7-2: As part of the planning described in Recommendation 7-1, particular attention is needed to address and provide resources for the readjustment needs of reserve-component service members and families.

Finding 7-3: Evaluation of both the support programs and the premise for their use appears to be limited.

Recommendation 7-3:

- **Evaluate the efficacy of the readjustment programs in place on the basis of clearly stated objectives.** Currently, such evaluations exist but are optional.
- **Carry out research into the needs of service members and their families during deployments and upon reintegration into the home environment. Use the findings to reevaluate programs and policies.**

Finding 7-4: It is crucial that service members returning from deployment have seamless access to health care and support services and that they know what services are available and how to access them. This is particularly important for those who will no longer be part of the active-duty forces.

Recommendation 7-4: As outlined by the National Science and Technology Council, the U.S. Department of Defense and U.S. Department of Veterans Affairs should coordinate plans to have reintegration support and health care services available to service members upon their return and be prepared to continue it while needs for such services remain widespread.

8

Protecting the Health of the Reserve Component

As the study team gathered information to address its charge, it became clear that several areas of the study focus warranted emphasis for the reserve forces. This chapter highlights particular needs for medical surveillance, record keeping, preventive measures, and reintegration support for the reserve components. In its 1996 report, *Health Consequences of Service During the Persian Gulf War: Recommendations for Research and Information Systems,* the Institute of Medicine (1996a) recognized the special needs and unique concerns of deployed members of the reserve forces. The report found that:

> National Guard and reserve component personnel may differ substantially from active duty personnel in average age, level of training, occupational specialties, family status, and readiness for deployment. Further, it is unclear whether either policies and procedures or the manner in which they are implemented differs between activated reserve or National Guard units and active duty troops for mobilization, deployment, demobilization, and return. All of these factors may affect the health consequences of deployment. (p. 30)

The committee recommended research

> to determine whether differences in personal characteristics or differences in policies and procedures for mobilization, deployment, demobilization, and return of reserves, National Guard, and regular troops are associated with different or adverse health consequences. If there are associations, strategies necessary to prevent or reduce these adverse health effects should be developed. (p. 30)

Those observations reflect the situation in 1995.

In 1999, more information about the reserve force is available. Published data and testimony from experts in the reserve force enabled the study team to document more clearly the distinctions between the reserve and active-duty forces in terms of access to health care, health surveillance programs, medical record keeping, preventive measures, and reintegration support. It has become apparent that the currently available resources are not adequate to ascertain the medical readiness of the reserve force, much less to provide the preventive services, health surveillance, and medical record keeping that the study team recommends for the total military force. The unique needs and issues of the reserve force mandate both a special chapter in this report and special attention to these concerns.

This chapter is focused on the reserve component with the specific objective of ensuring that the study recommendations are considered and implemented to the extent possible for reserve troops as well as for active-duty component troops. Since the reserve component constitutes almost 50 percent of the total military force of the United States and up to 41 percent of deployed forces in recent major deployments (Perry et al., 1999), the differences in medical protection, health consequences and treatment, and medical record keeping and surveillance between the reserves and active-duty forces must be addressed in any strategy to protect the health of U.S. forces. Differences must be eliminated whenever possible and given special attention when they result from the unique demographics of the reserve force.

DEMOGRAPHICS AND HEALTH ISSUES

Seven components constitute the reserve force. These include the Army National Guard, Army Reserve, Naval Reserve, Marine Corps Reserve, Air National Guard, Air Force Reserve, and Coast Guard Reserve. According to law,

> the purpose of each Reserve component is to provide trained units and qualified persons available for active duty in the armed forces, in times of war or national emergency, and at such other times as the national security may require, to fill the needs of the armed forces whenever, during and after the period needed to procure and train additional units and qualified persons to achieve the planned mobilization, more units and persons are needed than are in the regular components. (United States Code, 1998)

Categories of Reserve Forces

The reserve forces are not monolithic but have different categories with different circumstances and needs. Among the seven reserve components described above, there are three main categories: the Ready Reserve, the Standby Reserve, and the Retired Reserve. The Ready Reserve (1.4 million people in fiscal year 1998) is made up of the Selected Reserve, and the Individual Ready Reserve and Inactive National Guard (IRR/ING). The Selected Reserve are those best known to civilians. They are required to do 48 drills a year and to have at least 14 days of annual training. IRR/ING are also available to be called up, but they are not required to do the regular drilling and training required of the Selected Reserve. Because they are not part of regular units, they are even more difficult to reach for required programs, surveys, immunizations, and so forth. The Standby Reserve is a fairly small group of those who are temporarily disabled or who cannot perform their duties because of their essential government jobs, for example. A final category is the Retired Reserve, roughly 521,000 people in fiscal year 1998 and slightly more than a quarter of the total U.S. Department of Defense (DoD) retiree population (Kohner, 1999a).

Demographics

Both during and since the Gulf War, the demographics of service members in the reserve components have differed somewhat from those on active duty. In the Gulf War, Reserve units were 14.7 percent female, with 69.7 percent white, 20.8 percent black service members, and 9.5 percent service members of other races or ethnicities. The average age of reservists in 1991 was 30.4 years. The National Guard units deployed to the Gulf had 9.6 percent women, with 75.4 percent white, 18.3 percent black, and 6.3 percent other service members. The average age for the National Guard participants in 1991 was 32.6 years (Murphy et al., 1999). The proportion of both National Guard and Reserves with dependents was 51.7 percent (Dove et al., 1994a). Active-duty service members deployed to the Gulf War included 6.1 percent women, with 66.8 percent white, 23.2 percent black, and 10.0 percent other service members. The average age of active-duty troops was 27.4 years in 1991, and 50.4 percent had dependents (Dove et al., 1994b; Murphy et al., 1999). For more recent deployments, some demographic differences between reserve and active-duty members are greater. Roughly 70 percent of reserves deployed to Bosnia and Southwest Asia (since 1994 and 1995) have had dependents, whereas the proportion was 54 to 57 percent for active-duty troops (30 percent of reserves deployed to Haiti have had dependents). Women constituted 13 to 15 percent of reserve units sent to Haiti and Bosnia and 7.6 percent of those deployed to Southwest Asia, whereas women constituted 6 to 8 percent of the deployed active-duty forces (Perry et al., 1999).

Considering the military forces in their entirety, the average age of active duty service members is 32.4 years for officers and 26.2 years for enlisted members, whereas for the Selected Reserve it is 39.9 years for officers and 32.2 years for enlisted members. Women make up 14.1 percent of the total active-duty force and 15.8 percent of the Ready Reserve. Approximately 60 percent of both active-duty and reserve forces have dependents. (Kohner, 1999b).

Deployments of Reserve Forces

The reserve components play an increasingly critical role in the total armed forces of the United States. As noted in Chapter 7, National Guard and Reserves constituted a larger portion of the force deployed in the Gulf War than in any previous mobilizations. Of the 696,531 service members deployed to the Gulf War, 9.8 percent were members of the Reserves and 6.2 percent were members of the National Guard (Gray et al., 1998). Since then, reserve forces have increasingly been integrated into the total force. Although the active-duty component made up 51.2 percent of the total force in 1998, the Selected Reserve constituted 32.1 percent and the IRR/ING made up 16.7 percent. Some capabilities exist only in the reserve components, so reserves are mandatory assets for particular missions.

An individual joining a reserve component today should expect to be called up and deployed in support of a military operation anywhere in the world. The probability and frequency of deployment for reserve members are dependent on the type of reserve unit joined, the member's military specialty, and the requirements of the various military operations.

As an example, there are certain units and specialties, such as Civil Affairs/Psychological Operations, Intelligence, and transport units, which are predominantly in the reserve components and are titled "High demand/low density." There are relatively few of these units and specialties in the force structure, but due to the nature of recent military operations throughout the world, these units and specialties have been used extensively during the past several years. Some reserve members in these types of units, or with these specialties, have experienced more than one deployment since 1990 (Kohner, 1999c).

On any given day, reserve members are deployed all over the world. Before the call-ups for the conflict in Kosovo, roughly 30,000 reserve members were on active duty and were providing support to different missions including the Bosnia and Southwest Asia deployments (Kohner, 1999a). Reservists have constituted 3 percent of the forces deployed to Southwest Asia since October 1994, 18 percent of those deployed to Bosnia since December 1995, and 41 percent of the forces deployed to Haiti since September 1994 (Perry et al., 1999; data are current as of May and June 1999).

Health Problems in Reserves

Some data have indicated that after the deployment to the Gulf War the health toll was greater on reserve forces than on active-duty forces. The earliest investigations of reported health problems after the Gulf War were in response to symptoms reported in several different National Guard and Reserve units in Indiana, Pennsylvania, and the southeastern United States. In each case, these units came to the attention of the medical community because of reports of high rates of unexplained illnesses among members of the units (Institute of Medicine, 1996a).

In a large telephone interview survey of military personnel from Iowa, those who had deployed to the Gulf War reported a significantly higher prevalence of several medical and psychiatric symptoms compared with those who had served elsewhere during the Gulf War (Iowa Persian Gulf Study Group, 1997). Differences in reported prevalences of medical and psychiatric symptoms were more apparent in the National Guard and Reserve units than in the regular military. Among those deployed to the Gulf, National Guard and Reserve personnel were more likely to have symptoms of chronic fatigue or alcohol abuse than regular military personnel (Iowa Persian Gulf Study Group, 1997). In a cross-sectional survey of veterans 18 to 24 months after their return from the Gulf War, subjects reporting greater than five health symptoms on a health symptom checklist were more likely to be female, to be unemployed, to have more alcohol and drug problems, and to be Reserve and National Guard members (Wolfe et al., 1998). In contrast, a study of women who served in the Air Force during the Gulf War found that despite their younger age, active-duty women reported significantly more general health problems than those in the National Guard or Reserve (Pierce, 1997).

In the years following the Gulf War, both the U.S. Department of Veterans Affairs (VA) and DoD established health evaluation and treatment programs for Gulf War veterans with concerns about their health: together these programs are called the Persian Gulf War registry. National Guard and Reserve service members deployed to the Gulf were roughly twice as likely to have participated in the Persian Gulf War registry than their active-duty counterparts (Gray et al., 1998).

UNIQUE CIRCUMSTANCES

The circumstances of the reserve components create additional challenges for strategies to protect their health during and after deployments. Although they carry a serious obligation to maintain readiness and provide military service in time of national need, reserve forces spend most of their time as civilians, with civilian jobs and lives. This has both psychosocial and practical ramifications.

Cultural differences between the active-duty and reserve components are important. Active-duty personnel, by definition, work full-time for the military and are immersed in its culture. Increasingly frequent deployments for service members keep the potential for deployment a present possibility. Reserve members engage in frequent drills and in 2 weeks of training each year, but their full-time occupations are civilian. They are necessarily more fully integrated into civilian culture than the active-duty component is. When a deployment occurs, their lives are disrupted more dramatically, and the increasing pace of deployments for reserve forces has meant more disruption and tension with their employers (Brackett, 1999b).

Some of the stressors that were new to the Gulf War may also have had a greater effect on the deployed reserve forces. Rapid mobilization, easier access than in previous major conflicts to communications with friends and families and, therefore, to problems at home, and rapid demobilization were more disruptive for reservists and their families, since the reservists were being deployed from and returned to civilian life rather than to a military garrison setting (Institute of Medicine, 1996a). Since many reservists were activated to support units, this also created greater disruption, since in the Gulf War these units "had heavier workloads, more crowded and primitive living conditions, and less clearly defined roles and missions" (Institute of Medicine, 1996a, p. 60).

The manner in which health care is received is another important difference between reserve and active-duty personnel that leads to challenges for health protection. Although active-duty component service members receive all of their health care (except when they choose to use civilian providers and pay for health care themselves) from DoD, members of the reserve components receive most of their health care from civilian providers through their civilian employers' insurance. Only during periods when they are activated, such as during their 2 weeks of annual training or during a deployment, are they entitled to health care from DoD. If they become ill or are injured in the line of duty, special provisions for their care are made.

Because their medical care is provided outside the military system, medical records for reserve forces are not readily available to the military system. As in the military, most civilian medical records are still kept on paper. For a military physician to review a reservist's civilian medical record, he or she must be granted permission as well as the name and location of the reservist's provider. Such circumstances make it virtually impossible to easily consider reservists' health issues on a population basis, including monitoring of their health status over both the short and long term after a deployment. However, annually administering the Health Evaluation and Assessment Review (HEAR) to reserve members as recommended in Chapter 4 should help to provide population data for this group.

A related problem for both reserve and active-duty forces that is exacerbated for the reserve force is the carryover of medical records to VA and the capture of health information from the civilian sector. The creation of a true lifetime medical record is a challenge for all forces, but it is far more complicated for the reserve force members, who move more frequently than active-duty force troops among the civilian, DoD, and VA health care systems (National Science and Technology Council, 1998; Brackett, 1999a). Although the military is working toward a computer-based patient record for service members who use military treatment facilities, a lack of integration with civilian systems will pose a hurdle for the inclusion of medical records for reserve forces in this system. However, health history data from the Recruit Assessment Program (RAP) and health status information from the HEAR, and additional information from periods of deployment collected in a retrievable electronic form could be part of information carried over to the VA when reserves separate from the service.

Compounding the fact that reservists receive their care outside the military health system is the fact that the reservists' available time is very limited. Their weekend drills and annual training are meant to be training time rather than administrative or health care sessions. Thus, physical examinations, immunizations, health appraisals, and briefings on health risks all compete for time with training for their deployment occupations (Brackett, 1999a).

At the same time that there is an increase in the use of the reserve component, there are few resources for health surveillance. The lack of equipment and funds results in training compromises. When medical personnel attend weekend training, they have time for little other than giving required periodic physicals. When immunizations such as the anthrax vaccine must be carried out on a specific schedule, the training must be rescheduled. For some immunizations, such as with the hepatitis A vaccine, the funds for the vaccine and the medical personnel to administer it are so limited that immunization has been delayed. The requirements for "medical readiness" of the reserve forces are not being met because of limited funding and policies requiring that physical examinations be carried out by military care providers. Dental screening is an example of a requirement for an annual screening that must be done by military dentists, yet there are very few in the reserves, so this requirement is not met (Brackett, 1999a). The availability of medical personnel is a problem in the Army Reserves, since these troops are dispersed throughout the United States and a corpsman or medic is not attached to each unit as in the Air Force and Naval Reserves. The Army Reserves thus frequently do not get physicals within the period of time required by law or get them at the expense of sustainment of training and readiness (Woody, 1999).

IMPLEMENTATION OF REPORT RECOMMENDATIONS

Medical Surveillance

Given the special circumstances of the reserve forces, some of the study team's recommendations might prove challenging for implementation for the reserve component. In the area of medical surveillance, tools such as the RAP and the HEAR are important aspects of the effort to gather baseline health information on deployed forces and to be able to ascertain medical problems as they arise. The annual administration of the HEAR to reservists would raise several difficult issues, however. In addition to its added toll on training time and the logistical challenges of arranging for an additional 1.4 million people to take a survey every year, difficult questions will arise when the health risk survey identifies areas in which the reservist could benefit from medical care. He or she must still seek this care in the civilian sector. Despite these obstacles, the revision and use of the HEAR as described in Chapter 4 should be helpful both to the deployed forces and to the military. Better understanding of the health status (including reproductive health status) of the forces both before and after deployments should lead to improved care and perhaps to the prevention of exacerbation of medically unexplained physical symptoms.

Administration of the postdeployment health questionnaires as currently required is particularly problematic if it is not done before the reservists leave the theater of operation. Once they have returned home, it is extremely difficult to collect such information. If the pre- and postdeployment questionnaires are phased out because they are made unnecessary by the annual administration of the HEAR (as discussed in Chapter 4), the administration of the HEAR to the reserve forces as well will be even more crucial.

Overall, the recent additional requirements for health surveillance have been particularly burdensome for the reserve forces because of their limited time and resources. Although it is important that these steps be taken, it should be done by use of a reasoned strategy for the reserve forces that takes their circumstances into account and that provides sufficient resources for additional demands.

In November 1997, Secretary Cohen launched a Reserve Health Summit to make recommendations to improve the medical readiness of reserve component members (Woody, 1999). Among the recommendations generated by the summit was to conduct a phased study to identify reserve component member health risks, develop a focused reserve component health assessment tool, implement a pilot program with the tool to measure individual medical fitness, and implement use of the tool if successful. Use of the HEAR for reserves as recommended in this report should help to address the health information needs identified by the Reserve Health Summit.

Medical Record Keeping

One of the goals articulated by the National Science and Technology Council (1998) was to "ensure the accuracy, timeliness, security, and retrievability of information that must be entered into records or automated systems that document health history for active, guard, and reserve service members and veterans" (p. 18). Longitudinal record keeping is critical to monitoring the delayed and prolonged manifestations of the health effects of war. For reserve-force members who receive health care from civilian health care systems, data collected from the RAP and the HEAR will be of particular importance as well as that added from periods of deployment as a way to permit some health surveillance of this group before and after deployment. An attempt to develop a form for the required annual dental screening for use by civilian dentists that is compatible with the form used by the military dentists is an example of an effort to integrate military and civilian medical records for the reserve forces. This is one of the less complicated components of the medical record, yet it is not an easy one to achieve (Woody, 1999).

As discussed above, the primary reliance upon civilian medical care providers by reserve forces poses considerable challenges to maintaining medical records for reserve members. These challenges should not be written off as insurmountable, however, and concrete initiatives are needed, as discussed in Chapter

5, such as collecting data from the RAP and HEAR in retrievable, analyzable, electronic form.

Preventive Measures

Time and resource constraints for reserve forces also affect the preventive measures provided for them. Among the preventive measures discussed in this report, risk communication is particularly important. It poses different challenges for reserve forces because they are deployed from a very different context of employment and family. Information networks for reserve forces are likely to be somewhat different from those for active-duty forces, and rumors and misinformation may be more rampant. Less contact time between reserve forces and command leadership is available to develop the trust and credibility necessary for effective communication. Recognition of these differences by command leadership is critical for providing maximally effective risk communication.

Just as accession and retention standards are applied differently across the services, there are likely disparities in their application among the seven reserve components. This is also the case for the periodic physical examinations, which are assiduously performed for National Guard and Reserve pilots, but not as regularly performed for the geographically scattered Army Reserve. In 1997 a Reserve Health Summit considered alternatives to periodic physicals because compliance was sporadic and incomplete among the reserves (Woody, 1999). Rather than maintaining the current focus on illness, discussions from the summit point to a need to move toward the health assessment and prevention model being pursued in the civilian sector and the military health care system. Administration of the HEAR to reserve forces would reflect this change in emphasis. It is likely that the civilian lifestyle is, in general, less healthy from a diet and fitness perspective than the active duty lifestyle. To the extent that this is true, members of the reserve forces might benefit even more from an emphasis on preventive intervention.

Immunizations are difficult to accomplish because of time and resource constraints, as described earlier. Reserve forces have inadequate funding to ensure that immunization programs are both complete and administered according to necessary schedules (Brackett, 1999a).

Reintegration

Chapter 7 stresses the particular extent to which separation and reintegration pose challenges for the reserve component.

FINDINGS AND RECOMMENDATIONS

Finding 8-1: Several of the most important components of a strategy to protect the health of deployed forces (improved medical surveillance and care responsive to medically unexplained physical symptoms, record keeping, risk communication, preventive measures, and reintegration) pose particular challenges for the reserve component because of their quasicivilian status and geographically dispersed situation. Since the Ready Reserve now constitutes almost half of the total force and is a significant component of deployed forces, its needs cannot be ignored or postponed. Although their special circumstances make it impossible to mandate a health protection strategy identical to that used for active-duty forces, a coherent strategy should be developed to provide similar programs that work toward the same ends and that are provided adequate resources.

Recommendation 8-1: Include the reserves in the planning, coordination, and implementation of improved health surveillance, record keeping, and risk communication. Inform recruits about the operational tempo of the units they are likely to join. Develop a strategy for the reserve forces that takes into consideration their limited access to the military health care system before and after deployment but that recognizes their particular needs for health protection and that provides adequate resources to meet those needs. Include the following:

- **Administer the Recruit Assessment Program to members of the reserve components upon their entrance into the military, and annually administer the improved Health Enrollment Assessment Review to members of the reserve components.** (See Chapter 4, Recommendations 4-1 and 4-2a.)
- **Develop methods to gather and analyze retrievable, electronically stored health data on reservists. For example, ensure that data from the Recruit Assessment Program and the Health Evaluation and Assessment Review collected from reserves (as recommended in Chapter 4) are captured as part of a computerized record permitting retrievability and population-level analysis as well as the addition of new data from periods of deployment or activation.** (Chapter 5, Recommendation 5-6)
- **Plan and provide adequate resources for the readjustment needs of the reserve component.** (Chapter 7, Recommendations 7-1 and 7-2)

References

Abbey, S. E., and P. E. Garfinkel. 1991. Neurasthenia and Chronic Fatigue Syndrome: The Role of Culture in the Making of a Diagnosis. *American Journal of Psychiatry* 148(12):1638–46.

ACS Government Solutions Group. 1999. *PHCA ATIC Demonstrations Weekly Report. Demonstration March 24, 1999*. Provided July 27, 1999.

Alexander, R. W., L. A. Bradley, G. S. Alarcon, et al. 1998. Sexual and Physical Abuse in Women with Fibromyalgia: Association with Outpatient Health Care Utilization and Pain Medication Usage. *Arthritis and Rheumatism* 11(2):102–15.

Altheimer, E. L. 1999. Chief of Social Work Service, Veterans Affairs Medical Center, Little Rock, Ark., Written Communication, May 11, 1999.

American Psychiatric Association. 1980. *Diagnostic and Statistical Manual of Mental Disorders 3rd ed. (DSM-III)*. Washington, D.C.: APA.

American Psychiatric Association. 1994. *Diagnostic and Statistical Manual of Mental Disorders, 4th ed. (DSM-IV)*. 427–429. Washington, D.C.: APA.

Anderson, J. S., and C. E. Ferrans. 1997. The Quality of Life of Persons with Chronic Fatigue Syndrome. *Journal of Nervous and Mental Disease* 185(6):359–67.

Archibald, H. C., and R. D. Tuddenham. 1965. Persistent Stress Reaction After Combat: A 20-Year Follow-Up. *Archives of General Psychiatry* 12:475.

Armed Forces Pest Management Board. 1996. "Technical Information Memorandum No. 36. Personal Protective Techniques Against Insects and Other Arthropods of Military Significance." Walter Reed Army Medical Center, Washington, D.C.

Artiss, K. L. 1963. Human Behavior Under Stress: From Combat to Social Psychiatry. *Military Medicine* 128(10):1011–15.

Bailey, S. 1999a. DoD: Medicine at Crossroads. *U.S. Medicine* 35(1):20–1.

Bailey, S. 1999b. Keynote Address. Presentation at *Unexplained Symptoms After War and Terrorism: Building Toward Consensus. 13th Conference on Military Medicine*. May 24–26, 1999. Uniformed Services University of the Health Sciences (USUHS), Bethesda, Md.

Bakketeig, L. S., H. J. Hoffman, and E. E. Harley. 1979. The Tendency to Repeat Gestational Age and Birth Weight in Successive Births. *American Journal of Obstetrics and Gynecology* 135(8):1086–103.

Barnard, J. 1999. Program Manager, Family Readiness. U.S. Army Reserve Command. Ft. McPherson, GA. Written Communication (electronic mail), February 19, 1999.

Barsky, A. J. 1997. A 37-Year-Old Man with Multiple Somatic Complaints. *JAMA* 278(8):673–9.

Barsky, A. J. 1998. A Comprehensive Approach to the Chronically Somatizing Patient [editorial]. *Journal of Psychosomatic Research* 45(4):301–6.

Barsky, A. J., and J. F. Borus. 1999. Functional Somatic Symptoms. *Annals of Internal Medicine* 130:910–21.

Barsky, A. J., G. Wyshak, and G. L. Klerman. 1986. Medical and Psychiatric Determinants of Outpatient Medical Utilization. *Medical Care* 24(6):548–60.

Barsky, A. J., G. Wyshak, K. S. Latham, et al. 1991. Hypochondriacal Patients, Their Physicians, and Their Medical Care. *Journal of General Internal Medicine* 6(5): 413–9.

Bassett, N. 1998. Chief of Family Readiness, Air Force Reserve. Robins Air Force Base, Ga. Written Communication (electronic mail), December 8, 1998.

Bateman, H. 1999. Outlook: Our Crisis in Military Readiness Is Real and Growing. *Houston Chronicle,* April 16, 1999, sec. A: 33.

Bates, D. W., D. J. Cullen, N. Laird, et al. 1995. Incidence of Adverse Drug Events and Potential Adverse Drug Events. Implications for Prevention. ADE Prevention Study Group. *JAMA* 274(1):29–34.

Beebe, G. W., and J. W. Appel. 1958. Psychological Breakdown in Relation to Stress and Other Factors. In *Variation in Psychological Tolerance to Ground Combat in World War II, Final Report*, 88–131. Washington, D.C.: National Academy of Sciences.

Beebe, G. W., and M. E. DeBakey. 1952. Battle Casualties: Incidence, Mortality, and Logistic Considerations. Springfield, Ill.: Charles C. Thomas.

Belenky, G., and J. A. Martin. 1996a. The Future Practice of Combat Psychiatry. In *The Gulf War and Mental Health: A Comprehensive Guide*, ed. J. A. Martin, L.R. Sparacina, and G. Belenky, 179–90. Westport, Conn.: Praeger Publishers.

Belenky, G., J. A. Martin, and S. C. Marcy. 1996b. After-Action Critical Incident Stress Debriefings and Battle Reconstructions Following Combat. In *The Gulf War and Mental Health: A Comprehensive Guide*, ed. J. A. Martin, L. R. Sparacino, and G. Belenky, 105–13. Westport, Conn.: Praeger Publishers.

Benenson, A. S. 1995. *Control of Communicable Diseases Manual*. Washington, D.C.: American Public Health Association.

Bergmann, M. M., T. Byers, D. S. Freedman, et al. 1998. Validity of Self-Reported Diagnoses Leading to Hospitalization: A Comparison of Self-Reports with Hospital Records in a Prospective Study of American Adults. *American Journal of Epidemiology* 147(10):969–77.

Bigos, S. J., M. C. Battie, D. M. Spengler, et al. 1991. A Prospective Study of Work Perceptions and Psychosocial Factors Affecting the Report of Back Injury [published erratum appears in *Spine* 16(6):688, 1991]. *Spine* 16(1):1–6.

Birch and Davis. 1998. Immunization Coverage Studies and Analyses in the Military Services. White Paper, Armed Forces Epidemiology Board.

Black, D. W., A. Rathe, and R. B. Goldstein. 1990. Environmental Illness. A Controlled Study of 26 Subjects with "20th Century Disease." *JAMA* 264(24):3166–70.

Black, W. G. Jr. 1993. Military-Induced Family Separation: A Stress Reduction Intervention. *Social Work* 38(3):273–80.

Blake, D., T. M. Keane, P. R. Wine, et al. 1990. Prevalence of PTSD Symptoms in Combat Veterans Seeking Medical Treatment. *Journal of Traumatic Stress* 3:15–27.

Blanchard, E. B., K. A. Appelbaum, C. L. Radnitz, et al. 1990. Placebo-Controlled Evaluation of Abbreviated Progressive Muscle Relaxation and of Relaxation Combined with Cognitive Therapy in the Treatment of Tension Headache. *Journal of Consulting and Clinical Psychology* 58(2):210–5.

Block, A. R., E. F. Kremer, and M. Gaylor. 1980. Behavioral Treatment of Chronic Pain: The Spouse as a Discriminative Cue for Pain Behavior. *Pain* 9(2):243–52.

Blount, B. W., A. Curry Jr., and G. I. Lubin. 1992. Family Separations in the Military. *Military Medicine* 157(2):76–80.

Blumer, D., G. Montouris, and B. Hermann. 1995. Psychiatric Morbidity in Seizure Patients on a Neurodiagnostic Monitoring Unit. *Journal of Neuropsychiatry and Clinical Neurosciences* 7(4):445–56.

Bolton, J. 1999. Role of Laboratories in Military Public Health Surveillance. Presentation at *Strategies to Protect the Health of Deployed U.S. Forces: Medical Surveillance, Record Keeping, and Risk Reduction.* Workshop IV. January 14, 1999. Institute of Medicine, Washington, D.C.

Boss, L. P. 1997. Epidemic Hysteria: A Review of the Published Literature. *Epidemiologic Reviews* 19(2):233–43.

Boss, P. G., McCubbin H. I., and Lester G. 1979. The Corporate Executive Wife's Coping Patterns in Response to Routine Husband-Father Absence. *Family Process* 18: 79–86.

Brackett, S. 1999a. Health Surveillance of the Reserve Components. Presentation at *Strategies to Protect the Health of Deployed U.S. Forces: Medical Surveillance, Record Keeping, and Risk Reduction.* Workshop IV. January 13, 1999. Institute of Medicine, Washington, D.C.

Brackett, S. 1999b. Office of the Assistant Secretary of Defense for Health Affairs. Personal Communication, May 21, 1999.

Bray, R. M., R. P. Sanchez, M. L. Ornstein, et al. 1999. "1998 Department of Defense Survey of Health Related Behaviors Among Military Personnel." Research Triangle Institute, Research Triangle Park, N.C.

Bremner, J. D., P. Randall, T. M. Scott, et al. 1995. MRI-Based Measurement of Hippocampal Volume in Patients with Combat-Related Posttraumatic Stress Disorder. *American Journal of Psychiatry* 152(7):973–81.

Bremner, J. D., P. Randall, E. Vermetten, et al. 1997. Magnetic Resonance Imaging-Based Measurement of Hippocampal Volume in Posttraumatic Stress Disorder Related to Childhood Physical and Sexual Abuse—A Preliminary Report. *Biological Psychiatry* 41(1):23–32.

Brinton, L. A., L. J. Melton 3d, G. D. Malkasian Jr., et al. 1989. Cancer Risk After Evaluation for Infertility. *American Journal of Epidemiology* 129(4):712–22.

Buchwald, D., and D. Garrity. 1994. Comparison of Patients with Chronic Fatigue Syndrome, Fibromyalgia, and Multiple Chemical Sensitivities. *Archives of Internal Medicine* 154(18):2049–53.

Buckelew, S. P. 1989. Fibromyalgia: A Rehabilitation Approach. A Review. *American Journal of Physical Medicine and Rehabilitation* 68(1):37–42.

Buescher, P. A., K. P. Taylor, M. H. Davis, et al. 1993. The Quality of the New Birth Certificate Data: A Validation Study in North Carolina. *American Journal of Public Health* 83(8):1163–5.

Bush, R. A., T. C. Smith, D. E. Gee, et al. 1999. *Active Surveillance of Birth Defects Among U.S. Department of Defense Beneficiaries: Report of a Feasibility Study*. Naval Health Research Center, San Diego, Calif.

Buske-Kirschbaum, A., S. Jobst, D. Psych, et al. 1997. Attenuated Free Cortisol Response to Psychosocial Stress in Children with Atopic Dermatitis. *Psychosomatic Medicine* 59(4):419–26.

Calow, S., 139th Medical Group. "PM Lesson—U.S. Troops in Botswana, 1992." Available at http://139.161.16/lessons/reports/news2/sect4.htm. (accessed 17 May 1999).

Carucci, P. 1979. Reliability of Statistical and Medical Information Reported on Birth and Death Certificates. New York: New York State Department of Health Monograph 1979; 15:5–23.

Cash, J. M., L. J. Crofford, W. T. Gallucci, et al. 1992. Pituitary-Adrenal Axis Responsiveness to Ovine Corticotropin Releasing Hormone in Patients with Rheumatoid Arthritis Treated with Low Dose Prednisone. *Journal of Rheumatology* 19(11): 1692–6.

Cavanaugh, D. C., B. L. Elisberg, C. H. Llewellyn, et al. 1974. Plague Immunization,V. Indirect Evidence for Efficacy of the Plague Vaccine. *Journal of Infectious Diseases* 129(Suppl.):S37–S40.

Centers for Disease Control (CDC). 1988. Guidelines for Evaluating Surveillance Systems. *Morbidity and Mortality Weekly Report* 37(S-5):1–19.

Centers for Disease Control and Prevention (CDC). 1997. "Electronic Reporting of Laboratory Data for Public Health: Meeting Report and Recommendations." Available at http://www.phppo.cdc.gov/dls/. (accessed 15 July 1999).

Chester, A. C., and P. H. Levine. 1997. The Natural History of Concurrent Sick Building Syndrome and Chronic Fatigue Syndrome. *Journal of Psychiatric Research* 31(1): 51–7.

Clark, D. M., P. M. Salkovskis, A. Hackmann, et al. 1998. Two Psychological Treatments for Hypochondriasis. A Randomised Controlled Trial. *British Journal of Psychiatry* 173:218–25.

Clark, K. L., R. Mahmoud, M. R. Krauss, et al. 1999. Reducing Medical Attrition: The Role of the Accession Medical Standards Analysis and Research Activity. *Military Medicine* 164(7):485–87.

Classen, D. C., S. L. Pestotnik, R. S. Evans, et al. 1991. Computerized Surveillance of Adverse Drug Events in Hospital Patients [published erratum appears in *JAMA* 267(14):1922, 1992]. *JAMA* 266(20):2847–51.

Clauw, D. J., and G. P. Chrousos. 1997. Chronic Pain and Fatigue Syndromes: Overlapping Clinical and Neuroendocrine Features and Potential Pathogenic Mechanisms. *Neuroimmunomodulation* 4:134–53.

Clauw, D. J., M. Schmidt, D. Radulovic, et al. 1997. The Relationship Between Fibromyalgia and Interstitial Cystitis. *Journal of Psychiatric Research* 31(1):125–31.

Clines, T. 1998. Force Medical Protection. Presentation at *Strategies to Protect the Health of Deployed U.S. Forces: Medical Surveillance, Record Keeping, and Risk Reduction*. Workshop I. April 16, 1998. Institute of Medicine, Washington, D.C.

Commerce Business Daily (via GPO Access). 1999. "Broad Agency Announcement-Gulf War Illnesses Research: Force Health Protection-Deployment Health; Interactions of Drugs, Biologics and Chemicals in Service Members in Deployment Environments; Integrated Psychosocial and Neuroscience Research on Stress and Somatic Consequences; Innovative Biologically Based Toxicology Methods and Models for Assessing Mixed Chemical Exposures with Potential Neurotoxicological and Other Health Effects; Multidisciplinary Studies of Fibromyalgia, Chronic Fatigue Syndrome, and Chemical Sensitivities." Available at http://frwebgate.access.gpo.gov/cgi-bin/multidb.cgi.

Conner, D. 1999. Department of the Navy. Navy Personnel Command (Reserves). Millington, Tenn. Personal Communication, February 26, 1999.

Coryell, W., and S. G. Norten. 1981. Briquet's Syndrome (Somatization Disorder) and Primary Depression: Comparison of Background and Outcome. *Comprehensive Psychiatry* 22(3):249–56.

Costakos, D. T., L. A. Love, and R. S. Kirby. 1998. The Computerized Perinatal Database: Are the Data Reliable? *American Journal of Perinatology* 15(7):453–9.

Cothern, C. R., ed. 1996. *Handbook for Environmental Risk Decision Making: Values, Perceptions, and Ethics*. Boca Raton, Fla.: CRC Press.

Coyle, A. 1999. 11th Wing Personnel and Family Readiness NCO—Family Readiness Program. Bolling Air Force Base, Washington, D.C. Written Communication (electronic mail), February 12, 1999.

Craig, T. K., A. P. Boardman, K. Mills, et al. 1993. The South London Somatisation Study I: Longitudinal Course and the Influence of Early Life Experiences. *British Journal of Psychiatry* 163:579–88.

Craig, T. K., and G. W. Brown. 1984. Goal Frustration and Life Events in the Aetiology of Painful Gastrointestinal Disorder. *Journal of Psychosomatic Research* 28(5):411–21.

Craufurd, D. I., F. Creed, and M. I. Jayson. 1990. Life Events and Psychological Disturbance in Patients with Low-Back Pain. *Spine* 15(6):490–4.

Creed, F. 1981. Life Events and Appendicectomy. *Lancet* 1(8235):1381–5.

Crofford, L. J., S. R. Pillemer, K. T. Kalogeras, et al. 1994. Hypothalamic-Pituitary-Adrenal Axis Perturbations in Patients with Fibromyalgia. *Arthritis and Rheumatism* 37(11):1583–92.

Deale, A., T. Chalder, I. Marks, et al. 1997. Cognitive Behavior Therapy for Chronic Fatigue Syndrome: A Randomized Controlled Trial. *American Journal of Psychiatry* 154(3):408–14.

DeGuire, S., R. Gevirtz, Y. Kawahara, et al. 1992. Hyperventilation Syndrome and the Assessment of Treatment for Functional Cardiac Symptoms. *American Journal of Cardiology* 70(6):673–7.

Della Cava, M. 21 December 1998. With Busy Mission Over, Troops Reflect. *USA Today*, p. 17A.

Dellu, F., W. Mayo, M. Vallee, et al. 1994. Reactivity to Novelty During Youth as a Predictive Factor of Cognitive Impairment in the Elderly: A Longitudinal Study in Rats. *Brain Research* 653(1–2):51–6.

Demitrack, M. A., J. K. Dale, S. E. Straus, et al. 1991. Evidence for Impaired Activation of the Hypothalamic-Pituitary-Adrenal Axis in Patients with Chronic Fatigue Syndrome. *Journal of Clinical Endocrinology and Metabolism* 73(6):1224–34.

Depue, R. H., M. C. Pike, and B. E. Henderson. 1983. Estrogen Exposure During Gestation and Risk of Testicular Cancer. *Journal of the National Cancer Institute* 71(6): 1151–5.

Dhabhar, F. S., and B. S. McEwen. 1997. Acute Stress Enhances While Chronic Stress Suppresses Cell-Mediated Immunity in Vivo: A Potential Role for Leukocyte Trafficking. *Brain, Behavior, and Immunity* 11(4):286–306.

Dhabhar, F. S., and B. S. McEwen. 1999. Enhancing Versus Suppressive Effects of Stress Hormones on Skin Immune Function. *Proceedings of the National Academy of Sciences of the United States of America* 96(3):1059–64.

Dove, M., S. Butler, and S. Seggerman. 1994a. "Desert Shield/Desert Storm Participation Report (Reserves). Vol. 2." Defense Manpower Data Center, Seaside, Calif.

Dove, M., S. Butler, S. Seggerman, et al. 1994b. "Desert Shield/Desert Storm Participation Report (Active Duty). Vol. 1." Defense Manpower Data Center, Seaside, Calif.

Dworkin, S. F., M. Von Korff, and L. LeResche. 1990. Multiple Pains and Psychiatric Disturbance. An Epidemiologic Investigation. *Archives of General Psychiatry* 47(3): 239–44.

Egendorf, A. 1982. The Postwar Healing of Vietnam Veterans: Recent Research. *Hospital and Community Psychiatry* 33(11):901–8.

Egendorf, A., J. Farley, and A Remez. 1981. "Legacies of Vietnam: Dealing with the War: A View Based on Individual Lives of Vietnam Veterans." U.S. Government Printing Office, Washington, D.C.

Emery, E. S. 3rd, A. Eaton, J. K. Grether, et al. 1997. Assessment of Gestational Age Using Birth Certificate Data Compared with Medical Record Data. *Paediatric and Perinatal Epidemiology* 11(3):313–21.

Engel, C. C. Jr., and W. Katon. 1999. Commissioned Paper: Unexplained Physical Symptoms in Primary Care and the Community: What Might We Learn for Prevention in the Military? Paper prepared for the *Strategies to Protect the Health of Deployed U.S. Forces: Medical Surveillance, Medical Record Keeping, and Risk Reduction*. Institute of Medicine, Washington, D.C.

Engel, C. C. Jr., M. Roy, D. Kayanan, et al. 1998. Multidisciplinary Treatment of Persistent Symptoms After Gulf War Service. *Military Medicine* 163(4):202–8.

Escobar, J. I., J. M. Golding, R. L. Hough, et al. 1987. Somatization in the Community: Relationship to Disability and Use of Services. *American Journal of Public Health* 77(7):837–40.

Escobar, J. I., M. Rubio-Stipec, G. Canino, et al. 1989. Somatic Symptom Index (SSI): A New and Abridged Somatization Construct. Prevalence and Epidemiological Correlates in Two Large Community Samples. *Journal of Nervous and Mental Disease* 177(3):140–6.

Eskenazi, B. 1984. Behavioral Teratology. In *Perinatal Epidemiology*, ed. M. B. Brackem, 216–54. New York: Oxford University Press.

Evans, R. S., D. C. Classen, L. E. Stevens, et al. 1993. Using A Hospital Information System to Assess the Effects of Adverse Drug Events. *Proceedings of the Annual Symposium on Computer Applications in Medical Care* 161–5.

Federal Register. 1990. Informed Consent for Human Drugs and Biologics: Determination That Informed Consent Is Not Feasible. *Federal Register* 55(246):52814.

Federal Register. 1998. Informed Consent for Human Drugs and Biologics: Determination That Informed Consent Is Not Feasible. *Federal Register* 63(80):21957.

Feinstein, A. R. 1998. Nosologic Challenges of Diagnostic Criteria for a "New Illness." Presentation at *Conference on Federally Sponsored Gulf War Veterans' Illnesses Research*. 1998. Pentagon City, Va..

Figley, C. R. 1988. A Five-Phase Treatment of Post-Traumatic Stress Disorder in Families. *Journal of Traumatic Stress* 1(1):127–41.

Figley, C. R. 1993a. Weathering the Storm at Home: War-Related Family Stress and Coping. In *The Military Family in Peace and War*, ed. F. W. Kaslow and F. Whiteman, 173–90. New York: Springer Publishing.

Figley, C. R. 1993b. Coping with Stressors on the Home Front. *Journal of Social Issues* 49(4):51–71.

Figley, C. R. 1995. For Those Who Bore the Battle: Family-Centered Veterans' Services. In *The Legacy of Vietnam Veterans and Their Families—Survivors of War: Cata-*

lysts for Change, ed. D. K. Rhoades, M. R. Leaveck, and J.C. Hudson. Washington, D.C.: Agent Orange Class Assistance Program.

Fischhoff, B. 1995. Risk Perception and Communication Unplugged: Twenty Years of Process. *Risk Analysis* 15(2):137–45.

Flora, C. 1999. Associate Program Officer, Readjustment Counseling Service—VA Headquarters, Washington, D.C. Written Communication, April 15, 1999.

Flowers, R. 1998. Medical Doctrine for NBC Threats. Presentation at *Strategies to Protect the Health of Deployed U.S. Forces: Medical Surveillance, Record Keeping, and Risk Reduction*. Workshop III. October 1, 1998. Institute of Medicine, Washington, D.C.

Fonseca, V. P. 1998. Health Evalutation Assessment Review. Presentation at *Strategies to Protect the Health of Deployed U.S. Forces: Medical Surveillance, Record Keeping, and Risk Reduction*. Workshop I. April 16, 1998. Institute of Medicine, Washington, D.C.

Ford, J. D., P. Chandler, B. Thacker, et al. 1998. Family Systems Therapy After Operation Desert Storm with European-Theater Veterans. *Journal of Marital and Family Therapy* 24(2):243–50.

Ford, J., D. Shaw, S. Sennhauser, et al. 1993. Psychosocial Debriefing After Operation Desert Storm: Marital and Family Assessment and Intervention. *Journal of Social Issues* 49(4):73–102.

Fowles, J. B., E. Fowler, C. Craft, et al. 1997. Comparing Claims Data and Self-Reported Data with the Medical Record for Pap Smear Rates. *Evaluation and the Health Professions* 20(3):324–42.

Friedman, M. J., P. P. Schnurr, and A. McDonagh-Coyle. 1994. Post-Traumatic Stress Disorder in the Military Veteran. *Psychiatric Clinics of North America* 17(2):265–77.

Fukuda, K., R. Nisenbaum, G. Stewart, et al. 1998. Chronic Multisymptom Illness Affecting Air Force Veterans of the Gulf War. *JAMA* 280(11):981–88.

Fulcher, K. Y., and P. D. White. 1997. Randomised Controlled Trial of Graded Exercise in Patients with the Chronic Fatigue Syndrome. *British Medical Journal* 314(7095): 1647–52.

Futterman, S., and E. Pumpian-Mindlin. 1951. Traumatic War Neuroses Five Years Later. *American Journal of Psychiatry* 108:401.

Gambel, J. M. 1999. Department of Physical Medicine and Rehabilitation, Walter Reed Army Medical Center. Personal Communication, April 22, 1999.

Gambel, J. M., J. F. Brundage, R. J. Burge, et al. 1998. Survey of U.S. Army Soldiers' Knowledge, Attitudes, and Practices Regarding Personal Protection Measures to Prevent Arthropod-Related Diseases and Nuisance Bites. *Military Medicine* 163(10):695–701.

Gambel, J. M., J. J. Drabick, and L. Martinez-Lopez. 1999. Medical Surveillance of Multinational Peacekeepers Deployed in Support of the United Nations Mission in Haiti, June–October 1995. *International Journal of Epidemiology* 28(2):312–8.

Gambel, J. M., and R. G. Hibbs, Jr. 1996. U.S. Military Overseas Medical Research Laboratories. *Military Medicine* 161(11):638–45.

Garfield, R. M., and A. I. Neugut. 1997. The Human Consequences of War. In *War and Public Health*, ed. B. S. Levy and V. W. Sidel, 27–38. New York: Oxford University Press.

Gaydos, C. A., and J. C. Gaydos. 1995. Adenovirus Vaccines in the U.S. Military. *Military Medicine* 160(6):300–4.

GCPR Framework Project. 1999a. Project Management Plan (draft). May 6, 1999. v. 1.0. Washington, D.C. Available at http://www.ihs.gov/gcpr/gcpr/gcpr_documents_page.html (accessed September 3, 1999).

GCPR Framework Project. 1999b. GCPR Technical Press Kit: Framework Technical Highlights. August 16, 1999. v. 1.0. Washington, D.C.

GCPR Framework Project. 1999c. GCPR Technical Press Kit: Information Management and Modeling. August 16, 1999. v. 1.0. Washington, D.C.

GCPR Framework Project. 1999d. Project Management Plan (draft). Appendix B. Written Communication (electronic mail) from Jon Kempfer, TriCare Management Activity (webmaster). September 8, 1999.

Glass, A. J. 1966a. Army Psychiatry Before World War II. In *Neuropsychiatry in World War II, Zone of Interior,* Vol. 1., ed. A. J. Glass and R. Bernucci. 3–23. Washington, D.C.: Office of the Surgeon General, U.S. Army.

Glass, A. J. 1966b. Lessons Learned. In *Neuropsychiatry in World War II, Zone of Interior,* Vol. 1, ed. A. J. Glass and R. Bernucci, 735–59. Washington, D.C.: Office of the Surgeon General, U.S. Army.

Glass, A. J. 1973. Lessons Learned. In *Neuropsychiatry in World War II, Overseas Theaters,* Vol. 2, ed. A. J. Glass, 989–1027. Washington, D.C.: Office of the Surgeon General, U.S. Army.

Goldenberg, D. L. 1987. Fibromyalgia Syndrome. An Emerging but Controversial Condition. *JAMA* 257(20):2782–7.

Gomborone, J. E., D. A. Gorard, P. A. Dewsnap, et al. 1996. Prevalence of Irritable Bowel Syndrome in Chronic Fatigue. *Journal of the Royal College of Physicians of London* 30(6):512–3.

Gordon, N. P., R. A. Hiatt, and D. I. Lampert. 1993. Concordance of Self-Reported Data and Medical Record Audit for Six Cancer Screening Procedures. *Journal of the National Cancer Institute* 85(7):566–70.

Graham, J. D., and L. Rhomberg. 1996. How Risks Are Identified and Assessed. *Annals of the American Academy of Political Science* 545:15–24.

Gray, G. C., J. D. Callahan, A. W. Hawksworth, et al. 1999. Respiratory Diseases Among U.S. Military Personnel: Countering Emerging Threats. *Emerging Infectious Diseases* 5(3):379–87.

Gray, G. C., B. D. Coate, C. M. Anderson, H. K., et al. 1996. The Postwar Hospitalization Experience of U.S. Veterans of the Persian Gulf War. *New England Journal of Medicine* 335(20):1505–13.

Gray, G. C., A. W. Hawksworth, T. C. Smith, et al. 1998. Gulf War Veterans' Health Registries. Who Is Most Likely to Seek Evaluation? *American Journal of Epidemiology* 148(4):343–9.

Green, C. B. 1999. CENTCOM Perspective on Deployment Surveillance. Presentation at *Strategies to Protect the Health of Deployed U.S. Forces: Medical Surveillance, Record Keeping, and Risk Reduction.* 'Reality Check' Meeting. March 23, 1999. Institute of Medicine, Washington, D.C.

Green, D. C., J. M. Moore, M. M. Adams, et al. 1998. Are We Underestimating Rates of Vaginal Birth After Previous Cesarean Birth? The Validity of Delivery Methods from Birth Certificates. *American Journal of Epidemiology* 147(6):581–6.

Guevara, R., J. Butler, J. Plouffe, et al. 1996. The Reliability of ICD-9-CM Codes in Detecting Community-Acquired Streptococcus Pneumonia for Incidence and Vaccine Efficacy Studies. Presentation at *The 36th Interscience Conference on Antimicrobial Agents and Chemotherapy*. September 15–18, 1996. New Orleans, La.

Gureje, O., G. E. Simon, T. B. Ustun, et al. 1997. Somatization in Cross-Cultural Perspective: A World Health Organization Study in Primary Care. *American Journal of Psychiatry* 154(7):989–95.

Gureje, O., M. Von Korff, G. E. Simon, et al. 1998. Persistent Pain and Well-Being: A World Health Organization Study in Primary Care [published erratum appears in *JAMA* 280(13):1142, 1998]. *JAMA* 280(2):147–51.

Gurvits, T. V., M. E. Shenton, H. Hokama, et al. 1996. Magnetic Resonance Imaging Study of Hippocampal Volume in Chronic, Combat-Related Posttraumatic Stress Disorder. *Biological Psychiatry* 40(11):1091–9.

Gustafson, P. E. 1998. Gender Differences in Risk Perception: Theoretical and Methodological Perspectives. *Risk Analysis* 18(6):805–11.

Hadler, N. M. 1997. Fibromyalgia, Chronic Fatigue, and Other Iatrogenic Diagnostic Algorithms. Do Some Labels Escalate Illness in Vulnerable Patients? *Postgraduate Medicine* 102(2):161–2, 165–6, 171–2 passim.

Haley, R. W. 1997. Is Gulf War Syndrome Due to Stress? The Evidence Reexamined. *American Journal of Epidemiology* 146(9):695–703.

Halperin, W. 1992. Introduction. In *Public Health Surveillance*, ed. W. Halperin and E. Baker, Jr., xvii–xx. New York: Van Nostrand Reinhold.

Hamlet, M. P. 1987. An Overview of Medically Related Problems in the Cold Environment. *Military Medicine* 152(8):393–6.

Hammond, E. W. 1999. Paper Presentation: Paper on the G-CPR Project. Presentation at *Strategies to Protect the Health of Deployed U.S. Forces: Medical Surveillance, Record Keeping, and Risk Reduction.* Workshop IV. January 13, 1999. Institute of Medicine, Washington, D.C.

Harrison, L. H., and R. W. Pinner. 1998. Strategies to Protect the Health of Deployed U.S. Forces: Surveillance in the Military. *Paper prepared for Strategies to Protect the Health of Deployed U.S. Forces: Medical Surveillance, Medical Record Keeping, and Risk Reduction.* Institute of Medicine, Washington, D.C.

Haynes, R. B., D. L. Sackett, D. W. Taylor, et al. 1978. Increased Absenteeism from Work After Detection and Labeling of Hypertensive Patients. *New England Journal of Medicine* 299(14):741–4.

Hazen, S., and C. Llewellyn. 1991. Battle Fatigue Identification and Management for Military Medical Students. *Military Medicine* 156(6):263–7.

Health Insurance Portability and Accountability Act of 1996. 1996. P.L. 104-191. Available at http://thomas.loc.gov/cgi-bin/bdqu....3103:@@@L|TOM:/bss/d104query.html (accessed 4 August 1999).

Hellman, C. J., M. Budd, J. Borysenko, et al. 1990. A Study of the Effectiveness of Two Group Behavioral Medicine Interventions for Patients with Psychosomatic Complaints. *Behavioral Medicine* 16(4):165–73.

Helmkamp, J. C. 1994. United States Military Casualty Comparison During the Persian Gulf War. *Journal of Occupational Medicine* 36(6):609–15.

Higley, J. D., M. F. Hasert, S. J. Suomi, et al. 1991. Nonhuman Primate Model of Alcohol Abuse: Effects of Early Experience, Personality, and Stress on Alcohol Consumption. *Proceedings of the National Academy of Sciences of the United States of America* 88(16):7261–5.

Hill, R. 1949. *Families Under Stress.* New York: Harper and Brothers.

Hinds, M. W., J. W. Skaggs, and G. H. Bergeisen. 1985. Benefit–Cost Analysis of Active Surveillance of Primary Care Physicians for Hepatitis A. *American Journal of Public Health* 75(2):176–7.

Hobfoll, S. E., C. D. Spielberger, S. Breznitz, et al. 1991. War-Related Stress. Addressing the Stress of War and Other Traumatic Events. *American Psychologist* 46(8):848–55.

Holloway, H. 1999. Professor, Department of Psychiatry, Uniformed Services University of the Health Sciences, Bethesda, Md. Written Communication (electronic mail), January 26, 1999.

Holtzman, N. A., and M. J. Khoury. 1986. Monitoring for Congenital Malformations. *Annual Review of Public Health* 7:237–66.

Hotopf, M., R. Mayou, and S. Wessely. 1997. Childhood Risk Factors for Adult Medically Unexplained Symptoms: Results from a Prospective Cohort Study. Presentation at *44th Annual Meeting of the Academy of Psychosomatic Medicine*. November 20–23, 1997. Academy of Psychosomatic Medicine, Coronado, Calif.

Hudson, J. I., D. L. Goldenberg, H. G. Pope Jr., et al. 1992. Comorbidity of Fibromyalgia with Medical and Psychiatric Disorders. *American Journal of Medicine* 92(4):363–7.

Hunter, E. J. 1982. *Families Under the Flag*. New York: Praeger Publishers.

Hunter, E. J. 1984. Treating the Military Captive's Family. Chap. 8 in *The Military Family*, ed. F. W. Kaslow and R. I. Ridenour, 167–96. New York: Guilford Press.

Huycke, K. A., J. M. Gambel, B. P. Petruccelli, et al. 1997. Lessons Learned from Producing Health Information Booklets for Deploying U.S. Military Personnel. *Military Medicine* 162(3):209–14.

Hyams, K. C. 1998. Developing Case Definitions for Symptom-Based Conditions: The Problem of Specificity. *Epidemiologic Reviews* 20(2):148–56.

Hyams, K. C., K. Hanson, F. S. Wignall, et al. 1995. The Impact of Infectious Diseases on the Health of U.S. Troops Deployed to the Persian Gulf During Operations Desert Shield and Desert Storm. *Clinical Infectious Diseases* 20(6):1497–504.

Hyams, K. C., and F. M. Murphy. 1998. The Recruit Assessment Program. Presentation at *Strategies to Protect the Health of Deployed U.S. Forces: Medical Surveillance, Record Keeping, and Risk Reduction*. Workshop I. April 16, 1998. Institute of Medicine, Washington, D.C.

Hyams, K. C., F. S. Wignall, and R. Roswell. 1996. War Syndromes and Their Evaluation: From the U.S. Civil War to the Persian Gulf War. *Annals of Internal Medicine* 125(5):398–405.

Injury Prevention and Control Work Group. 1996. "Injuries in the Military: A Hidden Epidemic." (prepared for the Armed Forces Epidemiologic Board by the Injury Prevention and Control Work Group, with contributions from the DoD Injury Surveillance and Prevention Work Group), ed. B. H. Jones and B. C. Hansen. Falls Church, Va.: Armed Forces Epidemiologic Board.

Institute of Medicine. 1992. *Emerging Infections: Microbial Threats to Health in the United States*. Washington, D.C.: National Academy Press.

Institute of Medicine. 1996a. *Health Consequences of Service During the Persian Gulf War: Recommendations for Research and Information Systems*. Washington, D.C.: National Academy Press.

Institute of Medicine. 1996b. *Interactions of Drugs, Biologics, and Chemicals in U.S. Military Forces*. Washington, D.C.: National Academy Press.

Institute of Medicine. 1996c. *Evaluation of the Department of Defense Persian Gulf War Comprehensive Clinical Evaluation Program*. Washington, D.C.: National Academy Press.

Institute of Medicine. 1997. *The Computer-Based Patient Record: An Essential Technology for Health Care, Revised Edition.* 2nd ed. Washington, D.C.: National Academy Press.

Institute of Medicine. 1998. *Strategies to Protect the Health of Deployed U.S. Forces: Medical Surveillance, Record Keeping, and Risk Reduction,* Workshop III. October 1–2, 1998. Washington, D.C.

Institute of Medicine. 1999a. *Strategies to Protect the Health of Deployed U.S. Forces: Medical Surveillance, Record Keeping, and Risk Reduction,* Workshop IV. January 13–14, 1999. Washington, D.C.

Institute of Medicine. 1999b. *Strategies to Protect the Health of Deployed U.S. Forces: Medical Surveillance, Record Keeping, and Risk Reduction,* Workshop V ("Reality Check"). March 23–24, 1999. Washington, D.C.

Institute of Medicine. 1999c. *Chemical and Biological Terrorism: Research and Development to Improve Civilian Medical Response.* Washington, D.C.: National Academy Press.

Inzana, C. M., J. E. Driskell, E. Salas, et al. 1996. Effects of Preparatory Information on Enhancing Performance Under Stress. *Journal of Applied Psychology* 81(4):429–35.

Iowa Persian Gulf Study Group. 1997. Self-Reported Illness and Health Status Among Gulf War Veterans. A Population-Based Study. The Iowa Persian Gulf Study Group. *JAMA* 277(3):238–45.

Irish Times. 1999. "They Say Rest Is What Keeps You Ill." March 8, 1999. Available at http://www.ireland.com/scripts/search/highlight.plx?TextRes=%22They%20Say%20Rest%20is%20what%20keeps%20you%20ill%22&Path=/newspaper/features/1999/0308/fea2.htm. (accessed June 1999).

Irwin, C., S. A. Falsetti, R. B. Lydiard, et al. 1996. Comorbidity of Posttraumatic Stress Disorder and Irritable Bowel Syndrome. *Journal of Clinical Psychiatry* 57(12):576–8.

Jablonski, S. 1991. Syndrome: Le Mot de Jour. *American Journal of Medical Genetics* 39(3):342–6.

Jamison, R. N., and K. L. Virts. 1990. The Influence of Family Support on Chronic Pain. *Behavior Research and Therapy* 28(4):283–7.

Janca, A., J. D. Burke Jr., C. Isaac, et al. 1995. The World Health Organization Somatoform Disorders Schedule: A Preliminary Report on Design and Reliability. *European Psychiatry* 10:373–78.

Johnson, H., and D. Broder. 1991. Washington at War; Pentagon's Other Challenge: Major Troop Cuts. *Washington Post,* p. A22. 27 February 1991.

Johnson, J. 1998. What Does the Research on Informational Interventions to Reduce the Stress of Medical Procedures Tell Us About Communicating to Troops the Risks of Deployment? Paper prepared for *Strategies to Protect the Health of Deployed U.S. Forces: Medical Surveillance, Medical Record Keeping, and Risk Reduction.* Institute of Medicine, Washington, D.C.

Johnston, M. E., K. B. Langton, R. B. Haynes, et al. 1994. Effects of Computer-Based Clinical Decision Support Systems on Clinician Performance and Patient Outcome. A Critical Appraisal of Research. *Annals of Internal Medicine* 120(2):135–42.

Joint Chiefs of Staff. 1995. "Doctrine for Health Services Support in Joint Operations." Available at http://www.dtic.mil/doctrine/jel/new_pubs/jp4_02.pdf. (accessed 9 August 1999).

Joint Chiefs of Staff, Office of the Chairman. 1998. *Memorandum: Deployment Health Surveillance and Readiness,* MCM-251-98. Washington, D.C.

Jones, D. R. 1995. U.S. Air Force Combat Psychiatry. Chap. 8 in *Textbook of Military Medicine, Part I—War Psychiatry*, ed. F. D. Jones, L. R. Sparacino, V. L. Wilcox, J. M. Rothberg, and J. W. Stokes, 177–210. Washington, D.C.: Office of the Surgeon General, U.S. Army.

Jones, F. D. 1995a. Psychiatric Lessons of War. Chap. 1 in *Textbook of Military Medicine, Part I—War Psychiatry*, ed. F. D. Jones, L. R. Sparacino, V. L. Wilcox, J. M. Rothberg, and J. W. Stokes, 3–33. Washington, D.C.: Office of the Surgeon General, U.S. Army.

Jones, F. D. 1995b. Traditional Warfare Combat Stress Casualties. Chap. 2 in *Textbook of Military Medicine, Part I—War Psychiatry*, ed. L. R. Sparacino, V. L. Wilcox, J. M. Rothberg, J. W. Stokes, and F. D. Jones, 35–61. Washington, D.C.: Office of the Surgeon General, U.S. Army.

Jones, F. D. 1995c. Psychiatric Principles of Future Warfare. Chap. 5 in *Textbook of Military Medicine, Part I—War Psychiatry*, ed. L. R. Sparacino, V. L. Wilcox, J. M. Rothberg, J. W. Stokes, and F. D. Jones, 113–32. Washington, D.C.: Office of the Surgeon General, U.S. Army.

Joseph-Vanderpool, J. R., N. E. Rosenthal, G. P. Chrousos, et al. 1991. Abnormal Pituitary-Adrenal Responses to Corticotropin-Releasing Hormone in Patients with Seasonal Affective Disorder: Clinical and Pathophysiological Implications. *Journal of Clinical Endocrinology and Metabolism* 72(6):1382–7.

Kallen, B. 1988. *Epidemiology of Human Reproduction*. Boca Raton, FL: CRC Press.

Kaslow F. W., and Ridenour R. I. 1984. *The Military Family*. New York: Guilford Press.

Katon, W., D. Buchwald, G. Simon, et al. 1991a. Psychiatric Illness in Patients with Chronic Fatigue and Those with Rheumatoid Arthritis. *Journal of General Internal Medicine* 6(4):277–85.

Katon, W., K. Egan, and D. Miller. 1985. Chronic Pain: Lifetime Psychiatric Diagnoses and Family History. *American Journal of Psychiatry* 142(10):1156–60.

Katon, W., M. L. Hall, J. Russo, et al. 1988. Chest Pain: Relationship of Psychiatric Illness to Coronary Arteriographic Results. *American Journal of Medicine* 84(1):1–9.

Katon, W., A. Kleinman, and G. Rosen. 1982a. Depression and Somatization: A Review. Part I. *American Journal of Medicine* 72(1):127–35.

Katon, W., A. Kleinman, and G. Rosen. 1982b. Depression and Somatization: A Review. Part II. *American Journal of Medicine* 72(2):241–7.

Katon, W., E. Lin, M. Von Korff, et al. 1991a. Somatization: A Spectrum of Severity. *American Journal of Psychiatry* 148(1):34–40.

Katon, W., and J. Russo. 1992. Chronic Fatigue Syndrome Criteria. A Critique of the Requirement for Multiple Physical Complaints [see comments]. *Archives of Internal Medicine* 152(8):1604–9.

Keefe, F. J., J. Dunsmore, and R. Burnett. 1992. Behavioral and Cognitive-Behavioral Approaches to Chronic Pain: Recent Advances and Future Directions. *Journal of Consulting and Clinical Psychology* 60(4):528–36.

Kelley, P. W. 1999a. Role of Laboratories in Military Public Health Surveillance. Presentation at *Strategies to Protect the Health of Deployed U.S. Forces: Medical Surveillance, Record Keeping, and Risk Reduction*. Workshop IV. January 14, 1999. Institute of Medicine, Washington, D.C.

Kelley, P. W. 1999b. Director, Division of Preventive Medicine. Walter Reed Army Institute of Research. Written Communication (electronic mail), April 22, 1999.

Kellner, R. 1986. *Somatization and Hypochondriasis*. New York: Praeger.

Kellner, R. 1991. *Psychosomatic Syndromes and Somatic Symptoms*. Washington, D.C.: American Psychiatric Press.

Kellner, R., G. A. Fava, J. Lisansky, et al. 1986. Hypochondriacal Fears and Beliefs in DSM-III Melancholia. Changes with Amitriptyline. *Journal of Affective Disorders* 10(1):21–6.

Khoury, M. J., E. E. Calle, and R. M. Joesoef. 1989. Recurrence of Low Birth Weight in Siblings. *Journal of Clinical Epidemiology* 42(12):1171–8.

Kisely, S., D. Goldberg, and G. Simon. 1997. A Comparison Between Somatic Symptoms with and without Clear Organic Cause: Results of an International Study. *Psychological Medicine* 27(5):1011–9.

Kline, J., S. Stein, and M. Susser. 1989. Conception and Reproductive Loss: Probabilities. In *Conception to Birth: Epidemiology of Prenatal Development*, 43–68. New York: Oxford University Press.

Kohner, D. 1999a. The Reserve Components. Presentation at *Strategies to Protect the Health of Deployed U.S. Forces: Medical Surveillance, Record Keeping, and Risk Reduction*. Workshop IV. January 13, 1999. Institute of Medicine, Washington, D.C.

Kohner, D. 1999b. Office of the Assistant Secretary of Defense for Reserves Affairs. Written Communication (electronic mail). May 26, 1999.

Kohner, D. 1999c. Office of the Assistant Secretary of Defense for Reserves Affairs. Written Communication (electronic mail). July 30, 1999.

Koshes, R. J., S. A. Young, and J. W. Stokes. 1995. Debriefing Following Combat. Chap. 11 in *Textbook of Military Medicine, Part I—War Psychiatry*, ed. F.D. Jones, L.R. Sparacino, V.L. Wilcox, J.M. Rothberg, and J.W. Stokes, 271–90. Washington, D.C.: Office of the Surgeon General, U.S. Army.

Kouyanou, K., C. E. Pither, and S. Wessely. 1997. Iatrogenic Factors and Chronic Pain. *Psychosomatic Medicine* 59(6):597–604.

Kriegsman, D. M., B. W. Penninx, J. T. van Eijk, et al. 1996. Self-Reports and General Practitioner Information on the Presence of Chronic Diseases in Community Dwelling Elderly. A Study on the Accuracy of Patients' Self-Reports and on Determinants of Inaccuracy. *Journal of Clinical Epidemiology* 49(12):1407–17.

Kroenke, K. 1998a. Building-Related Illnesses. *New England Journal of Medicine* 338(15):1070–1.

Kroenke, K., M. E. Arrington, and A. D. Mangelsdorff. 1990. The Prevalence of Symptoms in Medical Outpatients and the Adequacy of Therapy. *Archives of Internal Medicine* 150(8):1685–9.

Kroenke, K., and A. D. Mangelsdorff. 1989. Common Symptoms in Ambulatory Care: Incidence, Evaluation, Therapy, and Outcome. *American Journal of Medicine* 86(3): 262–6.

Kroenke, K., R. L. Spitzer, F. V. deGruy 3rd, et al. 1998b. A Symptom Checklist to Screen for Somatoform Disorders in Primary Care. *Psychosomatics* 39(3):263–72.

Kroenke, K., R. L. Spitzer, J. B. Williams, et al. 1994. Physical Symptoms in Primary Care. Predictors of Psychiatric Disorders and Functional Impairment. *Archives of Family Medicine* 3(9):774–9.

Kulka, R. A., W. E. Schlenger, J. A. Fairbank, et al. 1990. *Trauma and the Vietnam War Generation: Report of Findings from the National Vietnam Veterans Readjustment Study*. New York: Brunner/Mazel, Inc.

Lancaster, J. 26 March 1992. Military Manpower Cuts Faulted: Key Lawmakers Worry About Effect on Morale, Unemployment Rolls. *Washington Post*, p. A23.

Landay, J. S. 2 June 1997. Reservists Buck Military Plan to Downsize Their Ranks. *Christian Science Monitor*, p. 3.

Lazarou, J., B. H. Pomeranz, and P. N. Corey. 1998. Incidence of Adverse Drug Reactions in Hospitalized Patients: A Meta-Analysis of Prospective Studies. *JAMA* 279(15):1200–5.

Leape, L. L., D. W. Bates, D. J. Cullen, et al. 1995. Systems Analysis of Adverse Drug Events. ADE Prevention Study Group. *JAMA* 274(1):35–43.

Leavitt, P. 14 February 1996. Casualties of Peace: Pentagon to Cut 16,000. *USA Today*, p. 3A.

Lee, F., J. M. Teich, C. D. Spurr, et al. 1996. Implementation of Physician Order Entry: User Satisfaction and Self-Reported Usage Patterns. *Journal of the American Medical Informatics Association* 3(1):42–55.

Leino, P., and G. Magni. 1993. Depressive and Distress Symptoms as Predictors of Low Back Pain, Neck-Shoulder Pain, and Other Musculoskeletal Morbidity: A 10-Year Follow-Up of Metal Industry Employees. *Pain* 53(1):89–94.

Lelliott, P. T., and P. Fenwick. 1991. Cerebral Pathology in Pseudoseizures. *Acta Neurologica Scandinavica* 83(2):129–32.

Leon, D. A., H. O. Lithell, D. Vagero, et al. 1998. Reduced Fetal Growth Rate and Increased Risk of Death from Ischaemic Heart Disease: Cohort Study of 15,000 Swedish Men and Women Born 1915–29. *British Medical Journal* 317(7153):241–5.

Lie, R. T., A. J. Wilcox, and R. Skjaerven. 1994. A Population-Based Study of the Risk of Recurrence of Birth Defects. *New England Journal of Medicine* 331(1):1–4.

Life Systems Inc. and GeoCenters Inc. for U.S. Army Center for Environmental Health Research. 1997. "Deployment Toxicology Research and Development Master Plan." U.S. Army Medical Research and Materiel Command, Fort Detrick, Md.

Linton, S. J. 1997. A Population-Based Study of the Relationship Between Sexual Abuse and Back Pain: Establishing a Link. *Pain* 73(1):47–53.

Litz, B. T., A. K. Moscowitz, M. J. Friedman, et al. 1995. "The Prevalence of PTSD in a National Sample of Persian Gulf Veterans: Comparison of Treatment-Seeking and Non-Treatment Samples." Unpublished manuscript Boston Department of Veteran's Affairs Medical Center.

Litz, B. T., S. M. Orsillo, M. Friedman, et al. 1997. Posttraumatic Stress Disorder Associated with Peacekeeping Duty in Somalia for U.S. Military Personnel [published erratum appears in *American Journal of Psychiatry* 154(5):722, 1997]. *American Journal of Psychiatry* 154(2):178–84.

Loeser, J. D., and Egan, K. J., ed. 1989. *Managing the Chronic Pain Patient: Theory and Practice at the University of Washington Multidisciplinary Pain Center*. New York: Raven Press.

Manning, F. J. 1994. Morale and Cohesion in Military Psychiatry. Chap. 1 in *Textbook of Military Medicine, Part I—Military Psychiatry: Preparing in Peace for War*, ed. F. D. Jones, L. R. Sparacino, V. L. Wilcox, and J. M. Rothberg, 1–18. Washington, D.C.: Office of the Surgeon General, U.S. Army.

Mareth, T. R., and A. E. Brooker. 1985. Combat Stress Reaction: A Concept in Evolution. *Military Medicine* 150(4):186–90.

Marshall, G.N., L.M. Davis, C.D. Sherbourne, et al. 1999. *A Review of the Scientific Literature as It Pertains to Gulf War Illnesses.* Vol. 4, *Stress*. Santa Monica, Calif.: RAND.

Martin, J. A., and W. R. Cline. 1996. Mental Health Lessons form the Persian Gulf War. In *The Gulf War and Mental Health: A Comprehensive Guide*, ed. J. A. Martin, L. R. Sparacino, and G. Belenky, 161–178. Westport, Conn.: Praeger.

Martin, P. R., P. R. Nathan, D. Milech, et al. 1989. Cognitive Therapy vs. Self-Management Training in the Treatment of Chronic Headaches. *British Journal of Clinical Psychology* 28 (Pt. 4):347–61.

Mason, D. 1991. Genetic Variation in the Stress Response: Susceptibility to Experimental Allergic Encephalomyelitis and Implications for Human Inflammatory Disease. *Immunology Today* 12(2):57–60.

Mateczun, J. M. 1995. U.S. Naval Combat Psychiatry. Chap. 9 in *Textbook of Military Medicine. Part I—War Psychiatry*, ed. F. D. Jones, L. R. Sparacino, V. L. Wilcox, J. M. Rothberg, and J. W. Stokes, 211–42. Washington, D.C.: Office of the Surgeon General, U.S. Army.

Mateczun, J. M., and E. K. Holmes. 1996. Return, Readjustment, and Reintegration: The Three R's of Family Reunion. In *Emotional Aftermath of the Persian Gulf War: Veterans, Families, Communities, and Nations*, ed. R. J. Ursano and A. E. Norwood, 369–92. Washington, D.C.: American Psychiatric Press.

Mayou, R. A., B. M. Bryant, D. Sanders, et al. 1997. A Controlled Trial of Cognitive Behavioural Therapy for Non-Cardiac Chest Pain. *Psychological Medicine* 27(5): 1021–31.

McCallum, D. B., S. L. Hammond, and V. T. Covello. 1991. Communicating About Environmental Risks: How the Public Uses and Perceives Information Sources. *Health Education Quarterly* 18(3):349–61.

McCormick, D. H. 26 March 1996. A Downsized, Down and Out Army. *Christian Science Monitor*, p. 19.

McCubbin, H. I., B. B. Dahl, and E. J. Hunter. 1976. *Families in the Military System*. Beverly Hills, Calif.: Sage.

McCubbin, H. I., B. B. Dahl, G. R. Lester, et al. 1975. The Returned Prisoner of War: Factors in Family Reintegration. *Journal of Marriage and the Family* 37(3): 471–78.

McCubbin, H. I., B. B. Dahl, P. Metres, et al. 1974. *Family Separation and Reunion: Families of Prisoners of War and Servicemen Missing in Action*, Cat. No. D-206:21; 74–70. Government Printing Office, Washington, D.C.

McDonald, C. J. 1976. Protocol-Based Computer Reminders, the Quality of Care and the Non-Perfectability of Man. *New England Journal of Medicine* 295(24):1351–5.

McDonald, C. J. 1999. Review of the GCPR Project. Presentation at *Strategies to Protect the Health of Deployed U.S. Forces: Medical Surveillance, Record Keeping, and Risk Reduction*. Workshop IV. January 13–14, 1999. Institute of Medicine, Washington, D.C.

McDonald, C. J., S. L. Hui, D. M. Smith, et al. 1984. Reminders to Physicians from an Introspective Computer Medical Record. A Two-Year Randomized Trial. *Annals of Internal Medicine* 100(1):130–8.

McDonald, C. J., S. Hui, and W. M. Tierney. 1992. Effects of Computer Reminders for Influenza Vaccination on Morbidity During Influenza Epidemics. *MD Computing* 9(5):304–12.

McDonald, C. J., J. M. Overhage, P. Dexter, et al. 1997. A Framework for Capturing Clinical Data Sets from Computerized Sources. *Annals of Internal Medicine* 127(8 Pt. 2):675–82.

McKee, K. T. Jr. 1999. U.S. Army Medical Research Institute of Infectious Diseases. Washington, D.C. Written Communication (electronic mail), June 28, 1999.

McKee, K. T. Jr., M. G. Kortepeter, and S. K. Ljaamo. 1998. Disease and Nonbattle Injury Among United States Soldiers Deployed in Bosnia-Herzegovina During 1997: Summary Primary Care Statistics for Operation Joint Guard. *Military Medicine* 163(11):733–42.

Meador, C. K. 1965. The Art and Science of Non-Disease. *New England Journal of Medicine* 272:92.

Meaney, M. J., D. H. Aitken, C. van Berkel, et al. 1988. Effect of Neonatal Handling on Age-Related Impairments Associated with the Hippocampus. *Science* 239(4841 Pt. 1):766–8.

Meaney, M. J., B. Tannenbaum, D. Francis, et al. 1994. Early Environmental Programming: Hypothalmic-Pituitary-Adrenal Responses to Stress. *Seminars in Neuroscience* 6:247–59.

Meirow, D., and J. G. Schenker. 1996. The Link Between Female Infertility and Cancer: Epidemiology and Possible Aetiologies. *Human Reproduction Update* 2(1):63–75.

Menzies, D. 1998. Building-Related Illnesses (editorial). *New England Journal of Medicine* 338(15):1071.

Menzies, D., and J. Bourbeau. 1997. Building-Related Illnesses. *New England Journal of Medicine* 337(21):1524–31.

Meyer, J. 1999. Office of the Assistant Secretary of Defense for Health Affairs. Washington, D.C. Written Communication (electronic mail), January 27, 1999.

Mitchell, J. T. 1983. When Disaster Strikes . . . the Critical Incident Stress Debriefing Process. *Journal of Emergency Medical Services (JEMS)* 8(1):36–9.

Moller, H., and N. E. Skakkebaek. 1999. Risk of Testicular Cancer in Subfertile Men: Case-Control Study. *British Medical Journal* 318(7183):559–62.

Murphy, D. L. 1999. Evaluation Specialist, Office of Educational Resources, Educational Research and Development, University of Texas Health Science Center at San Antonio. Written Communication, April 29, 1999.

Murphy, F. M., H. K. Kang, N. A. Dalager, et al. 1999. The Health Status of Gulf War Veterans: Lessons Learned from the Department of Veterans Affairs Health Registry. *Military Medicine* 164(5):327–31.

National Institutes of Health Technology Assessment Workshop Panel. 1994. The Persian Gulf Experience and Health. NIH Technology Assessment Workshop Panel. *JAMA* 272(5):391–6.

National Research Council. 1989. *Improving Risk Communication.* Washington, D.C.: National Academy Press.

National Research Council. 1997. *For the Record: Protecting Electronic Health Information.* Washington, D.C.: National Academy Press.

National Research Council. 1999a. *Strategies to Protect the Health of Deployed U.S. Forces: Analytical Framework for Assessing Risk.* Washington, D.C.: National Academy Press.

National Research Council. 1999b. *Strategies to Protect the Health of Deployed U.S. Forces: Detecting, Characterizing, and Documenting Exposures.* Washington, D.C.: National Academy Press.

National Research Council. 1999c. *Strategies to Protect the Health of Deployed U.S. Forces: Force Protection and Decontamination.* Washington, D.C.: National Academy Press.

National Science and Technology Council. 1998. "A National Obligation: Planning for Health Preparedness for and Readjustment of the Military, Veterans, and Their Families After Future Deployments." Washington, D.C.: Executive Office of the President.

Neeck, G., K. Federlin, V. Graef, et al. 1990. Adrenal Secretion of Cortisol in Patients with Rheumatoid Arthritis. *Journal of Rheumatology* 17(1):24–9.

Newhouse, J. P. and the Insurance Experiment Group. 1993. Free For All?: Lessons from the RAND Health Insurance Experiment. Cambridge, Mass.: Harvard University Press.

Nice, D. S., B. McDonald, and T. McMillian. 1981. The Families of U.S. Navy Prisoners of War from Vietnam Five Years After Reunion. *Journal of Marriage and the Family* 43(2):431–37.

Noy, S. 1987. Battle Intensity and the Length of Stay on the Battlefield as Determinants of the Type of Evacuation. *Military Medicine* 152(12):601–7.

Noyes, R., J. Reich, J. Clancy, et al. 1986. Reduction in Hypochondriasis with Treatment of Panic Disorder [published erratum appears in *British Journal of Psychiatry* 1987 150(Feb.):273]. *British Journal of Psychiatry* 149:631–5.

Office of the Special Assistant to the Deputy Secretary of Defense for Gulf War Illnesses. 1999. "Information Paper: Military Medical Recordkeeping During and After the Gulf War." Available at http://www.gulflink.osd.mil/mrk (accessed August 13, 1999).

Ogilvy-Lee, D. 1999. Chief, National Guard Bureau of Family Programs, Alexandria, Va. Written Communication (electronic mail), January 29, 1999.

Ognibene, A. J. 1982. Full-Scale Operations. Chapter 3. In *Internal Medicine in Vietnam* Vol. II*: General Medicine and Infectious Diseases*, ed. A. J. Ognibene and B. O'Neill, Jr., 63–65. Washington, D.C.: Office of the Surgeon General and Center of Military History.

Orr, S. P., R. K. Pitman, N. B. Lasko, et al. 1993. Psychophysiological Assessment of Posttraumatic Stress Disorder Imagery in World War II and Korean Combat Veterans. *Journal of Abnormal Psychology* 102(1):152–9.

Ostroski, M. 1999. Accession Medical Standards. Presentation at *Strategies to Protect the Health of Deployed U.S. Forces: Medical Surveillance, Record Keeping, and Risk Reduction*. Workshop IV. January 14, 1999. Institute of Medicine, Washington, D.C.

Page, D. 1999. Clinical Business Area. Presentation at *Strategies to Protect the Health of Deployed U.S. Forces: Medical Surveillance, Record Keeping, and Risk Reduction.* Workshop IV. January 13–14, 1999. Institute of Medicine, Washington, D.C.

Palmer, J. R., L. Rosenberg, and S. Shapiro. 1992. Reproductive Factors and Risk of Myocardial Infarction. *American Journal of Epidemiology* 136:404–16.

Parker, J. 1999. Policy Development for Vaccine Use. Presentation at *Strategies to Protect the Health of Deployed U.S. Forces: Medical Surveillance, Record Keeping, and Risk Reduction*. Workshop III. October 1, 1998. Institute of Medicine, Washington, D.C.

Parrish, K. 1993. Variations in the Accuracy of Obstetric Procedures and Diagnoses on Birth Records in Washington State, 1989. *American Journal of Epidemiology* 137(7):119–27.

Payne, A., and E. B. Blanchard. 1995. A Controlled Comparison of Cognitive Therapy and Self-Help Support Groups in the Treatment of Irritable Bowel Syndrome. *Journal of Consulting and Clinical Psychology* 63(5):779–86.

Peck, J. R., T. W. Smith, J. R. Ward, et al. 1989. Disability and Depression in Rheumatoid Arthritis. A Multi-Trait, Multi-Method Investigation. *Arthritis and Rheumatism* 32(9):1100–6.

Peebles-Kleiger, M. J., and J. H. Kleiger. 1994. Re-integration Stress for Desert Storm Families: Wartime Deployments and Family Trauma. *Journal of Traumatic Stress* 7(2):173–94.

Perry, N., M. Dove, and G. Marchi. 1999. Defense Manpower Data Center. Written Communication (electronic mail), May 27, 1999.

Persian Gulf Veterans Coordinating Board. 1999. "Comprehensive Risk Communication Plan for Gulf War Veterans." Clinical Working Group.

Piccinelli, M., and G. Simon. 1997. Gender and Cross-Cultural Differences in Somatic Symptoms Associated with Emotional Distress. An International Study in Primary Care. *Psychological Medicine* 27(2):433–44.

Pierce, P. F. 1997. Physical and Emotional Health of Gulf War Veteran Women. *Aviation Space and Environmental Medicine* 68(4):317–21.

Piper, J. M., E. F. Mitchel Jr., M. Snowden, et al. 1993. Validation of 1989 Tennessee Birth Certificates Using Maternal and Newborn Hospital Records. *American Journal of Epidemiology* 137(7):758–68.

Plesh, O., F. Wolfe, and N. Lane. 1996. The Relationship Between Fibromyalgia and Temporomandibular Disorders: Prevalence and Symptom Severity. *Journal of Rheumatology* 23(11):1948–52.

Presidential Advisory Committee on Gulf War Veterans' Illnesses. 1996a. "Interim Report." Washington, D.C.: U.S. Government Printing Office.

Presidential Advisory Committee on Gulf War Veterans' Illnesses. 1996b. "Final Report." Washington, D.C.: U.S. Government Printing Office.

Public Health Service. 1991. *Healthy People 2000: National Health Promotion and Disease Prevention Objectives—Full Report, with Commentary*, (DHHS Publication No. PHS 91-50212). U.S. Department of Health and Human Services, Washington, D.C.

Raine, T., S. Powell, and M. A. Krohn. 1994. The Risk of Repeating Low Birth Weight and the Role of Prenatal Care. *Obstetrics and Gynecology* 84(4):485–9.

Randolph, R. 1998. How Well Is Surveillance and Recordkeeping Taking Place with the Administration of the Anthrax Vaccine? Presentation at *Strategies to Protect the Health of Deployed U.S. Forces: Medical Surveillance, Record Keeping, and Risk Reduction*. Workshop III. October 2, 1998. Institute of Medicine, Washington, D.C.

Rathbone-McCuan, L. 1999. Professor of Social Work and Psychology and Director of Graduate Social Work Program, University of Missouri at Kansas City. Written Communication, April 29, 1999.

Ray, B. 1998. Program Manager for Deployment Programs and the Navy Ombudsman Program, Department of Navy. Navy Personnel Command. Millington, TN. Written Communication, July 28, 1998.

Ray, L. 1998. Medical Record Keeping: CHCS and CHCS II. Presentation at *Strategies to Protect the Health of Deployed U.S. Forces: Medical Surveillance, Record Keeping, and Risk Reduction*. Workshop I. April 16, 1998. Institute of Medicine, Washington, D.C.

Resnick, H. S., R. Yehuda, R. K. Pitman, et al. 1995. Effect of Previous Trauma on Acute Plasma Cortisol Level Following Rape. *American Journal of Psychiatry* 152(11): 1675–7.

Rettig, R. A. 1999. *Military Use of Drugs Not Yet Approved by the FDA for CW/BW Defense: Lessons from the Gulf War*. Santa Monica, Calif.: RAND.

Richard, K. 1988. The Occurrence of Maladaptive Health-Related Behaviors and Teacher-Related Conduct Problems in Children of Chronic Low Back Pain Patients. *Journal of Behavioral Medicine* 11:107–16.

Rock, N. L., Stokes J. W., R. J. Koshes, et al. 1995. U.S. Army Combat Stress Psychiatry. Chap. 7 in *Textbook of Military Medicine. Part I—War Psychiatry*, ed. F. D. Jones, L. R. Sparacino, V. L. Wilcox, J. M. Rothberg, and J. W. Stokes, 149–75. Washington, D.C.: Office of the Surgeon General, U.S. Army.

Rodell, D. 1999. Department of Social Work (DSW). Veterans Affairs Medical Center. Little Rock, Ark. Written Communication, May 4, 1999.

Russo, J., W. Katon, E. Lin, et al. 1997. Neuroticism and Extraversion as Predictors of Health Outcomes in Depressed Primary Care Patients. *Psychosomatics* 38(4):339–48.

Russo, J., W. Katon, M. Sullivan, et al. 1994. Severity of Somatization and Its Relationship to Psychiatric Disorders and Personality. *Psychosomatics* 35(6):546–56.

Salkovskis, P. M. 1989. Somatic Problems. In *Cognitive-Behavioral Approaches to Adult Psychiatric Disorders: A Practical Guide*, ed. K. Hawton, P. M. Salkovskis, J. W. Kirk, D. Clark, 235–76. Oxford: Oxford University Press.

Salmon, T. W. 1929. The Care and Treatment of Mental Diseases and War Neurosis ("Shell Shock") in the British Army. In *The Medical Department of the United States Army in the World War* (Vol. 10, *Neuropsychiatry)*, ed. P. Bailey, F. E. Williams, P. A. Komora, T. W. Salmon, and N. Fenton, 497–523. Washington, D.C.: Office of the Surgeon General, U.S. Army.

Schappert, S. M. 1992. National Ambulatory Medical Care Survey: 1989 Summary. *Vital Health Statistics* (110):1–80.

Schoendorf, K. C., J. D. Parker, L. Z. Batkhan, et al. 1993. Comparability of the Birth Certificate and 1988 Maternal and Infant Health Survey. *Vital Health Statistics* (116):1–19.

Schweitzer, R., B. Kelly, A. Foran, et al. 1995. Quality of Life in Chronic Fatigue Syndrome. *Social Science and Medicine* 41(10):1367–72.

Scurfield, R. M., and S. N. Tice. 1992. Interventions with Medical and Psychiatric Evacuees and Their Families: From Vietnam Through the Gulf War. *Military Medicine* 157(2):88–97.

Sharma, P., and S. K. Chaturvedi. 1995. Conversion Disorder Revisited. *Acta Psychiatrica Scandinavica* 92(4):301–4.

Sharpe, M. 1995. Cognitive Behavioural Therapies in the Treatment of Functional Somatic Symptoms. In *Treatment of Functional Somatic Symptoms*, ed. R. Mayou, C. Bass, and M. Sharpe, 122–43. Oxford: Oxford University Press.

Sharpe, M., K. Hawton, S. Simkin, et al. 1996. Cognitive Behaviour Therapy for the Chronic Fatigue Syndrome: A Randomized Controlled Trial. *British Medical Journal* 312(7022):22–6.

Sharpe, M., R. Peveler, and R. Mayou. 1992. The Psychological Treatment of Patients with Functional Somatic Symptoms: A Practical Guide. *Journal of Psychosomatic Research* 36(6):515–29.

Shea, S., W. DuMouchel, and L. Bahamonde. 1996. A Meta-Analysis of 16 Randomized Controlled Trials to Evaluate Computer-Based Clinical Reminder Systems for Preventive Care in the Ambulatory Setting. *Journal of the American Medical Informatics Association* 3(6):399–409.

Shiffman, RN, Liaw Y, Brandt CA, Corb, GJ. 1999. Computer-Based Guideline Implementation Systems: A Systematic Review of Functionality and Effectiveness. *Journal of the American Medical Informatics Association* 6(2):104–14.

Silver, F. W. 1996. Management of Conversion Disorder. *American Journal of Physical Medicine and Rehabilitation* 75(2):134–40.

Simon, G. E., W. Katon, and P. J. Sparks. 1990. Allergic to Life: Psychological Factors in Environmental Illness. *American Journal of Psychiatry* 147(7):901–6.

Simon, G. E., and M. VonKorff. 1991. Somatization and Psychiatric Disorder in the NIMH Epidemiologic Catchment Area Study. *American Journal of Psychiatry* 148(11):1494–500.

Skinner, J. B., A. Erskine, S. Pearce, et al. 1990. The Evaluation of a Cognitive Behavioural Treatment Programme in Outpatients with Chronic Pain. *Journal of Psychosomatic Research* 34(1):13–9.

Slovic, P. 1987. Perception of Risk. *Science* 236(4799):280–5.

Small, G. W., D. T. Feinberg, D. Steinberg, et al. 1994. A Sudden Outbreak of Illness Suggestive of Mass Hysteria in Schoolchildren. *Archives of Family Medicine* 3(8): 711–6.

Smith, G. R. Jr., R. A. Monson, and D. C. Ray. 1986a. Patients with Multiple Unexplained Symptoms. Their Characteristics, Functional Health, and Health Care Utilization. *Archives of Internal Medicine* 146(1):69–72.

Smith, G. R. Jr., R. A. Monson, and D. C. Ray. 1986b. Psychiatric Consultation in Somatization Disorder. A Randomized Controlled Study. *New England Journal of Medicine* 314(22):1407–13.

Snell, L. M., B. B. Little, K. A. Knoll, et al. 1992. Reliability of Birth Certificate Reporting of Congenital Anomalies. *American Journal of Perinatology* 9(3):219–22.

Speckens, A. E., A. M. van Hemert, P. Spinhoven, et al. 1995. Cognitive Behavioural Therapy for Medically Unexplained Physical Symptoms: A Randomised Controlled Trial. *British Medical Journal* 311(7016):1328–32.

Spiro, A., 3rd, P. P. Schnurr, and C. M. Aldwin. 1994. Combat-Related Posttraumatic Stress Disorder Symptoms in Older Men. *Psychology and Aging* 9(1):17–26.

Spitzer, R. L., J. B. Williams, K. Kroenke, et al. 1994. Utility of a New Procedure for Diagnosing Mental Disorders in Primary Care. The PRIME-MD 1000 Study. *JAMA* 272(22):1749–56.

St. Claire, N. 1998. Improving the Denominators for Medical Surveillance. Presentation at *Strategies to Protect the Health of Deployed U.S. Forces: Medical Surveillance, Record Keeping, and Risk Reduction*. Workshop III. October 2, 1998. Institute of Medicine, Washington, D.C.

Standaert, S. M., L. B. Lefkowitz, Jr., J. M. Horan, et al. 1995. The Reporting of Communicable Diseases: A Controlled Study of *Neisseria meningitidis* and *Haemophilus influenzae* Infections. *Clinical Infectious Diseases* 20(1):30–6.

Sternberg, E. M. 1998a. Host Neuroendocrine Factors in Susceptibility and Resistance to Inflammatory and Infectious Diseases: Implications for Unexplained Symptoms. Presentation at *Strategies to Protect the Health of Deployed U.S. Forces: Medical Surveillance, Record Keeping, and Risk Reduction*. Workshop II. July 15, 1998. Institute of Medicine, Washington, D.C.

Sternberg, E. M. 1998b. Neuroendocrine Responses and Susceptibility and Resistance to Inflammatory and Infectious Diseases: Implications for Unexplained Symptoms. Paper prepared for *Strategies to Protect the Health of Deployed U.S. Forces: Medical Surveillance, Medical Record Keeping, Risk Reduction*. Institute of Medicine, Washington, D.C.

Sternberg, E. M., J. M. Hill, G. P. Chrousos, et al. 1989a. Inflammatory Mediator-Induced Hypothalamic-Pituitary-Adrenal Axis Activation Is Defective in Streptococcal Cell Wall Arthritis-Susceptible Lewis Rats. *Proceedings of the National Academy of Sciences of the United States of America* 86(7):2374–8.

Sternberg, E. M., W. S. Young, 3d, R. Bernardini, et al. 1989b. A Central Nervous System Defect in Biosynthesis of Corticotropin-Releasing Hormone Is Associated with Susceptibility to Streptococcal Cell Wall-Induced Arthritis in Lewis Rats. *Proceedings of the National Academy of Sciences of the United States of America* 86(12): 4771–5.

Stokes, J. W. 1998. Combat Stress Control. Presentation at *Strategies to Protect the Health of Deployed U.S. Forces: Medical Surveillance, Record Keeping, and Risk Reduction*. Workshop II. July 15, 1998. Institute of Medicine, Washington, D.C.

Stokoe, C. 1999. Director, Naval Family Service Center, Norfolk, Va., Written Communication, January 6, 1999.

Stretch, R. H., D. H. Marlowe, K. M. Wright, et al. 1996. Post-Traumatic Stress Disorder Symptoms Among Gulf War Veterans. *Military Medicine* 161(7):407–10.

Struewing, J. P., and G. C. Gray. 1990. An Epidemic of Respiratory Complaints Exacerbated by Mass Psychogenic Illness in a Military Recruit Population. *American Journal of Epidemiology* 132(6):1120–9.

Stuart, J. A., and R. R. Halverson. 1997. The Psychological Status of U.S. Army Soldiers During Recent Military Operations. *Military Medicine* 162(11):737–43.

Sullivan, M. D., W. Katon, R. Dobie, et al. 1988. Disabling Tinnitus. Association with Affective Disorder. *General Hospital Psychiatry* 10(4):285–91.

Sullivan, M. D., and J. D. Loeser. 1992. The Diagnosis of Disability. Treating and Rating Disability in a Pain Clinic. *Archives of Internal Medicine* 152(9):1829–35.

Suls, J., and C. K. Wan. 1989. Effects of Sensory and Procedural Information on Coping with Stressful Medical Procedures and Pain: A Meta-Analysis. *Journal of Consulting and Clinical Psychology* 57(3):372–9.

Sutker, P. B., M. Uddo, K. Brailey, et al. 1993. War-Zone Trauma and Stress-Related Symptoms in Operation Desert Shield/Storm (ODS) Returnees. *Journal of Social Issues* 49(4):33–50.

Swartz, M., D. Hughes, L. George, et al. 1986. Developing a Screening Index for Community Studies of Somatization Disorder. *Journal of Psychiatric Research* 20(4): 335–43.

Swartz, M., R. Landerman, L. K. George, et al. 1991. Psychiatric Disorders in America: The Epidemiologic Catchment Area Study. *Somatization Disorder*, ed. L. N. Robins and D. A. Regier. New York: Free Press.

Tang, P. C., M. P. LaRosa, C. Newcomb, et al. 1999. Measuring the Effects of Reminders for Outpatient Influenza Immunizations at the Point of Clinical Opportunity. *Journal of the American Medical Informatics Association* 6(2):115–21.

Thacker, S. B., S. Redmond, R. B. Rothenberg, et al. 1986. A Controlled Trial of Disease Surveillance Strategies. *American Journal of Preventive Medicine* 2(6):345–50.

Thompson, D. F. 1999. Chief, Force Health Protection and Surveillance Branch, Brooks Air Force Base, Texas. Written Communication (electronic mail), June 10, 1999.

Tibbets, P. 1999a. Office of the Assistant Secretary of Defense for Health Affairs. Written Communication (electronic mail), August 17, 1999.

Tibbets, P. 1999b. Office of the Assistant Secretary of Defense for Health Affairs. Written Communication (electronic mail), August 19, 1999.

Tinney, G. 1998. Navy's Return and Reunion Programs. Presentation at *Strategies to Protect the Health of Deployed U.S. Forces: Medical Surveillance, Record Keeping, and Risk Reduction*. Workshop II. July 14, 1998. Institute of Medicine, Washington, D.C.

U.S. Army Center for Health Promotion and Preventive Medicine. 27 April 1998. Letter to Mazzuchi, J. F. Health Assessment of Military Personnel Deployed to Operation Joint Endeavor.

U.S. Army Combined Arms Command. 1991. "The Yellow Ribbon: Army Lessons From the Home Front." U.S. Army Combined Arms Command. Report No. 91-2, Fort Leavenworth, Kan.

U.S. Army Medical Department. 1997. "Data Collection Effort (DCE) of the Theater Medical Information Program (TMIP)." Available at http://139.161.168.16/lessons/reports/ameddbrd/tmip-dce/tmip-dce.htm. (accessed 17 May 1999).

U.S. Army Medical Surveillance Activity. 1999. "DMSS Online Data." Available at http://amsa.army.mil/amsa/amsa_home.htm. (accessed 8 June 1999).

U.S. Army Research Institute of Environmental Medicine and Walter Reed Army Institute of Research. 1994. "Sustaining Soldier Health and Performance in Southwest Asia: Guidance for Small Unit Leaders." 95-1. Natick, Mass./Fort Detrick, Md.

U.S. Department of Defense. 1986. Immunization Requirements. DoD Instruction Number 6205.2. Washington, D.C.: U.S. Department of Defense. 9 October 1986.

U.S. Department of Defense. 1991. "DoD Report on the Title III of the Persian Gulf Conflict and Supplemental Authorization and Personnel Benefits Act of 1991 (Public Law 102-25, Title III, Part B, Section 315)." Office of Family Policy, Support, and Services. Washington, D.C.

U.S. Department of Defense. 1993. Immunization Program for Biological Warfare Defense. DoD Directive Number 6205.3. Washington, D.C.: U.S. Department of Defense. 26 November 1993.

U.S. Department of Defense. 1994a. Physical Standards for Appointment, Enlistment, and Induction. DoD Directive Number 6130.3. Washington, D.C.: U.S. Department of Defense. 2 May 1994.

U.S. Department of Defense. 1994b. "Report of the Defense Science Board Task Force on Persian Gulf War Health Effects." Defense Science Board, Office of the Under Secretary of Defense for Acquisition and Technology, Washington, D.C.

U.S. Department of Defense. 1995. Treatment of Chemical Agent Casualties and Conventional Military Chemical Injuries, FM-8-285. U.S. Department of Defense: Washington, D.C. (Available at http://www.dtic.mil/doctrine/jel/new_pubs/jp4_02. pdf)

U.S. Department of Defense. 1996a. DoD Pest Management Program. DoD Instruction Number 4150.7. Washington, D.C.: U.S. Department of Defense. 22 April 1996.

U.S. Department of Defense. 1996b. Joint Vision 2010: America's Military: Preparing for Tomorrow. Washington, D.C.

U.S. Department of Defense. 1996c. *Armed Forces Institute of Pathology (AFIP)*, DoD Directive Number 5154.24, Washington, D.C.: U.S. Department of Defense. 28 October 1996.

U.S. Department of Defense. 1996d. Separation or Retirement for Physical Disability. DoD Directive Number 1332.18. Washington, D.C.: U.S. Department of Defense. 4 November 1996.

U.S. Department of Defense. 1996e. Physical Disability Evaluation. DoD Instruction Number 1332.38. Washington, D.C.: U.S. Department of Defense. 14 November 1996.

U.S. Department of Defense. 1997a. Implementation and Application of Joint Medical Surveillance for Deployments. DoD Instruction Number 6490.3. Washington, D.C.: U.S. Department of Defense. 7 August 1997.

U.S. Department of Defense. 1997b. Joint Medical Surveillance. DoD Directive Number 6490.2. Washington, D.C.: U.S. Department of Defense. 30 August 1997.

U.S. Department of Defense. 1997c. "Force Medical Protection, News Release No. 601-97." Available at http://defenselink.mil/news/Nov1997/b11061997_bt601-97.html. (accessed June 1999).

U.S. Department of Defense. 1998a. "Single Acquisition Management Plan (SAMP) v1.0 15 April 1998." Available at http://cba.ha.osd.mil/documents/documents-name.htm#O. (accessed June 1999).

U.S. Department of Defense. 1998b. "Capstone Requirements Document for the Theater Medical Information Program." Available at http://www.hirs.brooks.af.mil/mhss/tmip/DocHTML/CapstoneReq.htm. (accessed 2 June 1999).

U.S. Department of Defense. 1998c. "Theater Medical Information Program Briefing Overview." Available at http://www.hirs.brooks.af.mil/mhss/tmip/Pages/Overview/. (accessed April 1999).

U.S. Department of Defense. 1999a. Combat Stress Control (CSC) Programs. DoD Directive Number 6490.5. Washington, D.C.: U.S. Department of Defense. 23 February 1999.

U.S. Department of Defense. 1999b. "Military Health System Response to Institute of Medicine Request for Information Management and Technology Input to the Study on 'Strategies to Protect the Health of Deployed U.S. Forces: Medical Surveillance, Record Keeping, and Risk Reduction.' " Written communication (electronic mail) from MaryAnn Morreale, Office of the Assistant Secretary of Defense (Health Affairs), March 22, 1999.

U.S. Department of Defense. 1999c. "CHCS II Projects." Available at http://cba.ha.osd.mil/projects.htm. (accessed June 1999).

U.S. Department of Defense. 1999d. "CHCS II—PIC (Personal Information Carrier)." Available at http://cba.ha.osd.mil/projects/fhp/pic/pic-main.htm. (accessed 28 May 1999).

U.S. Department of Defense. 1999e. "CHCS II PHCA Preventive Health Care Application (Main Front)." Available at http://cba.ha.osd.mil/projects/fhp/phca/phca-main.htm. (accessed June 1999).

U.S. Department of Defense. 1999f. "Featured CHCS II Module: Preventive Health Care Application." Progress Notes (Newsletter). Available at http://cba.ha.osd.mil/ documents/newsletters/chcsii/news-progress-notes-spring-99.htm. (accessed 26 July 1999).

U.S. Department of the Air Force. 1995. Air Force Joint Instruction 48-110—Aerospace Medicine: Immunizations and Chemoprophylaxis (Army Regulation 40-562/ Bumedinst 6230.15/CG COMDINST M6230.4E) November 1, 1995. Immunizations and Chemoprophylaxis, p. 4. Available at: http://afpubs.hq.af.mil.

U.S. Department of the Army. 1990. Army Regulation 40-5. Medical Services: Preventive Medicine.

U.S. Department of the Army. 1993. Health Service Support in a Nuclear, Biological, and Chemical Environment. FM-8-10-7. Washington, D.C.

U.S. Department of the Army. 1994. "Leader's Manual for Combat Stress Control. FM 22-51." Washington, D.C.

U.S. Department of the Army. 1996. "NATO Handbook on the Medical Aspects of NBC Defensive Operations AMedP-6(B), FM 8–9." Washington, D.C. Available at http://155.217.58.58/cgi-bin/atdl.dll/fm/8-9/toc.htm

U.S. Department of the Navy. 1998. "SECNAVINST 6230.4." Department of the Navy (DON) Anthrax Vaccination Implementation Program (AVIP). Department of the Navy, Washington, D.C.

U.S. Department of Veterans Affairs. 1996. "VA Persian Gulf Expert Scientific Committee Report. Department of Veterans Affairs Secretary's Responses and Action Plan." February 1996.

U.S. Department of Veterans Affairs. 1998a. "Vet Center: Detailed History." Available at http://www.va.gov/ station/telehealth/Histdet.html. (accessed June 1999).

U.S. Department of Veterans Affairs. 1998b. "Vet Center: Eligibility Requirements." Available at http://www.va.gov/station/telehealth/Eligibility.html.

United States Code. 1998. "Purpose of Reserve Components. Title 10, Sec 10102." Available at http://www4.law.cornell.edu/uscode/10/10102.html. (accessed June 1999).

Van Dulmen, A. M., J. F. Fennis, and G. Bleijenberg. 1996. Cognitive-Behavioral Group Therapy for Irritable Bowel Syndrome: Effects and Long-Term Follow-Up. *Psychosomatic Medicine* 58(5):508–14.

Vogel, S. 19 December 1998. The E-Mail Connection: Loved Ones Logging on to Check with Sailors in the Gulf. *Washington Post*, p. A17.

Vogt, R. L., D. LaRue, D. N. Klaucke, et al. 1983. Comparison of an Active and Passive Surveillance System of Primary Care Providers for Hepatitis, Measles, Rubella, and Salmonellosis in Vermont. *American Journal of Public Health* 73(7):795–7.

Von Korff, M., L. Le Resche, and S. F. Dworkin. 1993. First Onset of Common Pain Symptoms: A Prospective Study of Depression as a Risk Factor. *Pain* 55(2):251–8.

Walker, E. A., W. Katon, J. Hansom, et al. 1992. Medical and Psychiatric Symptoms in Women with Childhood Sexual Abuse. *Psychosomatic Medicine* 54(6):658–64.

Walker, E. A., W. Katon, J. Harrop-Griffiths, et al. 1988. Relationship of Chronic Pelvic Pain to Psychiatric Diagnoses and Childhood Sexual Abuse. *American Journal of Psychiatry* 145(1):75–80.

Walker, E. A., D. Keegan, G. Gardner, et al. 1997. Psychosocial Factors in Fibromyalgia Compared with Rheumatoid Arthritis: II. Sexual, Physical, and Emotional Abuse and Neglect. *Psychosomatic Medicine* 59(6):572–77.

Walker, E. A., P. P. Roy-Byrne, and W. Katon. 1990a. Irritable Bowel Syndrome and Psychiatric Illness. *American Journal of Psychiatry* 147(5):565–72.

Walker, E. A., P. P. Roy-Byrne, W. Katon, et al. 1990b. Psychiatric Illness and Irritable Bowel Syndrome: A Comparison with Inflammatory Bowel Disease. *American Journal of Psychiatry* 147(12):1656–61.

Walker, E. A., and M. A. Stenchever. 1993. Sexual Victimization and Chronic Pelvic Pain. *Obstetrics and Gynecology Clinics of North America* 20(4):795–807.

Walter Reed Army Institute of Research. 1998. "Department of Defense Global Emerging Infections Surveillance and Response System. Addressing Emerging Infectious Disease Threats: A Strategic Plan for the Department of Defense." Washington, D.C.

Weinstein, M. C., D. M. Berwick, P. A. Goldman, et al. 1989. A Comparison of Three Psychiatric Screening Tests Using Receiver Operating Characteristic (ROC) Analysis. *Medical Care* 27(6):593–607.

Wenger, J., A. Hightower, L. Harrison, et al. 1988. Use of Discharge Diagnosis for Detection of Haemophilus Influenzae Disease. Presentation at *The 28th Interscience Conference on Antimicrobial Agents and Chemotherapy*. October 23–26, 1988. Los Angeles.

Wessely, S., S. Rose, and J. Bisson. 1997. A Systematic Review of Brief Psychological Interventions ("Debriefing") for the Treatment of Immediate Trauma Related Symptoms and the Prevention of Post Traumatic Stress Disorder. *Cochrane Review*. In: The Cochrane Library, Oxford.

Whayne, T. F., and M. E. DeBakey. 1958. *Cold Injury, Ground Type*, ed. J. B. Coates, E. M. McFetridge. Office of the Surgeon General, Department of the Army. U.S. Government Printing Office.

White House, Office of the Press Secretary. 1997. "Statement by the President: Special Report of Presidential Advisory Committee on Gulf War Veterans' Illnesses." Available at http://www.pub.whitehouse.gov/uri-res/I2R?urn:pdi://oma.eop.gov.us/1997/11/12/5.text.1. (accessed June 1999).

White, L. K., F. Williams, and B. G. Greenberg. 1961. The Ecology of Medical Care. *New England Journal of Medicine* 265(18):885–92.

Withers, B. G., R. L. Erickson, B. P. Petruccelli, et al. 1994. Preventing Disease and Non-Battle Injury in Deployed Units. *Military Medicine* 159(1):39–43.

Wolfe, J. 1991. War Zone Stress Among Returning Persian Gulf Troops: A Preliminary Report (pp. D3–D14). *Preliminary Report of a Reunion Survey of Desert Storm Returnees.* West Haven, Conn.: National Center for PTSD.

Wolfe, J., P. J. Brown, and J. M. Kelley. 1993. Reassessing War Stress: Exposure and the Persian Gulf War. *Journal of Social Issues* 49(4):15–31.

Wolfe, J., S. P. Proctor, J. D. Davis, et al. 1998. Health Symptoms Reported by Persian Gulf War Veterans Two Years After Return. *American Journal of Industrial Medicine* 33(2):104–13.

Wood S., J. Scarville, and K. S. Gravino. 1995. Waiting Wives: Separation and Reunion Among Army Wives. *Armed Forces and Society* 21(2):217–36.

Woody, K. 1999. Recruit Health Care Summit: Developing Real Solutions to Real Problems. Presentation at *Strategies to Protect the Health of Deployed U.S. Forces: Medical Surveillance, Record Keeping, and Risk Reduction.* Workshop IV. January 13, 1999. Institute of Medicine, Washington, D.C.

Wortzel, C. 1999. Medical Fitness Standards for Retention. Presentation at *Strategies to Protect the Health of Deployed U.S. Forces: Medical Surveillance, Record Keeping, and Risk Reduction.* Workshop IV. January 14, 1999. Institute of Medicine, Washington, D.C.

Yehuda, R., B. Kahana, K. Binder-Brynes, et al. 1995. Low Urinary Cortisol Excretion in Holocaust Survivors with Posttraumatic Stress Disorder. *American Journal of Psychiatry* 152(7):982–6.

Yerkes, S. A., and H. C. Holloway. 1996. War and Homecomings: The Stressors of War and of Returning from War. In *Emotional Aftermath of the Persian Gulf War: Veterans, Families, Communities, and Nations*, ed. R. J. Ursano and A. E. Norwood, 25–42. Washington, D.C.: American Psychiatric Press.

Zinsser, H. 1935. *Rats, Lice, and History*. Boston: Little, Brown, and Company.

APPENDIX A

Population and Need-Based Prevention of Unexplained Physical Symptoms in the Community

Charles C. Engel, Jr., and Wayne J. Katon[*]

SYNOPSIS

How might military medicine respond to existing research on the epidemiology, burden, natural history, and management of medically unexplained physical symptoms (MUPS) in primary care and the general population? This review of extensive published research suggests that MUPS are pervasive and contribute substantially to physical, social, occupational, and organizational impairment, psychosocial distress, unnecessary health care utilization and expenditures, and adverse health care outcomes. These studies suggest that the natural history of MUPS is influenced by a number of predisposing, precipitating, and perpetuating factors and that certain prognostic factors may help clinicians and policy makers estimate the outcomes and population needs.

We use the epidemiology of MUPS and the basic principles of population-based health care to construct an efficient MUPS prevention strategy that emphasizes a continuum of care. In the absence of randomized trial evidence of efficacy for any single multifaceted continuum of MUPS care, the prevention program suggested is conservative and reasonably achievable, lends itself to subsequent evaluation and improvement, and calls for a multifaceted, well-integrated, stepped care management approach involving

---

[*]Charles C. Engel, Jr., M.D., M.P.H., is Chief of the Gulf War Health Center at Walter Reed Army Medical Center in Washington, D.C., and Assistant Professor of Psychiatry at the Department of Psychiatry of the Uniformed Services University in Bethesda, Maryland. Wayne J. Katon, M.D., is Professor and Vice-Chair, Department of Psychiatry and Behavioral Sciences at the University of Washington School of Medicine.

The views expressed by Doctor Engel in this article are his own and do not reflect the official policy or position of the Department of the Army, the Department of Defense, or the U.S. Government.

- broad-based and low-intensity educational interventions delivered to every member of the military services and perhaps their family members;
- primary care-based collaborative and interdisciplinary practice teams that aim to improve short- and long-term health behaviors using a variety of behavioral strategies including education;
- information systems that use expert systems to process and feed back data obtained by using a health care-based health information system and a population survey-based health data monitoring system;
- specialized, multimodal services available for the intensive multidisciplinary management of disabling and otherwise treatment-refractory MUPS; and
- development of a "center of excellence" to lead clinical, research, and educational efforts related to MUPS in the military.

We suggest that future improvement efforts target military clinicians, military health care delivery, the military work environment, and existing methods for compensating and returning ill personnel to work.

No matter the overall process and structure of care provided for individuals with MUPS, physicians are urged to practice "person-centered" rather than "disease-centered" care. They cannot ignore their place as consultants to real people in real predicaments who are attempting to make difficult decisions potentially affecting their future health, career, relationships, and status. Hadler has stated that the role of physicians, "should be more than that of concerned citizens or even of patients' advocates; [to that] we can add the perspective of students of the human predicament."[58] The expanded notion of ill health as a human predicament is especially apropos in occupational and military medicine settings. Occupational and military physicians treat diseases, but of equal import is their obligation to study and prepare the workplace so those workers with illness-related work limitations can eventually make a successful return to productivity. Eventually, we are impressed that military medicine's innovations in this area may provide an important model for civilian health care organizations seeking solutions to the difficult challenge of MUPS.

UNDERSTANDING MEDICALLY UNEXPLAINED PHYSICAL SYMPTOMS

The absence of a discerned cause for physical symptoms is best viewed through the lens of the scientific uncertainty necessarily involved in any one-to-one doctor–patient visit. We will use "MUPS" in reference to *health care use for physical symptoms that are not clinically explained by a medical etiology*. MUPS can be broken down into a four-part process. First, an individual must *experience* the symptom. In a simplified way, this might be viewed as the biological part of the process. Presumably, for one to perceive a symptom, some neurophysiological event must bring it to awareness. The second step is *cognitive*, or related to how we think about the symptom. The person perceiving a symptom overlays some knowledge, biases, or beliefs that he or she has about the symptom and its cause, assigning it a level of medical importance. We do not seek care for most of the symptoms we experience, partly because we assign them some relatively low level of medical significance. When we seek care, we are taking a third and *behavioral* step that is mediated by our belief in the symptom's significance.

The fourth and final step is the purview of the clinician: he or she must decide the extent to which symptoms are explained by the patient's medical diagnoses. This is one of the most problematic aspects of MUPS. There is a clear potential for doctor–patient conflict in this formulation. Differing clinician and patient explanations for MUPS may be one of the most important contributors to the frustration that these symptoms create for clinicians[61,97,154] and the dissatisfaction with care that many affected patients describe. Add some reason for doctor–patient mistrust, and the relationship can become outwardly adversarial and result in mutual rejection.[120]

In occupational settings like the military, clinicians must provide care within the context of competing and sometimes unacknowledged obligations. The clinician is committed to the welfare of the employer, who is both paying the clinician's salary and providing medical benefits for the patient. This same clinician has a simultaneous duty to the health and well-being of the patient. Under these circumstances, the patient may fear that the clinician is being coerced to deny the reality of the medical problem in service to the employer's financial or political interests. The patient may feel that the clinician is more interested in keeping the patient on the job than in providing treatment. Alternatively, the clinician may suspect that the patient is exaggerating health concerns to obtain benefits. Conflicts such as these heighten doctor–patient mistrust, dampen rapport, and diminish the chance of a productive clinical encounter.

Symptom-based disorders are diagnoses based upon patient-reported physical symptoms rather than specific findings on clinical examination or diagnostic testing. Symptom-based disorders seldom offer clinicians and patients more than a label. In most instances, the prognosis, treatment, and factors that determine disability are remarkably similar across different symptom-based disorders. Observed differences are typically small and are attributable to differences in severity, the number of other symptoms involved with the syndrome, or differences in loss of functioning due to symptom location (e.g., lower-extremity joint pain impedes walking, whereas headache pain does not). The names of symptom-based disorders are usually based on hypothesized etiology (e.g., chronic Lyme disease), putative triggers (e.g., multiple chemical sensitivity), a central descriptive feature (e.g., chronic fatigue syndrome), or body region (e.g., temporomandibular disorder). Labels often use complicated terminology (e.g., fibromyalgia or myalgic encephalomyelitis) that suggests to patients, doctors, and the public that the syndrome is better understood than it actually is. Therefore, we will use the term *symptom-based disorder* to signify syndromes that are clinically diagnosed almost exclusively by using patients' verbal descriptions. Table A-1 displays some common examples of symptom-based disorders and illustrates that clinicians in nearly every specialty encounter them. Symptom-based disorders overlap extensively, manifest remarkably similar pathophysiology, risk factors, clinical course, and prognosis, and respond to similar rehabilitative treatment approaches.[17,23,54,67,118,158] Historically, physicians have tended to categorize MUPS and symptom-based disorders as psychiatric symptoms on the basis of exclusion. It seems most logical that only some MUPS are psychiatric in their origin.

TABLE A-1 Some Symptom-Based Diagnoses and the Specialties that Commonly Diagnose and Encounter Them

Specialty	Clinical Syndrome	Specialty	Clinical Syndrome
Orthopedics	Low back pain Patellofemoral syndrome	Dentistry	Temporomandibular dysfunction
Gynecology	Chronic pelvic pain Premenstrual syndrome	Rheumatology	Fibromyalgia Myofascial syndrome Siliconosis
Ear-Nose-Throat	Idiopathic tinnitus	Internal Medicine	Chronic fatigue syndrome
Neurology	Idiopathic dizziness Chronic headache	Infectious Diseases	Chronic Lyme disease Chronic Epstein-Barr virus Chronic brucellosis Chronic candidiasis
Urology	Chronic prostatitis Interstitial cystitis Urethral syndrome	Gastroenterology	Irritable bowel syndrome Gastroesophageal reflux
Anesthesiology	Chronic pain syndromes	Physical Medicine	Mild closed head injury
Cardiology	Atypical chest pain Idiopathic syncope Mitral valve prolapse	Occupational Medicine	Multiple chemical sensitivity Sick building syndrome
Pulmonary	Hyperventilation syndrome	Military Medicine	**Gulf War Syndrome**
Endocrinology	Hypoglycemia	Psychiatry	Somatoform disorders

EPIDEMIOLOGY OF SYMPTOMS AND SYMPTOM-BASED DISORDERS

Prevalence in the Community and Primary Care

Review of the epidemiology of unexplained physical symptoms necessarily involves discussion of the epidemiological literature on somatization and the somatoform disorders (e.g., conversion disorder, somatization disorder, or pain disorder). The central feature in the somatoform disorders, however, is the presence of MUPS. The absence of test abnormalities or objective physical examination findings means that a psychiatric etiology is presumed but that the actual etiology is a matter of debate. We advocate an atheoretical, nonetiological, and phenomenological understanding of MUPS since this formulation is intellectually honest and maximally acceptable to those affected.

Population-based surveys have shown that 85 to 95 percent of community respondents experience at least one physical symptom every 2 to 4 weeks although relatively few of these symptoms are reported to physicians.[161] The population-based Epidemiologic Catchment Area Study examined 13,538 respondents from four U.S. communities and found that 25 percent reported chest pain, 24 percent reported abdominal pain, 23 percent reported dizziness, 25 percent reported headache, 32 percent reported back pain, and 25 percent reported fatigue.[91] Thirty-one percent of symptoms were medically unexplained, and the type of symptom was unrelated to the absence of explanation. Eighty-four percent of symptoms caused respondents to seek health care, take a medicine, or curtail activities.[91] Over 4 percent of people had a lifetime history of multiple, chronic, unexplained symptoms and an exacerbation within the past year.[38,142]

Other studies have shown that MUPS are associated with a high proportion of populationwide disability and health care utilization, largely because they are so common.[39,74] For example, the 1989 National Ambulatory Medical Care Survey estimated that physical symptoms account for 57 percent of all U.S. ambulatory care visits including some 400 million clinic visits per annum.[127] Kroenke and Mangelsdorff[90] reviewed the medical records of 1,000 primary care-internal medicine patients over a 3-year period and determined the incidence, diagnostic findings, and outcomes of 14 common symptoms. At least one common symptom was present in 38 percent of patients, and only 16 percent of symptoms were felt to have an organic cause. Symptomatic patients were monitored for an average of 11 months, and for 47 percent of patients the symptom persisted throughout the follow-up period. Two-thirds of symptoms were evaluated beyond the initial history and physical examination, but only approximately 1 in 10 evaluations resulted in an organic diagnosis not apparent at the index visit. Subsequently, Kroenke et al.[88] completed an office-based survey of 410 primary care-internal medicine patients to determine the prevalence and adequacy of therapy for 15 common symptoms. Eighty-two percent of patients had one or more symptoms, and in 77 percent one or more of these symptoms had been reported to patients' physicians. However, only 39 percent of patients with fatigue, dyspnea, dizziness, insomnia, sexual dysfunction, depression, and anxiety reported any noticeable response to treatment. Most other primary care research suggests that etiologies are unknown for at least 25 to 30 percent of patients with either painful or nonpainful physical symptoms.[87,92,93]

An extensive scientific literature has shown that MUPS are strongly and consistently associated with psychosocial distress, psychiatric disorders, decreased quality of life, and increased health care utilization.[6,18,25,38,39,56,76,90,92,129,135] Depression and anxiety are consistently associated with MUPS across many studies that have used wide-ranging methodologies including cross-sectional,[135] case-control,[73,82,140,152,156] and longitudinal designs.[150] Some evidence suggests that associated high health care utilization leads to more harm and patient dissatisfaction than benefit.[86,145]

Natural History of MUPS

MUPS are characteristically chronic and intermittently relapsing, although the natural history is reasonably variable in severity and periodicity. Factors responsible for variability in clinical outcomes may be classified as predisposing, precipitating, and perpetuating factors.

Predisposing factors are characteristics of individuals that render them more vulnerable to MUPS and related morbidity. Important predisposing factors are heredity;[136,162] neurophysiological, neurotransmitter, and autonomic nervous system factors;[4,31,44,52,55,83,144] early life adversity (e.g., child maltreatment);[3,26,68,85,98,152,153,155] chronic medical illness;[2,12,66,121,147] or chronic distress or mental illness.[34,70] Predisposing factors may be either intrinsic (i.e., innate to the individual) or acquired (i.e., obtained during lifetime exposure or experience).

A *precipitating factor* is essentially a "straw that breaks the camel's back," initiating an acute episode of MUPS and related morbidity. Factors that precipitate MUPS include biological stressors,[15,134] psychosocial stressors,[27–29] acute psychiatric disorders,[111] and epidemic health concerns.[14,21,24,62,69,139]

Perpetuating factors are those that maintain, exacerbate, or prolong symptoms, distress, and disability after they occur. Perpetuating factors may occur independently of the original precipitants. They include harmful illness beliefs (beliefs that lead to a maladaptive response to the symptoms),[132] labeling effects (i.e., the adverse effects associated with viewing oneself as ill),[40,60,63,106] misinformation,[1,7,16,100,130,133] workplace and compensation factors,[11,59,128,141] and social support factors.[107]

Prognostic Factors: Prediction of Outcomes and Assessment of Future Needs

MUPS occur along a spectrum of severity and prognosis[74] ranging from mild and transient to chronic and disabling. *Prognostic factors* are individual, environmental, or population characteristics that may be used to predict symptom outcomes and estimate future treatment and resource needs. The prognostic spectrum of MUPS includes acute, recurrent, and chronic subtypes. *Acute MUPS* occurs in the absence of a previous pattern or history of MUPS and lasts a few months at most, and associated disability is often temporally associated with an acutely stressful life event. *Recurrent MUPS* is characterized by alternating symptomatic, asymptomatic, and mildly symptomatic periods. *Chronic MUPS* is a pattern of persistent unexplained physical symptoms associated with chronic disability, high health care utilization, and persistent problems with coping.

Empirically evaluated prognostic indicators for MUPS include (1) prior level of health care use, (2) psychiatric factors, (3) physical symptom factors, and (4) factors related to functioning. A high level of previous health care use suggests that a poor long-term outcome characterized by chronic MUPS is relatively likely.[78,136] A large number of prospective studies have consistently found that the presence of stressors, distress, and psychiatric disorders, especially when they are chronic, predict persistent MUPS and related disability.[9,13,22,29,57,65,105,109,119,126] A higher number of comorbid physical symptoms ("symptom count")[53] and longer symptom duration[13,22,89,95,148] also predict a poor outcome. Past poor functioning including occupational functioning suggests a poor prognosis.[37,50,94] A patient's historical level of functioning can serve as a marker for a myriad of issues that diminish the amount of reserve that an individual can muster when symptoms worsen.

PREVENTION OF SYMPTOMS AND SYMPTOM-BASED DISORDERS

The epidemiology of MUPS suggests that those individuals afflicted with the mysterious "Gulf War Syndrome" may represent only the most disabled, symptomatic, and distressed of ill Gulf War veterans. For each veteran who seeks care for Gulf War-related health concerns, there may be several others with fewer physical symptoms. In a less protean manner, perhaps, these individuals' symptoms are reducing their capacity to function, increasing their use of health care, and heightening their health-related worries. Left unmanaged, these milder syndromes may become subject to the adverse influences of the previously described predisposing, precipitating, and perpetuating factors.

Is it possible to prevent MUPS? Resources are limited, and the scope of the problem is wide. The success of any program of prevention will depend on the degree of effectiveness of existing interventions and the resources required to deliver them. It may be feasible to significantly reduce the organizational impact of MUPS among military personnel by using a coordinated combination of population-based and need-based strategies. We recommend the adoption of a "population-based health care" model that uses a stepped-care approach (Figure A-1) to achieve maximum overall efficiency and effectiveness.

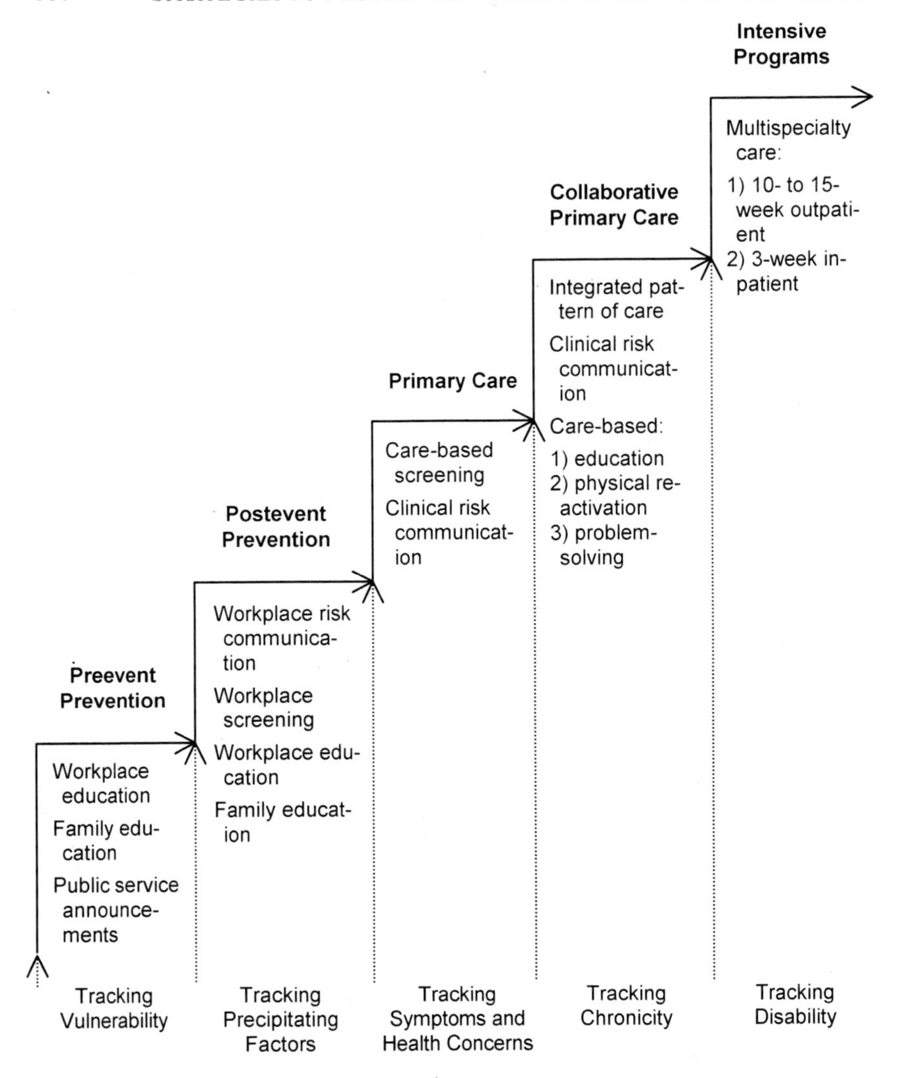

FIGURE A-1 A stepped-care approach to the population management of medically unexplained physical symptoms.

Advantages of Population-Based Intervention

Rose[123] has noted, "a large number of people exposed to a small risk may generate many more cases than a small number exposed to a high risk" (p. 24). Similarly, a large number of people exposed to a low-intensity preventive intervention can have a very large population effect (i.e., the effect of prevention summed across every person experiencing the intervention). Figure A-2 uses

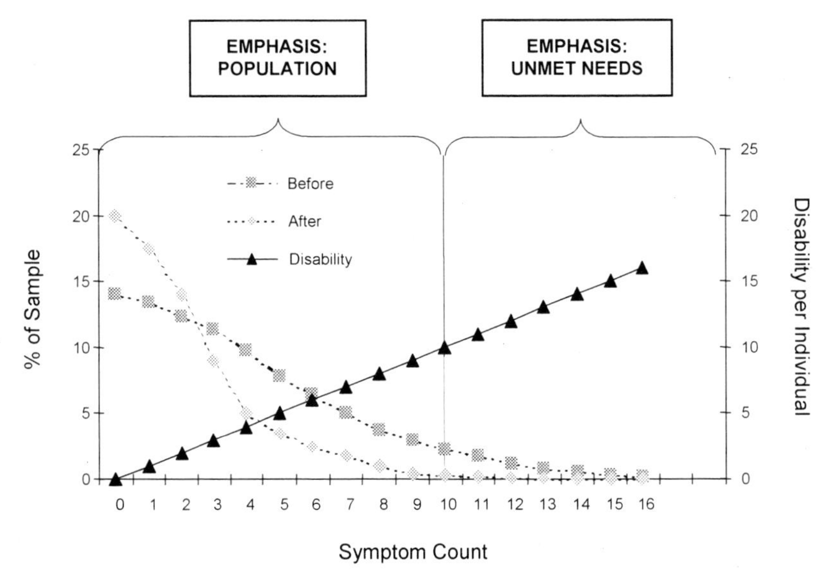

FIGURE A-2 Contrasting the population-based and needs-based approaches to reducing morbidity related to medically unexplained physical symptoms. Since disability (right vertical axis) is closely related to symptom count, population interventions that reduce symptoms a small amount per individual ("Before" = before intervention; "After" = after intervention) can prevent extensive disability when benefits are summed across the population. More intensive needs-based interventions can assist the relatively few individuals with repeated health care visits, multiple symptoms, and high levels of disability. Units of disability are hypothetical.

hypothetical data to illustrate that there is a graded and threshold-free relationship between symptom count and disability. Therefore, even among relatively healthy individuals, a small intervention benefit results in a small average individual improvement in functional status. Figure A-2 also shows that most of the population experiences relatively few symptoms and consequently little disability related to MUPS. When small reductions in individual disability occur across an entire population, the resulting societal benefits may be large and meaningful.

For the majority of people, MUPS come and go, usually without so much as a physician consultation. If these people are encouraged to seek health care for MUPS, it may increase the chance of long-term disability. This increase in disability may occur via mechanisms such as unnecessary worry, unnecessary avoidance of physical and social activities, unnecessary treatment, adverse effects of treatment, and provider errors.[42] "Medicalization" of otherwise minor and transient symptoms may also occur. This is a process similar to labeling, wherein the act of visiting a doctor for a symptom imbues the symptom with catastrophic meaning, thereby setting up a self-fulfilling expectation of future disability.

In sum, population-based approaches to MUPS have the advantages of universal exposure to an intervention and summation of the benefit per individual across an entire population. Since many individuals who would never have become ill necessarily receive intervention, population-based interventions must have a lower potential for harm than most interventions employed for the sick.

Advantages of Need-Based Intervention

Interventions that target the whole population can seldom address the unmet needs of the important minority suffering from many symptoms and extensive disability. Rose[123] described health care-based preventive approaches as "the high risk strategy" because the effort is to identify individuals at especially high health risk or with especially great need for health care. The time-limited nature of clinical practice requires that providers rapidly recognize patients who require special attention. In essence, the clinician must identify and dichotomously delineate people lying along the continuum of disability severity as either ill or not ill. The point at which people are deemed ill is more or less arbitrary but necessary to operationalize so that the process of care can proceed unhindered. Using the hypothetical data from Figure A-2, for example, the "cutoff point" for identification of individuals in need of clinical care is set at 10 symptoms.

This artificial dichotomy leads to the specific advantages and disadvantages of health care-based prevention strategies. The primary advantage is that intervention can be matched to the unique needs of a relatively few seriously ill individuals, an approach that is attractive and sensible to both ill patients and their providers. Another advantage is that intervention aimed at the ill is minimally intrusive or harmful for those who are not ill. Riskier, more intensive, or more invasive interventions may be justified for "high risk" or ill individuals because of the comparatively large potential for individual benefit and the reduced societal cost conferred by limiting the intervention to a few.

On the other hand, clinical strategies contribute disappointingly little to any overall reduction of population disability. This is because only a very small proportion of society is ever exposed to a clinically based intervention that targets an ill or needy population. For example, Figure A-2 suggests that relatively few individuals have 10 or more symptoms, and many who have fewer than 10 symptoms will manifest significant disability and unmet needs that would not be addressed by a clinical intervention.

In sum, the population-based and need-based prevention approaches both offer important advantages and suffer from unique limitations. The best approach to the prevention of MUPS therefore involves some combination of population-based and need-based prevention, intervention, and management.

Population-Based Care: Matching Resources to Needs

Population-based care aims to improve health outcomes through carefully structured clinical services linked through primary care to a population-based prevention plan. Population-based care is the development and implementation of a detailed plan that covers all people in a defined population who, despite population-based prevention, have developed a chronic or recurrent health condition or concern. Important symptoms are identified, a mechanism to track outcomes is devised, and a deliberate matching of appropriate resources to patients with unmet needs occurs.[151]

Katon and colleagues[81] have described how population-based care can reduce the prevalence of depression, and we advocate an analogous approach for MUPS. Critical is an understanding that various health care settings see different clinical populations with contrasting levels of MUPS severity and duration. More severely ill populations are encountered as the setting shifts from the community into higher levels of health care (e.g., tertiary care and inpatient hospital).

This is clearer when one considers the dynamics of illness in populations. Consider that the point prevalence (P) of some illness (i) is roughly equal to its incidence (I_i) times its average duration (D_i): $P_i \cong I_i * D_i$.[125] For intermittently relapsing illnesses such as MUPS, the duration of symptomatic illness can be approximated as the number of symptom episodes (N) times the average duration per symptom episode (D_e). Given some assumptions (beyond the scope of this discussion), the following can be shown:

$$P_i \cong I_i * D_e * N_i$$

This equation predicts that groups with more frequently episodic MUPS or MUPS of longer episode duration are overrepresented in populations because these characteristics elevate prevalence. The incidence of brief, nonrecurrent MUPS (e.g., acute back pain with a rapid resolution) may be relatively high compared with that of chronic MUPS. Even so, the long symptom duration and large number of episodes among those few individuals with an incident case of MUPS who develop chronic MUPS ensure that those with chronic MUPS are disproportionately represented in the population at any point in time. This overrepresentation of those with chronic and recurrent MUPS versus those with brief and acute MUPS is greater in specialty care than primary care and greater in referral facilities than local facilities. This occurs because local care and lower-intensity levels of care serve to "filter out" healthy and transiently ill individuals. Hence, the prevalence of chronic and recurrent illness is least in the general population, the greatest in specialty and tertiary referral settings, and intermediate in local and primary care settings.

The equation presented above suggests that the societal or organizational burden of MUPS may be reduced in at least three ways:

- incidence reduction or prevention of illness onset (primary prevention),

- duration reduction (secondary prevention), and
- relapse prevention (secondary prevention).

A fourth method of MUPS prevention (tertiary) targets the important morbid consequences of chronic MUPS: psychosocial distress, psychiatric disorders, and disability. From the equation, we would expect that the first three strategies might reduce the population prevalence of MUPS. The fourth approach may not alter the prevalence of MUPS but may still reduce the population burden of MUPS.

Implementing and Improving Population-Based Care

Wagner and coworkers[151] have described how to implement and improve population-based care. They describe three distinct organizational thrusts: information systems, practice design, and patient education.

Information Systems

Information systems (ISs) are computer-based systems used to capture data that can be used to inform clinicians regarding patient status, assist clinicians and medical executives interested in monitoring and improving the quality of care, and guide policy makers attempting to assess population needs and determine appropriate staffing levels. An IS for MUPS should use three components: a *health information system* (HIS) (a passive automated health surveillance system), a survey-based *health monitoring system* (HMS) (an active health surveillance system), and *expert computer systems* (ESs) (automated systems that generate useful reports for the identification of high-risk patients and evaluation of care, population health status, and clinical outcomes).

The schematic in Figure A-3 shows the interrelationship of IS components to various tools that may enhance the population-based care of MUPS. The HIS can record medical problem lists and measures of health care utilization (outpatient, inpatient, and pharmacy services and various procedures), health care costs, and presenting symptoms. These data, combined with HMS-based data on patient-reported physical symptoms, may be used to define MUPS for tracking purposes and to identify high-, intermediate-, and low-risk groups. Katon and colleagues[81] have suggested that the following elements are integral to any HIS that supports evidence-based interventions within a population-based health care system:

- regularly updated information on patients' primary care physician, place of care, and other contact information;
- current information on health care use including medication fills, procedures, laboratory results, primary care visits, and specialty care visits;
- a prioritized medical problem list; and

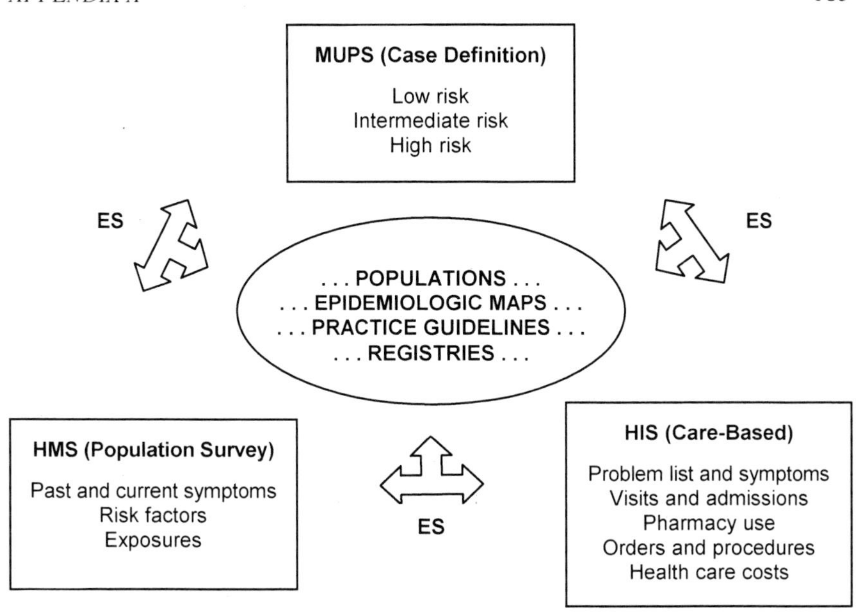

FIGURE A-3 Components of an IS used in population-based health care for MUPS and their relationship to one another. ES = expert computer systems, HIS = health information system, and HMS = health monitoring system

- other information relevant to establishing condition-specific patient registries for tracking and monitoring.[81]

The IS uses ESs to process raw data obtained with HMS and HIS, prepare these data for various uses, and deliver cleaned and collated data to appropriate users. ESs are programmed to generate tools that aid clinical management, patient follow-up, and treatment and policy decisions. Examples of ES tools include reports, reminders, clinical indicators, feedback systems, and guideline recommendations. ESs may be used to create registries, identify from a practice team panel patients who are likely to meet case criteria or who require intervention, monitor outcomes, compare outcomes for individual patients to those for groups of similar patients, and track the progress and relative prognosis of particular high-risk patients. An appropriate ES for MUPS might identify high-risk MUPS patients (for example, those with frequent visits or certain diagnostic codes from the International Classification of Diseases), remind clinicians of applicable guidelines and algorithms, identify relevant patient and family education tools, and implement screening scales or standard questions for consistent outcomes monitoring.[81] Eventually, it will become possible to compare the relative impact of primary care, specialty care, and quality of care on MUPS outcomes.

In the future, linking of the HIS and HMS with *administrative information systems* (AISs) (e.g., military personnel files containing dates of promotion, disciplinary actions, awards, deployments, and evaluations of performance) may allow careful empirical evaluation of whether risk factors and interventions alter militarily relevant MUPS outcomes. The combined use of ESs, HISs, HMSs, and AISs may provide for careful longitudinal tracking of the health status of individuals with MUPS who have recently deployed. Eventually, extensive empirical experience and understanding regarding the course of MUPS after deployments may be gained. IS data may be used to create population-based case registries and epidemiological maps showing the population distribution of people meeting case criteria. These individuals may be tracked for outcomes of potential interest such as long-term health care costs and service utilization, absenteeism, activity limitations recorded on military medical profiles, length of military career, rates of active duty reenlistment, promotion rates, and misconduct rates. Over time, refinements may be made to the existing case definition of MUPS so that it identifies individuals and groups at low, intermediate, and high risk of poor outcomes from MUPS. These data may also inform efforts to generate, implement, and evaluate pertinent clinical practice guidelines and best clinical practices.

Practice Design

Many have argued that the biggest barrier to quality clinical practice is the manner in which medical care is delivered.[161] Ambulatory care involves patients seeking care for a myriad of poorly understood psychosocial and medical reasons. In the traditional acute care approach, a physician quickly narrows to an often oversimplified "chief complaint," assesses only the most urgent medical needs, and then triages the patient to an appropriate level of care. Physicians managing acute medical problems are seldom practiced, skilled, or inclined to deliver preventive behavioral measures (e.g., dietary counseling, smoking cessation, and exercise prescription).

This approach fails to address the broad and often behaviorally based needs of people with chronic health conditions like MUPS. These individuals require systematic assessments, effective and targeted education, and sustained psychosocial support and follow-up aimed at maximizing long-term health and well-being. Their medical status may not become life threatening or severe enough to require acute medical attention until late in life or course of illness. By then, the opportunity to provide effective preventive measures has largely been lost.

The following are other barriers to the primary care management of MUPS:

- time restrictions and patient defensiveness;[113]
- high level of concern and low level of patient trust of military health care providers potentially responding to an organizational allegiance when caring for patients with MUPS after a deployment;
- reimbursement approaches that favor the use of invasive medical procedures over more behaviorally oriented rehabilitative care;[33]

- clinician perceptions of MUPS patients as frustrating, noncompliant, and undesirable;[61,97,112,154]
- inadequate coordination of care between primary and specialty care;[113]
- excessive reliance on physicians as the primary clinical facilitators of medical and behavioral change;
- disproportionate physician and media interest in disease-centered care featuring new technologies rather than patient-centered care stressing health behavior change; and
- an unwillingness or inability on the part of physicians to delegate crucial behavioral and educational aspects of the patient encounter that are best addressed by clinicians from nonmedical disciplines (e.g., nurses, psychologists, social workers, nutritionists, exercise physiologists, physical therapists).[151]

Improving primary care management of patients with MUPS requires far-reaching alterations in the culture, incentives, structure, and process of medical care as it is currently delivered. Given the demands on primary care, it seems unrealistic to expect that primary care physicians alone will comprehensively and intensively meet the diverse medical, educational, behavioral, and psychosocial needs of all MUPS patients. A more achievable goal is to develop a proximate, structured, collaborative, interdisciplinary, and multimodal process of primary care capable of reducing the burden of MUPS on primary care physicians. If primary care physicians can achieve success within the context of a reorganized clinic process, they may eventually find that behavioral management of MUPS and related distress and disability is rewarding and worthwhile.

Therefore, we recommend the development, implementation, and use of structured and carefully monitored health care programs that use *primary care practice teams*. Practice teams employ a wide range of nonphysician and physician providers collaborating together in a coordinated process of care. The team meets regularly to improve clinical coordination and intensify care-based efforts to inform patients about MUPS, prevent relapse of MUPS, increase physical activation, improve treatment adherence, respond to patient support needs, and hasten return to work.

Patient Education and Clinical Risk Communication

The range of patient education options is rapidly expanding. Carefully designed patient education materials are particularly important for those experiencing MUPS after deployments. Appropriate education materials can address harmful illness beliefs, the health effects of individual deployments, self-help strategies, the importance of managing disability and distress, the risks and limitations of extended diagnostic testing in "low-yield" clinical situations, and the ubiquitous nature of MUPS. Modalities available for disseminating patient information include brochures, mailings, books, videotapes, audiotapes, and waiting-room computers using self-guided learning approaches, as well as Internet-based learning technologies. Nonphysician specialists trained in patient education strategies and information technologies may assist patients with their questions in a manner that fosters trust and reduces distress regarding unlikely causes of symptoms. They may help patients troubleshoot attempts to initiate regimens of regular physical activity, take their medicines regularly, and so on.

Health risk communication is a discipline that addresses methods of enhancing bilateral communication in "low-trust, high-concern" situations. We have already described the insidious impact of the physician's competing and frequently unacknowledged obligation to the employer on the provider-patient encounter in occupational and military medicine. To date, risk communications experts have focused primarily on community-based methods of disseminating information and keeping communication constructive. However, risk communication approaches may be modified and applied to the low-trust, high-concern clinical encounter that occurs in occupational and military medicine settings. Risk communication imperatives are to carefully design and empirically test the impact of health risk messages. In clinical settings, we might ask: (1) Does a particular waiting room brochure foster patient trust in their physician? (2) Is there a way to restructure the clinical encounter that enhances communication between providers and patients under these tense situations? (3) What is the most effective way for a military physician to tell someone postdeployment that the person's symptoms are medically unexplained without fostering fear of a progressive illness due to some poorly understood military-related toxic exposure? *Clinical risk communication* might be defined as the application of health risk communication approaches in the interest of enhancing the overall effectiveness of occupational, military, and analogous medical encounters.

Stepped-Care Approach to Population MUPS Management

A critical focus of population-based care involves matching intervention intensity to the severity, duration, disability, and psychosocial needs of patients. The stepped administration of specific interventions (i.e., administration from least to most intensive) ensures that the individuals with the greatest need receive the most intensive and costly treatments. Figure A-1 summarizes the stepped approach that we currently envision. It employs five basic steps: preevent prevention, postevent prevention, routine primary care, collaborative primary care, and intensive multidisciplinary care. Note that a high level of clinical certainty and rigorous empirical evidence is not required to initiate this care model. The approach that we describe may be and should be incrementally updated and revised as necessary research is completed.

Step One: Preevent Primary Prevention

Currently, the primary prevention of MUPS is poorly understood, and resource-intensive attempts to implement unproven primary prevention strategies seem premature and unnecessarily costly. Nonetheless, populationwide primary preventive efforts to prevent the onset of MUPS as well as associated distress and disability are deserving of further attention and research. For example, "step one" approaches such as organizational policies and regulations or community- or workplace-level education involving literature, television, or other media segments require study and may have significant value. Unfortunately, the effectiveness of such efforts for MUPS is anecdotal and largely unknown. The routine administration of high-intensity step one prevention is likely to overextend costly resources to the majority of individuals who will never develop health concerns, making feasibility a major concern. Therefore, large resource expenditures may be difficult for policy makers to justify in the absence of experimental evidence supporting the efficacy of preevent prevention.

One promising primary prevention modality is education and related programs. For example, Symonds and colleagues[143] found that a low-intensity workplace intervention for back pain prevented subsequent sick leave. The intervention involved reattribution of back pain by use of an educational program. Pamphlets were distributed to all workers regardless of back pain history. The pamphlet highlighted the benign nature of low back pain and the importance of activity maintenance and early return to work as ways to successfully reduce morbidity. The investigators also found the program shifted worker beliefs about the causes of back pain. Similarly, military personnel, their families and significant others, their leaders, and health care personnel may benefit from brief, simple, education-oriented efforts that provide appropriate information regarding MUPS and their relationship to distress and treatable psychiatric disorders.

One potential way of narrowing the scope, increasing the feasibility, and reducing the cost of intensified step one prevention is to inform them by using IS technology. For example, smaller groups with predisposing MUPS factors may respond to a targeted intervention. ISs may help narrow the focus of intensified efforts to mitigate the impacts of these factors on subsequent development of MUPS and related morbidity.

Step Two: Postevent Primary Prevention

We suggest narrowing the focus of postevent prevention to specific units and associated families that have recently deployed or faced other events that might precipitate subsequent health concerns. Within these units smaller groups at especially elevated risk of MUPS may be identified on the basis of the presence or absence of past MUPS or other predisposing factors. The "real-time" availability of IS data has the potential to focus preventive efforts at identified points of organizational vulnerability.

Several candidates for postevent preventive efforts deserve further attention and evaluation. Workplace-based briefings may teach recently deployed personnel the associated possible or known health risks. Leadership efforts to normalize the workplace through an early return to work routines and previously scheduled activities may maximize postevent productivity. A feeling of chaos and loss of control are common immediately after a tactical deployment or a catastrophic event. A rapid return to routines may provide personnel with a familiar and predictable environment and a feeling of productivity. The availability of support meetings and meetings open to some larger community (so-called town hall meetings) may provide a forum for military and community leaders to learn of event-related community and family concerns. Similarly, town hall meetings offer opportunities for personnel and significant others to articulate and even ventilate important event-related health concerns. If the event or deployment involved sufficiently large numbers, telephone hot lines may be useful, too, providing personalized contact for people with questions, concerns, or previously undiscovered events or exposures.

A large anecdotal literature often promotes large-scale postevent debriefings. However, randomized trials of critical incident debriefings (CIDs) have shown limited efficacy, and at least one study has suggested that CIDs may actually increase the risk of postevent psychological distress.[159] A CID uses a structured debriefing format often led by mental health professionals with various levels of experience and expertise. Those exposed to the "critical incident" are encouraged to review the event in detail, focusing on current emotions and emotions during the incident. Efforts are made to inform people of the signs and symptoms of psychological trauma. CID is difficult and costly to successfully implement on any wide scale, may set up self-fulfilling expectations of subsequent psychological symptoms and disability, and is empirically unsupported from the experimental trials completed to date.

As in step one, caution is necessary when considering relatively high-intensity preventive measures for people who have yet to develop MUPS. A commonly considered step two approach is populationwide postevent screening. These efforts may positively reinforce or "medicalize" what are otherwise normal transient symptoms following such events. Even given IS data regarding predisposing and precipitating factors, it may be difficult to accurately predict who will develop MUPS and even harder to know who among individuals with MUPS will then develop disability and distress. Singling high-risk individuals out for a psychosocial intervention before the onset of symptoms and disability may unnecessarily and unfairly stigmatize or prematurely label many individuals. Most of those labeled immediately postdeployment will not develop symptoms or their symptoms will be time limited. Therefore, primary care-based screening for MUPS, tracking of outcomes of MUPS, and intensification of treatment for those with suboptimal outcomes is the most practical and least costly approach.

Step Three: Routine Primary Care

As noted, feasible primary prevention strategies for MUPS are, unfortunately, of a low intensity; therefore, we can expect that new cases of MUPS will regularly occur even after relatively successful population-based prevention programs. Virtually all individuals with MUPS will encounter primary health care. Therefore, a key to secondary prevention may involve early primary care recognition and timely management of MUPS to reduce the impact of precipitating and perpetuating factors on physical symptoms, emotional distress, and disability. IS technologies may remind primary care physicians which of their patients are most symptomatic, most concerned about their health, and most distressed regarding undiagnosed illness. Once these patients are identified, there are several ways that clinicians may mitigate the impacts of precipitating and perpetuating factors in an effort to prevent a chronic course. These are now reviewed.

Routine Primary Care Physician Management *First, do no harm.* Most patients with MUPS have had extensive diagnostic evaluations. Often, clinicians are aware at the time of initial history and physical that diagnostic testing offers a low yield or that anxiety or depression are important exacerbating factors. Studies suggest, however, that for patients with MUPS, clinical awareness is not well integrated into physicians' diagnostic and treatment practices.[8] As we have described, "shotgun" diagnostic testing under these circumstances can be harmful. Ordering unnecessary tests sends the wrong message to patients and promotes a passive patient mindset (e.g., "the doctor's in charge" and will "find it and fix it") that is counter to achieving behavioral activation goals and shifting some responsibility for wellness to the patient. Physicians are notoriously poor at making patients aware of the tests that they order, the rationale for ordering them, and the eventual results. One alternative to running new tests is for doctor and patient to carefully review past testing together, an approach that promotes clinician-patient collaboration and patient understanding. Sometimes, however, new diagnostic testing is necessary. A good rule of thumb for testing in patients with MUPS is to test only for classic constellations of symptoms or new objective signs.

Clinicians must take care not to present medications as a substitute for person-centered care for MUPS aimed at addressing health concerns and reducing disability. Although medical explanations for physical symptoms are often lacking, physicians often still place the patient on medications, even though medications are a relatively small part of the overall management of MUPS and unintended adverse effects often outweigh medication benefits. Sedatives are usually inappropriate unless insomnia is acute, stress related, and expected to abate within a short time. Narcotic analgesics usually do more harm than good, since they slow thinking, cause sedation, and reduce overall functioning. Both of these medication groups usually have adverse impacts on efforts to activate patients. Chronic administration of other central nervous system depressants such as so-called muscle relaxants is unadvised for similar reasons. Antidepressants, however, reduce the occurrence of MUPS among patients with chronic pain, panic disorder, dysthymic disorder, and major depressive disorder. In addition, reductions in depression and anxiety are critical to behavioral activation. It is important to carefully explain the rationale for antidepressants, or else patients will assume they were prescribed because the doctor thinks that the symptoms are "in the head," causing the patients to discontinue the medicine or see another doctor. All patients with MUPS should receive a complete and careful explanation of medication side effects, so that if they occur the clinician's credibility is enhanced and the chances of continued adherence is maximized.

Cure rarely; comfort always. Seldom is it possible to cure any chronic illness, and MUPS are no exception. Setting symptom eradication as a treatment goal will only lead to clinician and patient dissatisfaction. Clinicians intent on cures often feel as though they have nothing to offer patients with MUPS. They may devalue their role with patients with MUPS as "doing nothing" or "handholding." The importance of a supportive, empathic, and person-centered (rather than disease-centered) approach cannot be overemphasized.

Comforting patients with MUPS often entails reassurance. This means more than simply telling them that their symptoms are not serious. It involves elucidating harmful illness beliefs and directing education and advice to those beliefs. The following are common examples of harmful beliefs:

- "My symptoms are a sign of disease."
- "When I hurt it means I am seriously injuring myself" (e.g., "pinching a nerve").
- "When I have symptoms I can't make it without rest and a break from my responsibilities."

Clinicians can also learn the phrases that people with MUPS find belittling and avoid them. Similarly, they can learn some phrases that "join" the clinician and patient in a collaborative dialogue. For example, most individuals with MUPS describe their distress as secondary to symptoms. Although research is clear that distress increases the risk of subsequent physical symptoms and vice versa, it is best to adopt the patient's words and views regarding causation, no matter how faulty the clinician may think they are. Patients understandably react negatively to physician statements such as, "There's nothing physiologically wrong." Perhaps most physicians suffer from a good deal of overconfidence in their own clinical conclusions and would benefit from allowing their patients to have more input than they currently do.

Comforting involves office-based patient education and often centers on the health effects of adverse life events and toxic exposures, the impacts of anxiety and mood on physiology, symptoms, and functioning, the limits of medical testing, and the impacts of medication side effects on functioning. Self-help materials such as audiotapes and books about physical activation, relaxation techniques, and coping with chronic pain and similar symptom-based disorders are widely available.

Negotiate behavioral goals targeting illness and disability. Reducing disability requires specific changes in patient behavior. It requires patients to take an active, collaborative role in their treatment rather than a more traditional passive role ("fix me doc"). Provider-patient collaboration and negotiation of behavioral goals will usually prove to be more rewarding than striving for an elusive cure. Goals must be specific, incremental, realistic, and achievable, and they should center on observable or reportable behaviors. First and foremost, goals must be negotiated with the patient such that the patient "owns" the goals. If goals are simply clinician imposed, the patient may have no investment in them, view them as impossible, or covertly oppose them. It is often useful to have patients graph their incremental progress toward their goals and review the graphs with them at their follow-up appointments. Examples of good areas for goal formulation are occupational, household, or social task performance, physical activation, sleep hygiene, or medication adherence.

Hold the patient responsible for change, but avoid "the blame game." In disease-centered care, the patient is a passive participant. The patient is to "comply" with the doctor's "orders." The patient visits the doctor in search of answers, and the doctor is responsible for providing them. In person-centered care, the clinician must move out of the "answer man" role and join with the patient as a facilitator of behavioral change. The clinician negotiates the goals of treatment with the patient, helps him or her solve the problems "they" encounter, and carefully addresses the patient's expectations for quick or magical solutions. Simply acting as an "idea generator" for the obstacles that patients describe helps to facilitate behavioral gains. Clinicians must shift the responsibility for change to the patient, but they must also remain vigilant not to blame the patient for their lack of progress or their illness predicament.

Encourage physical and role reactivation. Regular exercise in tolerable doses helps patients with MUPS discharge distress, increase stamina, and improve functioning. Physical therapy programs of gradually increasing physical activity are sometimes useful for overcoming the deactivation and weight gain that occurs for many patients with MUPS. Usually, a physical therapist is not necessary to initiate reactivation strategies; these can be negotiated in the physician's office. Similarly, patients need encouragement to remain gainfully employed and active in supportive relationship roles. This reduces dependence and improves morale, self-confidence, and ability to meet expectations. In most occupational settings and especially in the military, reactivation strategies require careful coordination with employers or supervisors. The best reactivation plan will go awry if workplace supervisors are unaware of it or do not support it.

Involve social supports. Social supports may include family or close friends. Clinicians should encourage participation of support systems in nearly all aspects of care, provided that the patient approves of this. Family or friends can help clarify concerns, illness beliefs, symptoms, and deficits in functioning. Often, the patient's most important concerns are related to those closest to the patient, and their involvement in care can make or break the clinician's ability to successfully engage the patient in a constructive dialogue about the patient's health concerns. In occupational settings, the extent of involvement of the supervisor or employer must be similarly considered. "Collaboration" with the employer should seldom occur without the expressed (and usually written) permission and direct involvement of the patient. If organizational conditions, rules, or regulations pertain to employer or supervisor involvement, these should be clear and available to the patient from the time of the initial clinical contact or whenever it becomes apparent to either the patient or the clinician that employer involvement may occur.

Coordinate care with one designated clinician. Proper management of the delivery of care is both cost-effective and in the best interest of the patient. This is especially important for patients with many MUPS and those with chronic symptoms. In the absence of well-coordinated and centralized care, patients with multiple MUPS are likely to bounce from specialist to specialist, receive many unnecessary diagnostic procedures, and end up on multiple unnecessary medications. The key elements of coordinated care include (1) establishment of a relationship with a single primary care provider, (2) appointments at regular, time-contingent intervals of about every 4 to 6 weeks, (3) a brief physical examination at each visit to address new physical concerns, and (4) limits on patient-initiated visits for an exacerbation of otherwise chronic symptoms. Whenever possible negotiate an advance plan as to how symptom-contingent visits will be handled. If it is anticipated that this may become a problem, it is often sensible for clinician and patient to negotiate a written plan that both can refer to if limits become necessary. Some patients may fear that these limits mean that the doctor is angry with them or going to reject them. If the plan was previously negotiated and drafted in writing, these patient concerns may be tactfully addressed when they arise with minimal damage to the doctor–patient relationship. Consultants to the primary care physician must understand that they are to recommend care rather than assume it. Similarly, primary care clinicians should present consultants with a focused question. Consultants must understand their role and the key aspects of caring for patients with MUPS.

Anticipated and judicious mental health care referral. Psychiatric referral is frequently appropriate for those with MUPS, especially for patients who request it, have suffered a recent stressor, have a treatment-refractory psychiatric disorder, or describe suicidal or other clinically worrisome issues. However, most patients with MUPS do not require psychiatric treatment or psychological testing. Evidence suggests that a surprisingly large proportion of patients with

MUPS receive mental health referrals without an adequate explanation as to why they are needed.[86] In some cases, there is little doubt that a clinician desires primarily to "turf" (i.e., reject) a difficult patient. Not surprisingly, this message is seldom lost on the patient. Clinicians should not wait until the entire biomedical evaluation is complete and then obtain a referral because "potential medical causes are 'ruled out' and therefore the patient needs a psychiatrist." To prevent patients from experiencing mental health referral as rejection, it is usually best for clinicians to anticipate the potential need and introduce it early in a non-threatening way. Patients are best told that a frequent consequence of MUPS is disabling distress and that appropriate care can mitigate the impacts of their symptoms on their quality of life. It is important that primary care clinicians see patients after completion of the mental health referral to reduce the patient concerns that the doctor is rejecting or abandoning them. Primary care clinicians should ask patients how they experienced the consultation and contact the consultant directly for recommendations if possible.

Unfortunately, most mental health professionals have only infrequent exposure to patients with MUPS, are not skilled in their management, and do not readily appreciate the need to collaborate closely with primary care. Even when done under ideal conditions, less than half of referred patients ever obtain mental health evaluation. Patient defensiveness, excessive rejection fears, and social stigma associated with having a psychiatric disorder are among the significant obstacles to effective mental health consultation for patients with MUPS.[113]

Clinicians often obtain psychological tests such as the Minnesota Multiphasic Personality Inventory with the expectation that it will provide them with hard-and-fast evidence that MUPS are psychological rather than physical in origin. These tests can offer information regarding the relative style, quality, and success of patient coping and distress. However, they are not effective for diagnosing a psychological etiology for physical symptoms. Extensive psychological testing is not a panacea and may be quite threatening to patients when administered under any clinical circumstance, especially when the assessment may have occupational or military ramifications.

Teaching MUPS Management to Primary Care Physicians One reason that physicians minimize the importance of MUPS is their lack of awareness of and comfort with appropriate management strategies. Naturally, they focus on things they know how to treat, and most think there is nothing they can do about MUPS. It is important to enable them through proper educational experiences that focus on the basic primary care strategies described earlier.

MUPS-related clinical training experiences may add to the overall quality of patient care by improving the routine primary care management of associated, frequently unrecognized, and treatable psychiatric disorders. Research suggests that an excessively biomedical approach to MUPS or coexisting chronic medical illness markedly diminishes physician attention to psychosocial aspects of care such as recognition of treatable anxiety and depressive disorders. Kirmayer and Robbins[84] studied 685 patients presenting to a primary care clinic and found that approximately three-fourths of those with major depression or anxiety disorders complained exclusively of physical symptoms. Studies have shown that mentally ill patients with emotional complaints are usually detected, whereas those with only physical complaints are generally missed.[51]

Providers in medical settings may sometimes collude with patients in ways that undermine effective health care. For example, the provider may detect mental illness in a patient but fail to offer treatment because he or she senses that the patient might be unreceptive. Some clinicians are better than others at identifying treatable psychiatric disorders in their patients.[101] Conversely, distressed patients will more readily share their emotional concerns with those clinicians who are best at addressing them.[51] Appropriate medical education emphasizing communication skills, MUPS, and the recognition and treatment of anxiety and depressive disorders by primary care providers may improve clinical outcomes and provider confidence in addressing patients' psychosocial issues.

Efforts to improve physicians' communication skills are critical to improving the routine primary care management of MUPS. Too often clinicians fail to acknowledge to themselves and to their patients the high degree of uncertainty inherent in all clinical practice, perhaps especially for those patients in whom no explanation is found for physical symptoms. Clinicians must learn and relearn that the "absence of an explanation" is not synonymous with a "psychological explanation." A fundamental tenet in the art of caring for MUPS is to acknowledge the centrality of aversive symptoms to the patient's life before asking the patient to take responsibility for overcoming those symptoms. Often physicians admonish their patients to actively seek a state of health, and some even equip their patients with tools for seeking that health. However, unless they first validate, empathize, and even immerse themselves in the patient's physical symptoms and their sense of personal damage, sacrifice, and suffering, most patients will feel misunderstood. Some will feel that the physician is blaming them for their illness. A few patients will experience an unspoken challenge, the challenge to prove the reality of their suffering. In short, physicians must make it their routine clinical mission to develop an appreciation for the extent that each patient constructs his or her life around symptoms, suffering, and limitations, whether or not medical explanations are available. For example, Marple and colleagues[102] found that when physicians addressed patients' health worries and fears and understood the rationale behind their fears, their physical symptoms and functioning improved faster and the patient was more satisfied with care.

Physicians must develop strategies and experience explaining the limits of diagnostic testing and clinical treatments to their patients. Gallagher and coworkers[49] illustrated this in a recent study. Those investigators explored 39 internists' responses to a patient request for an expensive, unindicated diagnostic test. An actor was used to play out a standardized and blinded clinical scenario. Participating internists practiced in a health maintenance organization, and each encountered a young woman presenting with only chronic fatigue and no neurological symptoms. The patient desired magnetic resonance imaging (MRI) to rule out multiple sclerosis because of a friend's recent experience with the disease. Only 10 percent of internists asked about the friend's illness, but 8 percent ordered the MRI and 22 percent said they might in the future. Fifty-three percent referred the patient for a neurology consultation on the day of the visit, and all but 13 percent of internists said they might refer the patient in the future.[49] This study is but one of many that illustrate the need for greater clinician education regarding strategies for addressing patients who press for unnecessary diagnostic testing or treatments.

Step Four: Collaborative Interventions in Primary Care

To benefit patients, specialists and primary care providers need to learn and respect each others' ideas, share resources, and learn ways of successfully working together to develop consensus around common goals like the population-based care of patients with MUPS. Particularly important is the need to develop collaborative on-site programs of behavioral health care for primary care providers. Such programs can enhance patient adherence to behavioral approaches initiated in primary care. In addition, on-site consultation reduces stigma by presenting it as a routine part of the primary care experience rather than something mysterious and remote. On-site collaboration also provides primary care providers with satisfying opportunities to interface with and learn from specialists from the other disciplines rather than the more traditional approach of referring complex primary care patients to specialists "right when they get interesting."

Several groups have looked at primary care-based psychosocial interventions for persons with MUPS, distress, or both. Strategies have most commonly involved screening,[114–116] physician and patient education,[5] primary care-based mental health consultation,[72] interdisciplinary treatment teams,[108] and psychotherapy techniques adapted for primary care use.[20] Smith and colleagues[71,124,137] have found replicable reductions in the cost of care and even small improvements in health-related quality of life for patients with the most severe forms of MUPS (i.e., patients with somatization disorder) simply by sending a set of short, codified recommendations to patients' primary care providers advising them on how to manage them.

Katon and colleagues[79] completed a randomized trial of psychiatric consultation for "distressed high utilizers of primary care" at Group Health Cooperative of Puget Sound, a health maintenance organization serving over 350,000 enrollees in Washington State. Distressed high utilizers were defined as the top 10 percent of ambulatory care utilizers over the year prior to study who were identified as distressed either by their primary care physician or by high scores on a validated paper-and-pencil measure. This 10 percent of patients utilized approximately one-third of all outpatient visits, 26 percent of all prescriptions, and one-half of all inpatient hospital days. The intervention consisted of a structured psychiatric research interview followed by a 30-minute collaborative patient interview and treatment planning session involving the generalist, psychiatrist, and patient. Patients in the control group received usual primary care. Improvements in mental status or service utilization of intervention patients over that of controls could not be demonstrated. In retrospect, the intensity of the intervention was low, perhaps serving notice that MUPS involve many complex factors that are not responsive to a brief, one-time intervention that targets mainly psychiatric disorders. Prescription practices were marginally better for the intervention group, but subsequent antidepressant regimen adherence was generally poor for patients in both groups. There was no formalized mechanism for interdisciplinary collaboration after the initial consultation and no way of subsequently enhancing primary care clinicians' effectiveness or their adherence to the original collaborative care plan.[77]

More recently, primary care approaches to physically symptomatic and distressed primary care patients have focused on "multimodal" or "multifaceted" interventions. These are best administered in steps, so that the most intensive, expensive, or burdensome treatments are held in reserve for those who are otherwise treatment refractory. Components have included screening; on-site mental health consultation; cognitive-behavioral and problem-solving therapies aimed at medication adherence, depression, MUPS, physical activation, and relapse prevention; videotapes, pamphlets, and other education materials on self-care; structured follow-up strategies; and standardized written primary care instructions. Other efforts to enhance primary care clinicians' ability to tackle the multiple needs of their patients have employed "academic detailing," feedback to clinicians from their patients' automated pharmacy or health care utilization records, and case management.

Katon and colleagues[75,80] used a multifaceted approach to assist depressed primary care patients, an approach that can serve as a model for similar primary care-based MUPS interventions. Elements of their intervention targeted the patient, the physician, and the process of health care delivery. Elements that targeted patients were reading materials on depression, antidepressants, simple self-administered cognitive-behavioral techniques for managing depression, and a videotape on similar topics for viewing with spouses. Elements that targeted primary care physicians were didactics on antidepressants and behavioral treatment of depression, case-based consultation for each depressed patient, and ongoing interaction and feedback between the psychologist and primary care physicians. Elements that targeted the process of care were extensive and manualized. These included behavioral therapy done in the primary care setting. Behavioral therapy aimed at teaching patients depression self-management skills, improving medication regimen adherence, and preventing future relapses. Psychologist contacts were scheduled and occurred in the primary care setting. These contacts involved skills training, education, and homework. Relaxation training, assertiveness training, problem-solving training, and collaborative psychologist-patient development of a relapse prevention plan were done. Additional telephone contacts with the psychologist occurred after completion of primary care-setting contacts. Symptom monitoring occurred by a standardized measure and a checklist. The psychologist screened and documented antidepressant side effects, dosing, and adherence. During weekly interdisciplinary team meetings, a psychiatrist reviewed antidepressant-related information and overall treatment progress. The psychiatrist would advise medication alterations as indicated, and the psychologist communicated these recommendations to the primary care physician, who would carry them out. This integrated process of care was carefully monitored for integrity by using a numeric rating system. These integrity ratings were monitored and used to provide regular clinician feedback.

Katon and coworkers[75] compared this collaborative interdisciplinary intervention to usual care for depressed primary care patients using a randomized controlled design. As long as 4 months after completion of the intervention, intervention patients with major depression reported greater satisfaction with care, adherence to the medication regimen, and improvement in depressive symptoms than major depression patients receiving usual care. The results of the intervention were less clearly favorable among patients with minor depression (significantly improved antidepressant regimen adherence and perceived antidepressant helpfulness, but there were no significant differences between the groups regarding depression symptoms or satisfaction with depression care).[75] Other analyses of these data have found evidence of improvements in physical symptoms. Analyses of cost-effectiveness found that the intervention was more costly than usual care for patients with both major and minor depression. However, for the major depression patients, the multifaceted intervention offered significantly greater cost-effectiveness than usual primary care.[149]

Given the added expense associated with collaborative models, we suggest that they be held in reserve for patients for whom routine primary care management strategies for MUPS fail. Symptom duration is a key step four indicator to monitor using IS-generated reports. When a patient's symptoms reach some threshold of extended duration, more intensive collaborative efforts may be proactively introduced.

Step Five: Specialized Intensive Multimodal Care

There are several excellent examples on which to model tertiary prevention programs for patients with MUPS who fail to improve in response to collaborative primary care approaches. These programs are multimodal and multidisciplinary, occur in specialized (i.e., non-primary care) settings, and involve either a 3- to 4-week inpatient or intensive outpatient program or a 10- to 15-week program of weekly or biweekly individual or group visits. These programs emphasize carefully planned psychosocial elements that address the chronic nature of reduced functioning and the factors that reinforce it.

Usually, psychosocial and medical care is combined with a highly structured and generally supervised physical activation or exercise plan. These programs view disability as a behavior amenable to modification regardless of its biomedical etiology. Engel and colleagues[36] have described such a program for veterans with MUPS after service in the Gulf War. The intervention, called the

Specialized Care Program (SCP), is a 3-week intensive outpatient program modeled directly after the University of Washington's Multidisciplinary Pain Center.[99] Their preliminary data suggest that treated patients make mild to moderate gains in multiple domains including functional status and health-related quality of life, psychosocial distress, physical symptoms, and physical health concerns.[35]

Bonica at the University of Washington was among the first to apply a multidisciplinary approach to the treatment of chronic pain patients in the late 1950s.[99] Since then, the approach has gained relatively wide acceptance for work-impaired chronic pain patients, especially those with back pain and fibromyalgia. A recent meta-analysis of 65 controlled studies of multidisciplinary interventions for chronic pain patients noted improvements in return to work rates, pain, mood, and health care utilization.[43] The authors were cautious in their conclusions, noting that the level of methodological rigor for most studies was low.

IS-generated reports may monitor the patient population for individuals who develop chronic MUPS-related disability. If patients are recognized early and enrolled in specialized intensive multimodal care for MUPS, the chances of satisfactorily returning them to work may be maximized.

Components of Specialized Services The following sections review the common components of most intensive programs and the research that supports their efficacy.

Cognitive-behavioral therapy. Until recently, most approaches to patients with treatment-refractory chronic pain or other persistent disabling MUPS have involved an intensive burst of multimodal care delivered over several weeks, usually in an inpatient setting. Perhaps not surprisingly, given the general shift in emphasis from inpatient care to less expensive outpatient approaches, recent studies have evaluated less intensive but more longitudinal treatment strategies. The best studied of these involve combined cognitive-behavioral therapy (CBT) and physical reactivation. CBT used in this context aims to help patients test and appropriately adjust harmful beliefs that they may have regarding the cause of their symptoms and the ways of treating their symptoms. Empirical trials have shown the benefits of CBT for a range of MUPS including chronic fatigue,[131] irritable bowel syndrome,[117,146] temporomandibular disorders,[32] burning mouth syndrome,[10] hypochondriasis,[157] and multiple MUPS.[64,96,138]

Wessely's group[30] in London found that 63 percent of patients with chronic fatigue syndrome (CFS) showed significant improvement in their physical functioning after random assignment to CBT and physical activation, whereas only 19 percent assigned to relaxation training showed significant improvement. Improvements were enhanced over the 6 months following treatment. Significant improvements among CBT-physical activation recipients over those among the relaxation group were also noted in work and social adjustment, symptoms of fatigue, fatigue-related problems, and progress toward individualized long-term goals. Of note, improvements in distress and depression were only slightly better in the CBT-physical activation group, and the differences were not statistically significant.

Sharpe and colleagues[131] completed a randomized trial of CBT for patients with CFS by comparing it with usual medical care. They found that 73 percent of patients assigned to CBT rated their outcome as satisfactory or better, whereas only 27 percent of the usual care group gave such a rating, a difference that was highly statistically significant. Sixty-three percent of the CBT group improved in their work functioning, whereas only 20 percent of the usual care group improved in their work functioning. Functioning, fatigue, and depression but not anxiety were also significantly improved. As one would hypothesize under a model of treatment with CBT, illness beliefs and coping were more positively altered for those assigned to CBT than for those assigned to usual care. As was observed in the previously described CBT-physical activation trial, outcomes continued to improve for months after the completion of the intervention.[131]

Physical activation and exercise. Exercise is known to have important physical and psychological impacts upon health and well-being.[104,160] Using a randomized design, Fulcher and White[48] examined the impact of a gradually increasing program of supervised aerobic exercise for patients with CFS, comparing this approach to stretching and relaxation. After 12 weekly sessions, 51 percent of those assigned to exercise rated themselves globally as "much better" or "very much better," whereas 27 percent of the stretching and relaxation group gave such a rating, a statistically significant difference, and improvements were stable over the subsequent several months. Fatigue, physical functioning, and fitness were also significantly better in the exercise group.[48] Similar findings after exercise programs have been noted for other chronic or symptom-based disorders such as post-polio syndrome,[41] chronic low back pain,[46,47] depressive disorders,[160] fibromyalgia,[103] and "effort syndrome."[110]

Return-to-work strategies. Challenges exist around when and how to return workers with MUPS to work. There is general agreement that an early return to work is important to maintain role functioning and reduce chronic disability. There is evidence in the low back pain literature that a return to modified work can be successful.[45] Currently, the Army employs a profiling system of temporary or permanent work restrictions for those with diminished occupational functioning because of illness. Unfortunately, this approach may actually reinforce disability unless it is used in combination with a carefully supervised and graduated but relatively rapid return-to-work plan that is introduced to the worker very early in the rehabilitation process. For example, a 1-year follow-up of the use of work restrictions for nonspecific low back pain indicated they actually diminished the likelihood of return to work and did not reduce subsequent work absence or recurrences of back pain.[19] A supervised and graduated return-to-work approach may be especially important in the military when aerobic physical conditioning such as long-distance running is required. A "profile" brands the worker as a problem to supervisors and coworkers. The loss of physical conditioning and endurance that occurs in response to persistent physical symptoms and resulting deactivation requires time and a graduated program to reverse. Abrupt and haphazard return of personnel to full physical duties and the expectation that they will immediately perform at the same levels as others in their unit will commonly produce failure and an increased sense of defeat for the worker. In contrast, a rapid return of workers to their full levels of supervisory and other nonphysical roles is indicated to reinforce organizational expectations that a rapid return to productivity is expected. Likewise, worker productivity helps bolster self-esteem and a sense of accomplishment.

Obstacles to Specialized Services The greatest obstacle to the development of specialized care for patients with MUPS is the perception on the part of administrators, policy makers, and clinicians that MUPS are neither disabling nor important. Although explanations of "stress" or "somatization" for unexplained physical symptoms serve an important clinical purpose for many MUPS patients, they are often used to minimize the needs of affected patients. Another barrier at present is the lack of an institutionalized niche for specialized care for MUPS, especially after combat and deployments. Both primary and tertiary care of MUPS is, as we have shown, interdisciplinary and requires the collaboration of many clinicians such as generalists, psychiatrists, psychologists, physiatrists, anesthesiologists, nurses, social workers, physical therapists, occupational therapists, and dietitians. In the current health care environment, each of these clinicians is responsible to a department head, and departments are demarcated along specialty lines. Interdisciplinary care of MUPS is a lesser priority for each of these departments than illnesses that fall more clearly within their specialty purview. When competing clinical demands are high, the argument that patients with MUPS suffer more from "nothing" than "something" seems compelling organizationally.

Another important obstacle to intensive models of MUPS care is the conventional sense that such care is too costly. Currently, it is not known whether the extra costs associated with appropriate intervention are offset by longer-term decreases in health care use and improvements in occupational functioning. Most patients referred to intensive MUPS care, however, are using unusually large amounts of health care and are functioning poorly, so the potential for gains appears to be great. Left untreated, patients with MUPS remain costly to society. For the military, MUPS seem certain to occur after future wars, and excellence in this aspect of patient care may pay public relations dividends as well as improve the care of affected veterans. Further research on the cost-effectiveness of specialized services for patients with treatment-refractory MUPS is needed to rigorously examine these issues.

CONCLUSIONS

Hadler[58] has described four major areas in which occupational physicians might contribute to the care of workers: clinical, educational, research, and policy making. We adhere to his comprehensive outline and offer our own thoughts and a few of his in concluding this review of MUPS and their relevance for the military and perhaps other employers.

First, physicians caring for workers with MUPS must foster improved worker adaptation to illness *as the worker experiences it*. Hadler has urged physicians to try to understand the "sociopolitical arena" in which illness occurs. We urge clinicians to go several steps further and design a system of care that is responsive to people and their subjective health concerns rather than diseases per se.

Second, physicians caring for workers with MUPS must develop appropriate educational experiences for other providers and for affected workers and their significant others. Clinician education should emphasize the psychosocial and behavioral contexts of illness and disability rather than only simplistic biomedical perspectives. Providers must become more sophisticated regarding the ways that environmental factors may shape behavioral responses to symptoms and to ill health.

Third, physicians caring for workers with MUPS must develop short-, intermediate-, and long-term clinical research and policy research agendas with explicit goals and objectives. These research agendas must address important military health practice and policy questions. Research into biological mechanisms, although important for understanding one basis of unexplained symptoms, is costly. History suggests that mechanistic research is slow to yield immediate answers of importance to workers, patients, and organizations. Rather, epidemiological research is necessary to aid policy makers' attempts to comprehend the societal and military burdens of MUPS and the historical relevance of MUPS to diverse deployments.[122] Hadler has recommended research on the impact of job demands on physical and emotional health and workers' health perceptions, and this remains an area of need. Where, how, and why veterans with postdeployment health concerns seek their care and their satisfaction with that care is currently completely unknown within the military and is of great importance to prevention, treatment, and risk communication efforts.

Fourth, we suggest that physicians and policy makers move as rapidly as possible toward population-based models of health care and create system incentives for local-level development of novel interdisciplinary approaches to MUPS, interventions that span the spectrum of precare, primary care, collaborative primary care, and intensive specialty care. Physicians and policy makers must consider human factors whenever they are engaged in workplace structure and task design, since in the end, new technologies are effective only if the people who operate them are functioning well. Physicians and policy makers should carefully consider the impact of the prevailing military and U.S. Department of Veterans Affairs disability compensation system on incentives for workers to improve their health.

Given the necessary breadth of efforts to prevent MUPS in the military, we suggest the development of a "center of excellence" to lead clinical, research, and educational efforts related to MUPS in the military. A center of excellence could initiate and monitor efforts to implement clinical, educational, and research agendas pertaining to MUPS. When appropriate, the center could provide input to military policy makers interested in ensuring that they consider the impact of MUPS as they design, monitor, and adjust military health policy. A center of excellence would centralize U.S. Department of Defense responsibility in this arena and enhance organizational accountability. Eventually, military medicine's innovations may provide an important model for civilian health care organizations seeking solutions to the difficult challenge of medically unexplained physical symptoms.

REFERENCES

1. Abbey SE, Garfinkel PE. Neurasthenia and chronic fatigue syndrome: The role of culture in the making of a diagnosis. *American Journal of Psychiatry* 1991; 148(12):1638–46.
2. Adler RH, Zlot S, Hurny C, Minder C. Engel's "Psychogenic Pain and the Pain-Prone Patient:" A retrospective, controlled clinical study. *Psychosomatic Medicine* 1989;51(1):87–101.
3. Alexander RW, Bradley LA, Alarcon GS, et al. Sexual and physical abuse in women with fibromyalgia: Association with outpatient health care utilization and pain medication usage. *Arthritis Care Research* 1998;11(2):102–15.
4. Almy TP. Experimental studies on the irritable colon. *American Journal of Medicine* 1951;10:60–7.
5. Andersen SM, Harthorn BH. Changing the psychiatric knowledge of primary care physicians. The effects of a brief intervention on clinical diagnosis and treatment. *General Hospital Psychiatry* 1990;12(3):177–90.
6. Anderson JS, Ferrans CE. The quality of life of persons with chronic fatigue syndrome. *Journal of Nervous and Mental Disease* 1997;185(6):359–67.
7. Angell M. Breast implants—protection or paternalism? *New England Journal of Medicine* 1992;326(25):1695–6.
8. Barsky AJ, Delamater BA, Clancy SA, Antman EM, Ahern DK. Somatized psychiatric disorder presenting as palpitations. *Archives of Internal Medicine* 1996; 156(10):1102–8.
9. Beitman BD, Kushner MG, Basha I, Lamberti J, Mukerji V, Bartels K. Follow-up status of patients with angiographically normal coronary arteries and panic disorder. *JAMA* 1991;265(12):1545–9.
10. Bergdahl J, Anneroth G, Perris H. Cognitive therapy in the treatment of patients with resistant burning mouth syndrome: A controlled study. *Journal of Oral Pathology and Medicine* 1995;24(5):213–5.
11. Bigos SJ, Battie MC, Spengler DM, et al. A prospective study of work perceptions and psychosocial factors affecting the report of back injury. *Spine* 1991;16(1):1–6.
12. Blumer D, Montouris G, Hermann B. Psychiatric morbidity in seizure patients on a neurodiagnostic monitoring unit. *Journal of Neuropsychiatry and Clinical Neurosciences* 1995;7(4):445–56.
13. Bombardier CH, Buchwald D. Outcome and prognosis of patients with chronic fatigue vs. chronic fatigue syndrome. *Archives of Internal Medicine* 1995;155(19): 2105–10.
14. Boxer PA. Indoor air quality: A psychosocial perspective. *Journal of Occupational Medicine* 1990;32(5):425–8.

15. Bridges KW, Goldberg DP. Somatic presentation of DSM III psychiatric disorders in primary care. *Journal of Psychosomatic Research* 1985;29(6):563–9.
16. Brown J, Chapman S, Lupton D. Infinitesimal risk as public health crisis: News media coverage of a doctor–patient HIV contact tracing investigation. *Social Science and Medicine* 1996;43(12):1685–95.
17. Buchwald D, Garrity D. Comparison of patients with chronic fatigue syndrome, fibromyalgia, and multiple chemical sensitivities. *Archives of Internal Medicine* 1994;154(18):2049–53.
18. Buchwald D, Umali P, Umali J, Kith P, Pearlman T, Komaroff AL. Chronic fatigue and the chronic fatigue syndrome: Prevalence in a Pacific Northwest health care system. *Annals of Internal Medicine* 1995;123(2):81–8.
19. Burton AK, Erg E. Back injury and work loss. Biomechanical and psychosocial influences. *Spine* 1997;22(21):2575–80.
20. Catalan J, Gath DH, Anastasiades P, Bond SA, Day A, Hall L. Evaluation of a brief psychological treatment for emotional disorders in primary care. *Psychological Medicine* 1991;21(4):1013–8.
21. Chester AC, Levine PH. The natural history of concurrent sick building syndrome and chronic fatigue syndrome. *Journal of Psychiatric Research* 1997;31(1):51–7.
22. Clark MR, Katon W, Russo J, Kith P, Sintay M, Buchwald D. Chronic fatigue: Risk factors for symptom persistence in a 2 1/2-year follow-up study. *American Journal of Medicine* 1995;98(2):187–95.
23. Clauw DJ, Schmidt M, Radulovic D, Singer A, Katz P, Bresette J. The relationship between fibromyalgia and interstitial cystitis. *Journal of Psychiatric Research* 1997;31(1):125–31.
24. Colligan M, Pennebaker J, Murphy. *Mass Psychogenic Illness: A Social Psychological Analysis*. Hillsdale, N.J.: Lawrence Erlbaum Associates; 1982.
25. Coryell W, Norten SG. Briquet's syndrome (somatization disorder) and primary depression: Comparison of background and outcome. *Comprehensive Psychiatry* 1981;22(3):249–56.
26. Craig TK, Boardman AP, Mills K, Daly-Jones O, Drake H. The South London Somatisation Study. I: Longitudinal course and the influence of early life experiences. *British Journal of Psychiatry* 1993;163:579–88.
27. Craig TK, Brown GW. Goal frustration and life events in the aetiology of painful gastrointestinal disorder. *Journal of Psychosomatic Research* 1984;28(5):411–21.
28. Craufurd DI, Creed F, Jayson MI. Life events and psychological disturbance in patients with low-back pain. *Spine* 1990;15(6):490–4.
29. Creed F. Life events and appendectomy. *Lancet* 1981;1(8235):1381–5.
30. Deale A, Chalder T, Marks I, Wessely S. Cognitive behavior therapy for chronic fatigue syndrome: A randomized controlled trial. *American Journal of Psychiatry* 1997;154(3):408–14.
31. Drake MEJ, Padamadan H, Pakalnis A. EEG frequency analysis in conversion and somatoform disorder. *Clinical Electroencephalography* 1988;19(3):123–8.
32. Dworkin SF, Turner JA, Wilson L, et al. Brief group cognitive-behavioral intervention for temporomandibular disorders. *Pain* 1994;59(2):175–87.
33. Eisenberg L. Treating depression and anxiety in primary care. Closing the gap between knowledge and practice. *New England Journal of Medicine* 1992;326(16):1080–4.
34. Engel CC Jr. A collaborative primary care-mental health program in the military. *Federal Practitioner* 1994;11(11):18–29.

35. Engel CC Jr., Liu X, Miller R, et al. A 3-week intensive outpatient behavioral medicine intervention for veterans with persistent, unexplained post-war symptoms (slide presentation). The Society of Behavioral Medicine, 19th Annual Scientific Sessions, New Orleans, 1998.
36. Engel CC Jr., Roy M, Kayanan D, Ursano R. Multidisciplinary treatment of persistent symptoms after Gulf War service. *Military Medicine* 1998;163(4):202–8.
37. Engel CC Jr., von Korff M, Katon WJ. Back pain in primary care: Predictors of high health-care costs. *Pain* 1996;65(2–3):197–204.
38. Escobar JI, Golding JM, Hough RL, Karno M, Burnam MA, Wells KB. Somatization in the community: Relationship to disability and use of services. *American Journal of Public Health* 1987;77(7):837–40.
39. Escobar JI, Rubio-Stipec M, Canino GJ, Karno M. Somatic symptom index (SSI): A new and abridged somatization construct. *Journal of Nervous and Mental Diseases* 1989;177(3):140–6.
40. Feinstein AR. Nosologic Challenges of Diagnostic Criteria for a "New Illness." Conference on Federally Sponsored Gulf War Veterans' Illnesses Research: June, 1998; Pentagon City, Va.
41. Feldman RM, Soskolne CL. The use of nonfatiguing strengthening exercises in post-polio syndrome. *Birth Defects Original Article Series* 1987;23(4):335–41.
42. Fisher ES, Welch HG. Avoiding the unintended consequences of growth in medical care: How might more be worse? *JAMA* 1999;281(5):446–53.
43. Flor-H, Fydrich T, Turk DC. Efficacy of multidisciplinary pain treatment centers: A meta-analytic review. *Pain* 1992;49:221–30.
44. Flor-Henry P, Fromm-Auch D, Tapper M, Schopflocher D. A neuropsychological study of the stable syndrome of hysteria. *Biological Psychiatry* 1981;16(7):601–26.
45. Frank JW, Brooker AS, DeMaio SE, et al. Disability resulting from occupational low back pain. Part II: What do we know about secondary prevention? A review of the scientific evidence on prevention after disability begins. *Spine* 1996;21(24): 2918–29.
46. Frost H, Klaber Moffett JA, Moser JS, Fairbank JC. Randomised controlled trial for evaluation of fitness programme for patients with chronic low back pain. *BMJ* 1995;310(6973):151–4.
47. Frost H, Lamb SE, Klaber Moffett JA, Fairbank JC, Moser JS. A fitness programme for patients with chronic low back pain: 2-year follow-up of a randomised controlled trial. *Pain* 1998;75(2–3):273–9.
48. Fulcher KY, White PD. Randomised controlled trial of graded exercise in patients with the chronic fatigue syndrome. *BMJ* 1997;314(7095):1647–52.
49. Gallagher TH, Lo B, Chesney M, Christensen K. How do physicians respond to patient's requests for costly, unindicated services? *Journal of General Internal Medicine* 1997;12(11):663–8.
50. Gatchel RJ, Polatin PB, Kinney RK. Predicting outcome of chronic back pain using clinical predictors of psychopathology: A prospective analysis. *Health Psychology* 1995;14(5):415–20.
51. Goldberg D. Reasons for misdiagnosis. Sartorius N, Goldberg D, de Girolamo G, Costa e Silva J-G, Lecrubier Y, Wittchen U., Editors. *Psychological Disorders in General Medical Settings*. Lewiston, N.Y.: Hogrefe and Huber; 1990:139–45.
52. Goldenberg DL. Fibromyalgia syndrome. An emerging but controversial condition. [Review]. *JAMA* 1987;257(20):2782–7.

53. Goldman SL, Kraemer DT, Salovey P. Beliefs about mood moderate the relationship of stress to illness and symptom reporting. *Journal of Psychosomatic Research* 1996;41(2):115–28.
54. Gomborone JE, Gorard DA, Dewsnap PA, Libby GW, Farthing MJ. Prevalence of irritable bowel syndrome in chronic fatigue. *Journal of the Royal College of Physicians of London* 1996;30(6):512–3.
55. Gordon E, Kraiuhin C, Kelly P, Meares R, Howson A. A neurophysiological study of somatization disorder. *Comprehensive Psychiatry* 1986;27(4):295–301.
56. Gureje O, Von Korff M, Simon GE, Gater R. Persistent pain and well-being: A World Health Organization study in primary care. *JAMA* 1998;280(2):147–51.
57. Gwee KA, Graham JC, McKendrick MW, et al. Psychometric scores and persistence of irritable bowel after infectious diarrhoea. *Lancet* 1996; 347(8995):150–3.
58. Hadler NM. Occupational illness. The issue of causality. *Journal of Occupational Medicine* 1984;26(8):587–93.
59. Hadler NM. If you have to prove you are ill, you can't get well. *Spine* 1996;21(20): 2397–2400.
60. Hadler NM. Fibromyalgia, chronic fatigue, and other iatrogenic diagnostic algorithms. Do some labels escalate illness in vulnerable patients? [see comments]. [Review] [46 refs]. *Postgraduate Medicine* 1997;102(2):161–2, 165–6, 171–2 passim.
61. Hahn SR, Thompson KS, Wills TA, Stern V, Budner NS. The difficult doctor–patient relationship: Somatization, personality and psychopathology. *Journal of Clinical Epidemiology* 1994;47(6):647–57.
62. Hall EM, Johnson JV. A case study of stress and mass psychogenic illness in industrial workers. *Journal of Occupational Medicine* 1989;31(3):243–50.
63. Haynes RB, Sackett DL, Taylor DW, Gibson ES, Johnson AL. Increased absenteeism from work after detection and labeling of hypertensive patients. *New England Journal of Medicine* 1978;299(14):741–4.
64. Hellman CJ, Budd M, Borysenko J, McClelland DC, Benson H. A study of the effectiveness of two group behavioral medicine interventions for patients with psychosomatic complaints. *Behavioral Medicine* 1990;16(4):165–73.
65. Hotopf M, Mayou R, Wadsworth M, Wessely S. Temporal relationships between physical symptoms and psychiatric disorder. Results from a national birth cohort. *British Journal of Psychiatry* 1998;173:255–61.
66. Hotopf M, Mayou R, Wessely S. Childhood risk factors for adult medically unexplained symptoms: Results from a prospective cohort study. 44th Annual Meeting of the Academy of Psychosomatic Medicine 1998.
67. Hyams KC. Developing case definitions for symptom-based conditions: The problem of specificity. *Epidemiological Reviews* 1998;20(2):148–56.
68. Irwin C, Falsetti SA, Lydiard RB, Ballenger JC, Brock CD, Brener W. Comorbidity of posttraumatic stress disorder and irritable bowel syndrome. *Journal of Clinical Psychiatry* 1996;57(12):576–8.
69. Johanning E, Auger PL, Reijula K. Building-related illnesses. *New England Journal of Medicine* 1998;338(15):1070; discussion 1071.
70. Kaplan DS, Masand PS, Gupta S. The relationship of irritable bowel syndrome (IBS) and panic disorder. *Annals of Clinical Psychiatry* 1996;8(2):81–8.
71. Kashner TM, Rost K, Smith GR, Lewis S. An analysis of panel data. The impact of a psychiatric consultation letter on the expenditures and outcomes of care for patients with somatization disorder. *Medical Care* 1992;30(9):811–21.
72. Kates N. Psychiatric consultation in the family physician's office. Advantages and hidden benefits. *General Hospital Psychiatry* 1988;10(6):431–7.

73. Katon W, Hall ML, Russo J, et al. Chest pain: Relationship of psychiatric illness to coronary arteriographic results. *American Journal of Medicine* 1988;84(1):1–9.
74. Katon W, Lin E, Von Korff M, Russo J, Lipscomb P, Bush T. Somatization: A spectrum of severity. *American Journal of Psychiatry* 1991;148(1):34–40.
75. Katon W, Robinson P, Von Korff M, et al. A multifaceted intervention to improve treatment of depression in primary care. *Archives of General Psychiatry* 1996; 53(10):924–32.
76. Katon W, Russo J. Chronic fatigue syndrome criteria. A critique of the requirement for multiple physical complaints. *Archives of Internal Medicine* 1992;152(8):1604–9.
77. Katon W, Von Korff M, Lin E, Bush T, Ormel J. Adequacy and duration of antidepressant treatment in primary care. *Medical Care* 1992;30(1):67–76.
78. Katon W, Von Korff M, Lin E, et al. Distressed high utilizers of medical care. DSM-III-R diagnoses and treatment needs. *General Hospital Psychiatry* 1990; 12(6):355–62.
79. Katon W, Von Korff M, Lin E, et al. A randomized trial of psychiatric consultation with distressed high utilizers. *General Hospital Psychiatry* 1992;14(2):86–98.
80. Katon W, Von Korff M, Lin E, et al. Collaborative management to achieve treatment guidelines. Impact on depression in primary care. *JAMA* 1995;273(13):1026–31.
81. Katon W, Von Korff M, Lin E, et al. Population-based care of depression: Effective disease management strategies to decrease prevalence. *General Hospital Psychiatry* 1997;19(3):169–78.
82. Katon WJ, Buchwald DS, Simon GE, Russo JE, Mease PJ. Psychiatric illness in patients with chronic fatigue and those with rheumatoid arthritis. *Journal of General Internal Medicine* 1991;6(4):277–85.
83. Katon WJ, Sullivan M. Antidepressant treatment of functional somatic symptoms. Mayou RA, Bass C, Sharpe M, Editors. *Treatment of Functional Somatic Symptoms*. New York: Oxford University Press; 1995.
84. Kirmayer LJ, Robbins JM. Three forms of somatization in primary care: Prevalence, co-occurrence, and sociodemographic characteristics. *Journal of Nervous and Mental Disease* 1991;179(11):647–55.
85. Koss MP, Koss PG, Woodruff WJ. Deleterious effects of criminal victimization on women's health and medical utilization. *Archives of Internal Medicine* 1991; 151(2):342–7.
86. Kouyanou K, Pither CE, Wessely S. Iatrogenic factors and chronic pain. *Psychosomatic Medicine* 1997;59(6):597–604.
87. Kroenke K. Symptoms in medical patients: An untended field. *American Journal of Medicine* 1992;92(1A):3S–6S.
88. Kroenke K, Arrington ME, Mangelsdorff AD. The prevalence of symptoms in medical outpatients and the adequacy of therapy. *Archives of Internal Medicine* 1990;150(8):1685–9.
89. Kroenke K, Jackson JL, Chamberlin J. Depressive and anxiety disorders in patients presenting with physical complaints: Clinical predictors and outcome. *American Journal of Medicine* 1997;103(5):339–47.
90. Kroenke K, Mangelsdorff AD. Common symptoms in ambulatory care: Incidence, evaluation, therapy, and outcome. *American Journal of Medicine* 1989;86(3):262–6.
91. Kroenke K, Price RK. Symptoms in the community. Prevalence, classification, and psychiatric comorbidity. *Archives of Internal Medicine* 1993;153(21):2474–80.

92. Kroenke K, Spitzer RL, deGruy FV3rd, et al. Multisomatoform disorder. An alternative to undifferentiated somatoform disorder for the somatizing patient in primary care. *Archives of General Psychiatry* 1997;54(4):352–8.
93. Kroenke K, Spitzer RL, Williams JB, et al. Physical symptoms in primary care. Predictors of psychiatric disorders and functional impairment. *Archives of Family Medicine* 1994;3(9):774–9.
94. Kroenke K, Wood DR, Mangelsdorff AD, Meier NJ, Powell JB. Chronic fatigue in primary care. Prevalence, patient characteristics, and outcome. *JAMA* 1988;260(7):929–34.
95. Lembo T, Fullerton S, Diehl D, et al. Symptom duration in patients with irritable bowel syndrome. *American Journal of Gastroenterology* 1996;91(5):898–905.
96. Lidbeck J. Group therapy for somatization disorders in general practice: Effectiveness of a short cognitive-behavioural treatment model. *Acta Psychiatrica Scandinavica* 1997;96(1):14–24.
97. Lin EH, Katon W, Von Korff M, et al. Frustrating patients: Physician and patient perspectives among distressed high users of medical services. *Journal of General Internal Medicine* 1991;6(3):241–6.
98. Linton SJ. A population-based study of the relationship between sexual abuse and back pain: Establishing a link. *Pain* 1997;73(1):47–53.
99. Loeser JD, Egan KJ, Editors. *Managing the Chronic Pain Patient: Theory and Practice at the University of Washington Multidisciplinary Pain Center.* New York: Raven Press; 1989.
100. Loeser JD, Sullivan M. Doctors, diagnosis, and disability: A disastrous diversion. *Clinical Orthopaedics and Related Research* 1997(336):61–6.
101. Marks JN, Goldberg DP, Hillier VF. Determinants of the ability of general practitioners to detect psychiatric illness. *Psychological Medicine* 1979;9(2):337–53.
102. Marple RL, Kroenke K, Lucey CR, Wilder J, Lucas CA. Concerns and expectations in patients presenting with physical complaints. Frequency, physician perceptions and actions, and 2-week outcome. *Archives of Internal Medicine* 1997;157(13):1482–8.
103. McCain GA, Bell DA, Mai FM, Halliday PD. A controlled study of the effects of a supervised cardiovascular fitness training program on the manifestations of primary fibromyalgia. *Arthritis and Rheumatism* 1988;31(9):1135–41.
104. McCully KK, Sisto SA, Natelson BH. Use of exercise for treatment of chronic fatigue syndrome. *Sports Medicine* 1996;21(1):35–48.
105. McDonald AJ, Bauchier PAD. Non-organic gastro-intestinal illness: A medical and psychiatric study. *British Journal of Psychiatry* 1980;136:1276–83.
106. Meador CK. The art and science of non-disease. *New England Journal of Medicine* 1965;272:92.
107. Murray J, Corney R. Not a medical problem? An intensive study of the attitudes and illness behaviour of low attenders with psychosocial difficulties. *Social Psychiatry and Psychiatric Epidemiology* 1990;25(3):159–64.
108. National Institute of Mental Health. Mental disorder and primary medical care: An analytical review of the literature. DHEW Publication No. (ADM) 78-661. Washington, D.C.: Superintendent of Documents, U.S. Government Printing Office; 1979.
109. Neitzert CS, Davis C, Kennedy SH. Personality factors related to the prevalence of somatic symptoms and medical complaints in a healthy student population. *British Journal of Medical Psychology* 1997;70(Pt. 1):93–101.
110. Newham D, Edwards RH. Effort syndromes. *Physiotherapy* 1979;65(2):52–6.

111. Noyes R, Reich J, Clancy J, O'Gorman TW. Reduction in hypochondriasis with treatment of panic disorder. *British Journal of Psychiatry* 1986;149:631–5.
112. Olfson M. Primary care patients who refuse specialized mental health services. *Archives of Internal Medicine* 1991;151(1):129–32.
113. Orleans CT, George LK, Houpt JL, Brodie HK. How primary care physicians treat psychiatric disorders: A national survey of family practitioners. *American Journal of Psychiatry* 1985:142(1):52–7.
114. Ormel J, Giel R. Medical effects of nonrecognition of affective disorders in primary care. Sartorius N, Goldberg D, de Girolamo G, Costa e Silva J-G, Lecrubier Y, Wittchen U., Editors. *Psychological Disorders in General Medical Settings.* Lewiston, N.Y.: Hogrefe and Huber; 1990:146–58.
115. Ormel J, Koeter MW, van den Brink W, van de Willege G. Recognition, management, and course of anxiety and depression in general practice. *Archives of General Psychiatry* 1991:48(8):700–6.
116. Ormel J, van den Brink W, Giel MWJ, van der Meer K, van de Willige G, Wilmink FW. Recognition, management and outcome of psychological disorders in primary care: A naturalistic follow-up study. *Psychological Medicine* 1990;20:909–23.
117. Payne A, Blanchard EB. A controlled comparison of cognitive therapy and self-help support groups in the treatment of irritable bowel syndrome. *Journal of Consulting and Clinical Psychology* 1995;63(5):779–86.
118. Plesh O, Wolfe F, Lane N. The relationship between fibromyalgia and temporomandibular disorders: Prevalence and symptom severity. *Journal of Rheumatology* 1996;23(11):1948–52.
119. Potts SG, Bass CM. Psychological morbidity in patients with chest pain and normal or near- normal coronary arteries: A long-term follow-up study. *Psychological Medicine* 1995;25(2):339–47.
120. Quill TE. Somatization disorder. One of medicine's blind spots. *JAMA* 1985; 254(21):3075–9.
121. Richard K. The occurrence of maladaptive health-related behaviors and teacher-related conduct problems in children of chronic low back pain patients. *Journal of Behavioral Medicine* 1988;11:107–116.
122. Robins LN. Psychiatric epidemiology. *Archives of General Psychiatry* 1978;35: 697–702.
123. Rose G. *The Strategy of Preventive Medicine*. New York: Oxford University Press; 1992.
124. Rost K, Kashner TM, Smith RGJ. Effectiveness of psychiatric intervention with somatization disorder patients: Improved outcomes at reduced costs. *General Hospital Psychiatry* 1994;16(6):381–7.
125. Rothman KJ, Greenland S. Measures of disease frequency. Rothman KJ, Greenland S, editors. *Modern Epidemiology*. 2nd ed. Philadelphia: Lippincott-Raven Publishers; 1998.
126. Russo J, Katon W, Clark M, Kith P, Sintay M, Buchwald D. Longitudinal changes associated with improvement in chronic fatigue patients. *Journal of Psychosomatic Research* 1998;45(1 Spec. No.):67–76.
127. Schappert SM. National Ambulatory Medical Care Survey: 1989 Summary. *Vital Health Statistics* 1992;13(110)1–80.
128. Schrader H, Obelieniene D, Bovim G, et al. Natural evolution of late whiplash syndrome outside the medicolegal context. *Lancet* 1996;347(9010):1207–11.
129. Schweitzer R, Kelly B, Foran A, Terry D, Whiting J. Quality of life in chronic fatigue syndrome. *Social Science and Medicine* 1995;41(10):1367–72.

130. Sharpe M, Hawton K, Seagroatt V, Pasvol G. Follow up of patients presenting with fatigue to an infectious diseases clinic. *BMJ* 1992;305(6846):147–52.
131. Sharpe M, Hawton K, Simkin S, et al. Cognitive behaviour therapy for the chronic fatigue syndrome: A randomized controlled trial. *BMJ* 1996;312(7022):22–6.
132. Sharpe MC. Cognitive-behavioral therapy for patients with chronic fatigue syndrome: How? In: MA Demitrack; SE Abbey (Eds.). Chronic Fatigue Syndrome: An Integrative Approach to Evaluation and Treatment. New York: Guilford Press; 1996:240–262.
133. Shuchman M, Wilkes MS. Medical scientists and health news reporting: A case of miscommunication. *Annals of Internal Medicine* 1997;126(12):976–82.
134. Silver FW. Management of conversion disorder. *American Journal of Physical Medicine and Rehabilitation* 1996;75(2):134–40.
135. Simon GE, VonKorff M. Somatization and psychiatric disorder in the NIMH Epidemiologic Catchment Area study. *American Journal of Psychiatry* 1991;148(11): 1494–1500.
136. Smith GR Jr. *Somatization Disorder in the Medical Setting.* Washington, D.C.: American Psychiatric Press; 1991.
137. Smith GR Jr., Monson RA, Ray DC. Psychiatric consultation in somatization disorder. A randomized controlled study. *New England Journal of Medicine* 1986; 314(22):1407–13.
138. Speckens AE, van Hemert AM, Spinhoven P, Hawton KE, Bolk JH, Rooijmans HG. Cognitive behavioural therapy for medically unexplained physical symptoms: A randomised controlled trial. *BMJ* 1995;311(7016):1328–32.
139. Struewing JP, Gray GC. An epidemic of respiratory complaints exacerbated by mass psychogenic illness in a military recruit population. *American Journal of Epidemiology* 1990;132(6):1120–9.
140. Sullivan MD, Katon W, Dobie R, Sakai C, Russo J, Harrop-Griffiths J. Disabling tinnitus. Association with affective disorder. *General Hospital Psychiatry* 1988; 10(4):285–91.
141. Sullivan MD, Loeser JD. The diagnosis of disability. Treating and rating disability in a pain clinic. *Archives of Internal Medicine* 1992;152(9):1829–35.
142. Swartz M, Landerman R, George LK, Blazer DG, Escobar J. Somatization disorder. Robins LN, Regier DA, Editors. *Psychiatric Disorders in America: The Epidemiologic Catchment Area Study*. New York: Free Press; 1991.
143. Symonds TL, Burton AK, Tillotson KM, Main CJ. Absence resulting from low back trouble can be reduced by psychosocial intervention at the work place. *Spine* 1995;20(24):2738–45.
144. Thompson WG. *Gut Reactions: Understanding the Symptoms of the Digestive Tract.* New York: Plenum; 1989.
145. Twemlow SW, Bradshaw SLJ, Coyne L, Lerma BH. Patterns of utilization of medical care and perceptions of the relationship between doctor and patient with chronic illness including chronic fatigue syndrome. *Psychological Reports* 1997; 80(2):643–58.
146. van Dulmen AM, Fennis JF, Bleijenberg G. Cognitive-behavioral group therapy for irritable bowel syndrome: Effects and long-term follow-up. *Psychosomatic Medicine* 1996;58(5):508–14.
147. Vaughan KB, Lanzetta JT. The effect of modification of expressive displays on vicarious emotional arousal. *Journal of Experimental Social Psychology* 1981; 17(1):16–30.

148. Vercoulen JH, Swanink CM, Fennis JF, Galama JM, van der Meer JW, Bleijenberg G. Prognosis in chronic fatigue syndrome: A prospective study on the natural course. *Journal of Neurology, Neurosurgery and Psychiatry* 1996;60(5):489–94.
149. Von Korff M, Katon W, Bush T, et al. Treatment costs, cost offset, and cost-effectiveness of collaborative management of depression. *Psychosomatic Medicine* 1998;60(2):143–9.
150. Von Korff M, Le Resche L, Dworkin SF. First onset of common pain symptoms: A prospective study of depression as a risk factor. *Pain* 1993;55(2):251–8.
151. Wagner EH, Austin BT, Von Korff M. Organizing care for patients with chronic illness. *Milbank Quarterly* 1996;74(4):511–44.
152. Walker E, Katon W, Harrop-Griffiths J, Holm L, Russo J, Hickok LR. Relationship of chronic pelvic pain to psychiatric diagnoses and childhood sexual abuse. *American Journal of Psychiatry* 1988;145(1):75–80.
153. Walker EA, Katon WJ, Hansom J, Harrop-Griffiths, Holm L, Jones ML, Hickok L, Jemelka RP. Medical and psychiatric symptoms in women with childhood sexual abuse. *Psychosomatic Medicine* 1992;54(6):658–64.
154. Walker EA, Katon WJ, Keegan D, Gardner G, Sullivan M. Predictors of physician frustration in the care of patients with rheumatological complaints [see comments]. *General Hospital Psychiatry* 1997;19(5):315–23.
155. Walker EA, Keegan D, Gardner G, Sullivan M, Bernstein D, Katon WJ. Psychosocial factors in fibromyalgia compared with rheumatoid arthritis: II. Sexual, physical, and emotional abuse and neglect. *Psychosomatic Medicine* 1997;59(6):572–7.
156. Walker EA, Roy-Byrne PP, Katon WJ, Li L, Amos D, Jiranek G. Psychiatric illness and irritable bowel syndrome: A comparison with inflammatory bowel disease. *American Journal of Psychiatry* 1990;147(12):1656–61.
157. Warwick HM, Clark DM, Cobb AM, Salkovskis PM. A controlled trial of cognitive-behavioural treatment of hypochondriasis. *British Journal of Psychiatry* 1996; 169(2):189–95.
158. Wessely S, Nimnuan C, Sharpe M. Functional somatic syndromes—one or many? *Lancet* In Press.
159. Wessely S, Rose S, Bisson J. Brief psychological interventions ("debriefing") for treating immediate trauma-related symptoms and preventing post-traumatic stess disorder (Cochrane Review). In: *The Cochrane Library* 1999; Oxford: Update Software.
160. Weyerer S, Kupfer B. Physical exercise and psychological health. *Sports Medicine* 1994;17(2):108–16.
161. White KL, Williams F, Greenberg BG. The ecology of medical care. *New England Journal of Medicine* 1961;265(18):885–92.
162. Woodman CL, Breen K, Noyes RJ, et al. The relationship between irritable bowel syndrome and psychiatric illness. A family study. *Psychosomatics* 1998;39(1):45–54.

APPENDIX B

Statement of Task

Major Unit: Institute of Medicine
Division, Office, or Board: Medical Follow-Up Agency
Subject: Strategies to Protect the Health of Deployed U.S. Forces, Subtask 2.4
Staff Officer Name: Lois Joellenbeck

Statement of Task: The project will advise DoD [U.S. Department of Defense] on a long-term strategy for protecting the health of our nation's military personnel when deployed to unfamiliar environments. Drawing on the lessons of previous conflicts, it will advise the DoD with regard to a strategy for managing the health and exposure issues faced during deployments; these include infectious agents, vaccines, drug interactions, and stress. It also will include adverse reactions to chemical or biological warfare agents and other substances. The project will address the problem of limited and variable data in the past, and in the development of a prospective strategy for improved handling of health and exposure issues in future deployments.

Subtask 2.4 concerns medical protection, health consequences and treatment, and medical record keeping. Specific issues to be addressed include:

- Prevention of adverse health outcomes that could result from exposures to threats and risks including chemical warfare and biological warfare, infectious disease, psychological stress, heat and cold injuries, unintentional injuries;
- Requirements for compliance with active duty retention standards;
- Pre-deployment screening, physical evaluation, risk education for troops and medical personnel;
- Vaccine and other prophylactic agents;

• Improvements in risk communication with military personnel in order to minimize stress casualties among exposed, or potentially exposed personnel;

• Improvements in the reintegration of all troops to the home environment;

• Treatment of the health consequences of prevention failures, including battle injuries, DNBI [disease and non-battle injury], acute management, and long term follow-up;

• Surveillance for short- and long-term outcomes, to include adverse reproductive outcomes; and

• Improvement in keeping medical records, perhaps using entirely new technology, in documenting exposures, treatment, tracking of individuals through the medical evacuation system, and health/administrative outcomes.

Sponsor(s): Department of Defense

Date of Statement: 11/21/97

APPENDIX C

Roster and Biographies of Study Team

PRINCIPAL INVESTIGATORS

Samuel B. Guze, M.D.
Spencer T. Olin Professor of Psychiatry
Washington University School of Medicine

Philip K. Russell, M.D.
Professor Emeritus
Department of International Health
Johns Hopkins School of Public Health

ADVISORS

Arthur J. Barsky, M.D.
Professor of Psychiatry
Harvard Medical School
Brigham and Women's Hospital

Dan G. Blazer, M.D., Ph.D., M.P.H.
Dean of Medical Education
Professor of Psychiatry and Community and Family Medicine
Duke University Medical Center

Germaine M. Buck, Ph.D.
Associate Professor
Department of Social and Preventive Medicine
University at Buffalo
State of New York

Charles C. J. Carpenter, M.D.
Professor of Medicine
The Miriam Hospital
Brown University

John A. Fairbank (through 9/98)
Associate Professor
Department of Psychiatry and Behavioral Sciences
Duke University

Kenneth W. Goodman, Ph.D.
Director, Forum for Bioethics and Philosophy
University of Miami

Sanford S. Leffingwell, M.D., M.P.H.
Occupational and Environmental Health Consultant
HLM Consultants
Atlanta, GA

Bruce S. McEwen, Ph.D.
Professor and Head
Harold and Margaret Milliken Hatch Laboratory of Neuroendocrinology
Rockefeller University

G. Marie Swanson, Ph.D., M.P.H.
Director, Cancer Center
Professor of Family Practice and Medicine
Michigan State University

Paul C. Tang, M.D.
Medical Director, Clinical Informatics
Palo Alto Medical Foundation
Vice President, Epic Research Institute, Epic Systems

Frank W. Weathers, Ph.D.
Assistant Professor of Psychology
Department of Psychology
Auburn University

Neil D. Weinstein, Ph.D.
Professor
Departments of Human Ecology and Psychology
Cook College
Rutgers University

BIOGRAPHIES

Principal Investigators

Samuel B. Guze, M.D. Dr. Guze is Spencer T. Olin Professor and former Head of the Department of Psychiatry at Washington University School of Medicine. He served as Vice Chancellor for Medical Affairs and President of the Washington University Medical Center from 1971 to 1989. His areas of expertise include psychiatry and psychiatric epidemiology, internal medicine, neurobiology, and medical center administration. He served in the Army Medical Corps after World War II, separating from service as a Captain. He has served on Extramural Scientific Advisory Boards of the National Institute of Mental Health and of the National Institute of Alcohol Abuse and Alcoholism and currently chairs the American Psychiatric Association Council on Research. He received the Samuel Hamilton Medal and the Paul Hoch Award Medal from the American Psychopathological Association, the Gold Medal Research Award from the Society of Biological Psychiatry, the Achievement Award from the American Academy of Clinical Psychiatrists, and the Distinguished Public Service Award from the Department of Health and Human Services. He is a fellow of the American College of Physicians, the American Psychiatric Association, the American Association for the Advancement of Science, and the Royal College of Psychiatrists. He is a senior member of the Institute of Medicine.

Philip K. Russell, M.D. Dr. Russell recently retired as Professor in the Department of International Health of the Johns Hopkins University School of Hygiene and Public Health. From 1959 to 1990 he served in the U.S. Army Medical Corps, retiring as a Major General and Assistant Surgeon General for Research and Development. He has expertise in infectious diseases, tropical medicine, virology, immunology, and vaccines. He has served on the Board of Scientific Counselors for the Centers for Disease Control and Prevention's Center for Infectious Diseases, the Scientific Advisory Group of Experts for the World Health Organization Programme on Vaccine Development, the Presidential Advisory Committee on Human Radiation Experiments, Defense Science Board task forces on chemical weapons and on biological defense, and on numerous National Academy of Sciences committees, including the Committee on R&D Needs for Improving Civilian Medical Responses to Chemical and Biological Terrorism Incidents; Committee on Interactions of Drugs, Biologics, and Chemicals in Deployed U.S. Military Forces; Committee to Review the Health Consequences of Service During the Persian Gulf War; Committee on Microbial Threats to Health; and Committee on Issues and Priorities for New Vaccine Development. He has received the Order of Military Medical Merit and the Distinguished Service Medal and is a fellow of the American Academy of Microbiology and the Infectious Diseases Society of America.

Advisors

Arthur J. Barsky, III, M.D. Dr. Barsky is currently Professor in the Department of Psychiatry at the Harvard Medical School and Psychiatrist at Brigham and Women's Hospital in Boston, where he supervises the Psychiatric Consultation Liaison Service and is Director of Psychosomatic Research. His research interests include somatoform disorders, interindividual variability in symptom reporting among the medically ill, and psychiatric and psychosocial aspects of chronic medical illness. He sits on the editorial boards of the *Harvard Review of Psychiatry* and the *Somatization Newsletter*.

Dan G. Blazer, M.D., Ph.D., M.P.H. Dr. Blazer is Dean of Medical Education at the Duke University School of Medicine, where he serves as J.P. Gibbons Professor of Psychiatry and Behavioral Sciences and Professor of Community and Family Medicine. He is also Adjunct Professor in the Department of Epidemiology at the University of North Carolina School of Public Health. Dr. Blazer is the author or editor of over 20 books and author or coauthor of over 200 peer-reviewed articles on topics including depression, epidemiology, and consultation liaison psychiatry. He has served on several Institute of Medicine committees, recently chairing the Committee on the Evaluation of the Department of Defense Comprehensive Clinical Evaluation Program. He is a fellow of the American College of Psychiatry and the American Psychiatric Association and a member of the Institute of Medicine.

Germaine M. Buck, Ph.D. Dr. Buck is currently Associate Professor in the Department of Social and Preventive Medicine, School of Medicine and Biomedical Sciences, State University of New York at Buffalo. She is an epidemiologist with expertise in reproductive and perinatal outcomes, particularly following environmental exposures. Dr. Buck serves on the Committee on Toxicology, Board on Environmental Studies and Toxicology, and on the Board of the Medical Follow-Up Agency, Institute of Medicine. She is a board member of the American College of Epidemiology.

Charles C. J. Carpenter, M.D. Dr. Carpenter is Professor of Medicine at Brown University School of Medicine and Director of the International Health Institute at Brown University. He has over 30 years of clinical and research experience in infectious diseases and internal medicine. He currently chairs the Office of AIDS Research Advisory Committee for the National Institutes of Health and is president of the Johns Hopkins Medical and Surgical Association. Dr. Carpenter is a master in the American College of Physicians and a senior member of the Institute of Medicine.

Kenneth W. Goodman, Ph.D. Dr. Goodman is founder and director of the University of Miami Forum for Bioethics and Philosophy and co-director of the university's Programs in Business, Governmental and Professional Ethics. He has appointments in the university's departments of Philosophy, Medicine, and Epidemiology and Public Health and the School of Nursing. His research interests are in ethics in epidemiology and public health and ethics in medical informatics. He founded and has chaired the American Medical Informatics Association's Ethical, Legal and Social Issues Working Group and is a member of the American College of Epidemiology's Ethics and Standards of Practice Committee.

Sanford S. Leffingwell, M.D., M.P.H. Dr. Leffingwell is an occupational and environmental medicine consultant with HLM Consultants in Atlanta, Georgia. From 1985 to 1995, he served as medical epidemiologist for the Chemical Demilitarization Program with the Centers for Disease Control and Prevention, a group that provides congressionally mandated oversight of the Army's chemical weapons disposal activities. Dr. Leffingwell also served as a member of the U.S. negotiating team for a bilateral (U.S. and U.S.S.R.) Chemical Weapons Treaty and was a member of the U.S. Medical Delegation to provide technical assistance to Japan regarding medical management of people injured in the 1995 subway nerve agent incident. He serves on the National Research Council Standing Committee on Program and Technical Review of the U.S. Army Chemical and Biological Defense Command (CBDCOM Committee) and the Committee on Chronic Reference Doses for Selected Chemical Warfare Agents.

Bruce S. McEwen, Ph.D. Dr. McEwen is Professor and Head of the Harold and Margaret Milliken Hatch Laboratory of Neuroendocrinology at Rockefeller

University. His research interests include the nonreproductive actions of sex hormones, stress effects on the structure and function of the brain, and adrenal steroids and the plasticity of brain and behavior. He is a member of the MacArthur Foundation Network on Socioeconomic Status and Health and has developed a new formulation of how stress affects health. Dr. McEwen is a member of the National Academy of Sciences and immediate Past President of the Society for Neuroscience.

G. Marie Swanson, Ph.D., M.P.H. Dr. Swanson is Director of the Cancer Center and Professor in the departments of Family Practice and Medicine in the College of Human Medicine at Michigan State University. Her major areas of research are cancer and chronic disease epidemiology, with particular emphasis upon primary prevention, occupational and environmental risk factors, chronic disease comorbidity, and high-risk populations. She also has expertise in population-based medical surveillance for epidemiologic and clinical research. She serves on the National Board of the American Cancer Society and on the editorial boards of the *Journal of the National Cancer Institute* and *Cancer Epidemiology, Biomarkers, and Prevention.* Dr. Swanson is past President of the Michigan Division of the American Cancer Society, a Fellow and former President of the American College of Epidemiology, a Fellow of the American Association for the Advancement of Science, and the 1996 recipient of the St. George Medal of the American Cancer Society.

Paul C. Tang, M.D. Dr. Tang is Medical Director of Clinical Informatics at the Palo Alto Medical Foundation, and Vice President of Epic Research West, Epic Systems. He serves on the boards of directors of the American College of Medical Informatics and the American Medical Informatics Association and is a past Chairman of the Board of Directors of the Computer-Based Patient Record Institute. His research interests include computer-based patient record systems, clinical decision support, and patient and consumer health information.

Frank W. Weathers, Ph.D. Dr. Weathers is Assistant Professor in the Department of Psychology at Auburn University. From 1989 to 1997 he served as Staff Psychologist at the National Center for Posttraumatic Stress Disorder at the Boston Veterans' Affairs Medical Center. His research interests include assessment and treatment of posttraumatic stress disorder and social information processing in anxiety, depression, and personality disorders. He is the recipient of the Chaim Danieli Young Professional Award from the International Society for Traumatic Stress Studies.

Neil D. Weinstein, Ph.D. Dr. Weinstein is Professor in the departments of Human Ecology and Psychology and former chair of the Department of Human Ecology at Cook College, Rutgers University. His research is directed at health and environmental psychology, with an emphasis on risk perceptions, risk communication, and health behavior. Dr. Weinstein serves on the editorial boards of the *Journal of Applied Social Psychology*, the *British Journal of Health Psychology*, *Health Psychology*, and the *Journal of Environmental Psychology*. He has advised or served on numerous national advisory and review panels on risk communication and is a Fellow of the American Psychological Association in both the Division of Health Psychology and the Division of Population and Environment.

APPENDIX D

Principal Investigators' and Advisors' Meeting Dates and Locations

January 13, 1998—St. Louis, Mo.
March 2, 1998—Washington, D.C.
April 16, 1998—Washington, D.C. (Workshop)
May 6, 1998—Washington, D.C.
July 14–15, 1998—Washington, D.C. (Workshop)
October 1–2, 1998—Washington, D.C. (Workshop)
January 13–14, 1999—Washington, D.C. (Workshop)
March 23–24, 1999—Washington, D.C. (Workshop)
May 5–6, 1999—Woods Hole, Mass.

APPENDIX E

Workshop Agendas

WORKSHOP I—APRIL 16, 1998
Mirage Room I, Holiday Inn Georgetown

AGENDA

8:15 **Introduction of the Study and the Purpose of the Workshop**
Philip Russell, M.D.
Johns Hopkins School of Public Health
Samuel Guze, M.D.
Washington University

8:30 **Force Medical Protection**
LTC Tom Clines, USA
Medical Readiness Division
The Joint Staff, J-4

8:45 **Health Enrollment Assessment Review (HEAR)**
Maj Vincent Fonseca, USAF, MC
Office for Prevention and Health Service Assessment

9:05 **Pre- and Postdeployment Questionnaires**
Maj Sheila Kinty, USAF, BSC
Director, Deployment Surveillance Team

9:20 **Proposed Recruit Assessment Program**
CAPT Craig Hyams, MC, USN
Naval Medical Research Institute
Frances Murphy, M.D., M.P.H.
Department of Veterans Affairs

9:40 **Break**

9:50 **Global Epidemiologic Tracking System**
Maj Kevin Hall, USAF, MC
Office of the Command Surgeon, Langley AFB

10:05 **Current Deployment Surveillance Practices in Bosnia and SW Asia**
LTC(P) Robert F. DeFraites, MC, USA
Office of the Army Surgeon General

10:35 **DMSS/DMED and Progress Toward Integrated Medical Surveillance**
John F. Brundage, M.D., M.P.H., (COL, Ret.)
Henry M. Jackson Foundation

11:00 **Break**

11:10 **Panel Discussion on Medical Surveillance Issues**

LTC Catherine Bonnefil, AN, USA
USACHPPM

John F. Brundage, M.D., M.P.H., (COL, Ret)
Henry Jackson Foundation

LTC Tom Clines, USA
J-4, Medical Readiness Division

LTC(P) Robert F. DeFraites, MC, USA
Office of the Army Surgeon General

Maj Vincent Fonseca, USAF, MC
Ofc. for Prevention and Health Svc. Assessment

Maj Kevin Hall, USAF, MC
Ofc. of the Command Surgeon, Langley AFB

Capt Samuel Hall, USAF, BSC
Ofc. for Prevention and Health Svc. Assessment

CDR Kevin R. Hanson, MC, USN
USUHS-PMB

CAPT Craig Hyams, MC, USN
NMRI

COL Bruce H. Jones, MC, USA
USACHPPM

LTC(P) Patrick W. Kelley, MC, USA
WRAIR

Maj Sheila Kinty, USAF, BSC
Clinical Business Area/CHCSII

Frances Murphy, M.D., M.P.H.
Department of Veterans Affairs

12:30 **Working Lunch—continuing discussion**

1:20 **Medical Recordkeeping-CHCS and CHCSII**
Col Lynn Ray, USAF, BSC
CHCS II Program Manager

1:40 **Medical Recordkeeping—CPR and GCPR**

Col Lynn Ray, USAF, BSC
CHCS II Program Manager

Robert Kolodner, M.D.
Department of Veterans Affairs

2:00 **Force Health Protection and the Portable Information Carrier**

Col Lynn Ray, USAF, BSC
CHCS II Program Manager

LTC Mark Lyford, USA
Theater Information Management Program

2:20 **Panel Discussion on Medical Recordkeeping Issues**

MAJ Catherine Beck, MS, USA
TATRC

Robert Kolodner, M.D.
Department of Veterans Affairs

Maj Kevin Hall, USAF, MC
Ofc. of the Command Surgeon, Langley AFB

LTC Mark Lyford, USA
Theatre Information Management Program

Col Lynn Ray, USAF, BSC
CHCS II Program Manager

3:15 **Open Portion of Meeting Adjourned**

WORKSHOP II—JULY 14–15, 1998

Mirage Room I, Holiday Inn Georgetown

AGENDA

8:15 **Introduction of the Study and the Purpose of the Workshop**

Samuel Guze, M.D.
Washington University

Philip Russell, M.D.
Johns Hopkins School of Public Health

I. What do we know about unexplained physical symptoms and how they might be prevented?

Unexplained Physical Symptoms in Primary Care and the Community: What Might We Learn for Prevention in the Military?
(presented July 15 for schedule conflict reasons)

8:30 **Medically Unexplained Symptoms in Survivors of Community Disasters**

Carol North, M.D.
Washington University

8:55 **Somatic and Psychosomatic Consequences of Technological Disasters**
Evelyn Bromet Ph.D.
SUNY Stony Brook

9:20 **War Syndromes and Their Evaluation**
CAPT Craig Hyams, MC, USN
Naval Medical Research Institute

9:45 **War Syndromes Since 1900: An Ongoing Study**
Dr. Edgar Jones
University of London

10:10 **Break**

10:20 **Relationship of Psychological Symptoms and Self-Reported Exposure to Gulf War Health Problems: Preliminary Findings**
Jessica Wolfe, Ph.D.
VA Medical Center, Boston

10:45 **The Prewar Health Care Seeking Patterns of Soldiers Who Develop Unexplained Illnesses**
Dick Miller, M.D.
Medical Follow-up Agency

11:00 **Current Early Testing Practices in the Military**
LTC Margot Krauss, MC, USA
Walter Reed Army Institute of Research

Dr. Imelda Idar
Office of Naval Training

CDR Glenna Tinney
Navy Bureau of Medicine and Surgery

12:00 **Stressful Events and Factors That Modify or Amplify Their Impact**
Bruce Dohrenwend Ph.D.
New York State Psychiatric Institute and Columbia University

12:30 **Working Lunch—provided**

1:15 **Can We Predict the Development of Medically Unexplained Illnesses? Psychological, Medical, and Public Policy Challenges**
Terry Keane, Ph.D.
VA Medical Center, Boston

1:40 **Summary from USUHS conference, *"Pathways, Dynamics, and Relationships Involved in the Somatic Consequences and Symptomatic Responses to Stress—The Directions of Future Research."***

Ann Norwood, M.D.
Uniformed Services University of the Health Sciences

II. Examining Opportunities for Prevention/Intervention in the Military Setting

A. Induction/Start of Basic Training

2:00 **Panel Discussion**

- What appears to be the epidemiology of unexplained symptoms?
- To what extent is it possible to identify people at high risk of developing unexplained illnesses?
- What screening tests might be appropriate for the military?
- How many people might be identified as at higher risk?
- What prevention efforts might be directed at those at higher risk?
- What additional data are needed?

3:00 **Break**

E. Tertiary Prevention-What is known about treatment?

3:15 **Multidisciplinary Treatment of Persistent Symptoms After Gulf War Service**
Charles Engel, Jr., M.D., M.P.H.
Walter Reed Army Medical Center
Uniformed Services University of the Health Sciences

3:35 **Treating Medically Unexplained Symptoms: The Real and Potential Contributions of Cognitive-Behavioral Therapy**
Arthur Nezu, Ph.D.
Allegheny University of the Health Sciences

3:55 **Treating Medically Unexplained Symptoms: Linking Physiologic Mechanisms to More Effective Treatments**
Daniel Clauw, M.D.
Georgetown University Medical Center

4:15 **Panel Discussion**

- What has been learned about tertiary prevention of unexplained symptoms?
- What additional research is needed?
- Are any additional methods of treatment being explored?

5:15 **Adjourn**

AGENDA CONTINUED
July 15, 1998

8:10 **Reintroduction to the Workshop, quick recap of July 14**
Dr. Samuel Guze

8:20 **Unexplained Physical Symptoms in Primary Care and the Community: What Might We Learn for Prevention in the Military?**
Wayne Katon, M.D.
University of Washington

8:45 **Host Neuroendocrine Factors in Susceptibility and Resistance to Inflammatory and Infectious Diseases: Implications for Unexplained Symptoms**
Esther Sternberg, M.D.
National Institute of Mental Health

9:10 **Neuroendocrinology of Stress and Related Pathophysiology**
George Chrousos, M.D.
National Institute of Child Health and Human Development

9:35 **Panel Discussion-Physiologic Measures**

- What implications do these presentations on the physiologic factors and unexplained illnesses provide for prevention in the military setting?
- What additional data are needed?

10:30 **Break**

II. Examining Opportunities for Prevention/Intervention in the Military Setting (continued)
B. Predeployment (Routinely or Immediate-Predeployment)

10:40 **Risk Communication**

What Are Current Risk Communication Practices in the Military, and What Is Known of Their Efficacy?
Kevin Delaney
U.S. Army Center for Health Promotion and Preventive Medicine

11:05 **What Does the Research on Informational Interventions to Reduce the Stress of Medical Procedures Tell Us About Communicating to Troops the Risks of Deployment?**
Jean Johnson Ph.D., R.N., F.A.A.N.
University of Rochester

11:30 **Communicating with Veterans Exposed to Depleted Uranium**
Kathleen McPhaul, M.P.H., R.N.
University of Maryland

11:55 **Panel Discussion-Risk Communication**

- What type and how much information would be helpful in communicating to troops the risks of deployment?
- What changes in risk communication methods are feasible within the deployment setting?
- What are current risk communication training procedures for commanders?
- What changes in communications from leaders are envisaged after hazardous exposures in future deployments?
- What additional data are needed?

12:40 **Working Lunch—continued discussion**

C. During Deployment

What Are Current Military Practices to Measure or Counteract Stress During Deployment?

1:15 **Combat Stress Teams**
COL James Stokes
Army Medical Department Center and School

1:40 **Measuring Operational Physical Signs of Stress**
MAJ Spencer Campbell
WRAIR

D. Redeployment (Return to U.S.)

2:05 **How Does the Military Currently Prepare Troops for Reintegration/Reunion?**

Army Practices
LTC James Jackson
Army Community Service

Navy Practices
CDR Glenna Tinney
Navy Bureau of Medicine and Surgery

2:35 **Panel Discussion-Prevention during and after deployment**

- Are current measures taken to prevent acute casualties also preventive for unexplained physical outcomes? Do any data exist to address this topic?
- What types of data are needed to better understand any relationship between stress during deployment and unexplained illnesses?
- What types of data are needed to better understand any relationship between reintegration difficulties and unexplained illnesses?
- What additional preventive measures might be explored?

3:20 **Break**

3:30 **Concluding Discussions-What Additional Issues Should Be Considered for Action or Research for Preventing Unexplained Symptoms in Deployed Populations?**

4:00 **Public Portion of Meeting Adjourned**
Start of closed meeting

5:00 **Adjourn**

WORKSHOP III—OCTOBER 1–2, 1998

Workshop on Medical Protection from Chemical and Biological Warfare Agents and Follow-Up Workshop on Medical Surveillance

Green Building, Washington, D.C.

AGENDA

8:00 **Introduction of the Study and the Purpose of the Workshop**

Philip Russell, M.D.	*Samuel Guze, M.D.*
Johns Hopkins School of Public Health	*Washington University*

8:15 **Medical Doctrine for NBC Threats**
Mr. Roy Flowers
Technical Publications Writer
AMEDD Center and School

8:45 **Medical Protection from Chemical Warfare Agents**
COL James Little
Commander, U.S. Army Medical Research Institute of Chemical Defense

9:15 **Discussion of Medical Doctrine and Protection from CW**

10:00 **Break**

Medical Protection from Biological Warfare Agents

10:15 **Threat, Training, and Treatment**
COL Gerald Parker
Commander, U.S. Army Medical Research Institute of Infectious Disease

10:45 **Medical Product Development**
LTC Robert Borowski
Deputy Program Manager for Medical Systems
Joint Program Office for Biological Defense

11:15 **Policy Development for Vaccine Use**
Major General John Parker
Commander, U.S. Army Medical Research and Materiel Command

Discussion of Medical Doctrine and Protection from BW

12:30 **Working Lunch-continuing discussion**

After Lunch-Medical Surveillance Portion of Agenda

1:30 **Presentation of Paper on Medical Surveillance in the Military (follow-up to IOM Workshop held April 16, 1998)**
Lee H. Harrison, M.D.
University of Pittsburgh
Robert Pinner, M.D.
Centers for Disease Control and Prevention

Panel Discussion of Medical Surveillance Issues

3:00 **Break**

3:15 **Continued Discussion of Medical Surveillance Issues**
Surveillance Systems and Illness Registries After Future Deployments

5:00 **Adjourn**

AGENDA CONTINUED
Friday, October 2

8:30 **Improving the Denominators for Medical Surveillance**
Norma St. Claire
Director, Joint Requirements and Integration
Office of the Secretary of Defense for Personnel and Readiness

Questions and Discussion

9:30 **How Well Is Surveillance and Record Keeping Taking Place with the Administration of the Anthrax Vaccine?**
LTC Randy Randolph
DOD Anthrax Program
Office of the Army Surgeon General

Questions and Discussion

10:30 **Open Meeting Adjourned**

WORKSHOP IV—JANUARY 13–14, 1999
The Cecil and Ida Green Building, Washington, D.C.

AGENDA

8:00 **Introduction of the Study and the Purpose of the Workshop**
Samuel Guze, M.D.
Washington University
Philip Russell, M.D.
Johns Hopkins School of Public Health

8:05 **Medical Record Keeping—Update on Progress**

GCPR
Robert Kolodner, M.D.
Department of Veterans Affairs
Maureen Coyle
Department of Veterans Affairs

CHCSII and PIC
Col Deborah Page
Director, Force Health Protection
CHCS II Program Office

9:00 **Paper Presentation:**
Clement McDonald, M.D.
Regenstrief Institute for Health Care
Edward Hammond, Ph.D.
Duke University Medical Center

9:45 **Discussion**

11:15 **Break**

11:30 **Medical Recordkeeping as Described in, "A National Obligation: Planning for Health Preparedness for and Readjustment of the Military, Veterans, and Their Families After Future Deployments"**
LTC Mary Ann Morreale
Military Health System Technology Interagency Sharing
Office of the Assistant Secretary of Defense for Health Affairs

12:15 **Lunch**

1:00 **Reserve Issues**

Background, Medical Surveillance, and Health Care
Mr. Dan Kohner
CAPT Sheila Brackett
Col Kathleen Woody
Office of the Assistant Secretary of Defense for Reserve Affairs

Reintegration of Reserve Component Members into the Home Environment upon Redeployment
LTC Jane Meyer
Office of the Assistant Secretary of Defense for Reserve Affairs

Discussion

3:00 **Break**

3:15 **Preventing Medically Unexplained Physical Symptoms**
Paper Presentation: Unexplained Physical Symptoms in Primary Care and the Community: What Might We Learn for Prevention in the Military?
LTC Charles C. Engel, Jr., M.D., M.P.H.
Walter Reed Army Medical Center
Uniformed Services University

Paper Presentation: Can We Predict the Development of Medically Unexplained Illnesses? Psychological, Medical, and Public Policy Challenges
Terry Keane, Ph.D.
VA Medical Center, Boston

Discussion of Possibilities for Prevention

5:30 **Adjourn for the day**

AGENDA CONTINUED
Thursday, January 14, 1999

8:30 **Discussion of "A National Obligation: Planning for Health Preparedness for and Readjustment of the Military, Veterans, and Their Families After Future Deployments"**

Research
Dr. Tim Gerrity
Special Assistant to Chief Research and Development Officer
Department of Veterans Affairs

Discussion

9:00 **Deployment Health**
CAPT David Trump
Program Director, Preventive Medicine and Surveillance
Office of the Assistant Secretary of Defense for Health Affairs

Discussion

9:30 **Risk Communication**
Dr. Max Lum
Director, Office of Health Communications
National Institute of Occupational Safety and Health

Implementation of Risk Communication Changes Within the Military
Input from: *Kevin Delaney*
Risk Communication Team
Center for Health Promotion and Preventive Medicine
(unable to attend due to inclement weather)

Lt Col Steve Williams
Office of the Special Assistant for Gulf War Illnesses

Discussion

10:45 **Break**

11:00 **Accession Standards**
Col Michael Ostroski
Directorate for Accession Policy

Retention Standards
Ms. Tina Wortzel
Office of the Army Surgeon General

12:00 **Lunch**

12:45 **Role of Laboratories in Military Public Health Surveillance**
COL Patrick Kelley
Walter Reed Army Institute of Research

COL James Bolton
U.S. Army Medical Command

1:45 **End of open portion of meeting**

"REALITY CHECK" MEETING—MARCH 23–24, 1999

The Cecil and Ida Green Building, Washington, D.C.

AGENDA

8:00 **Introduction of the Study and the Purpose of the Meeting**
Philip Russell, M.D.
Johns Hopkins School of Public Health
Samuel Guze, M.D.
Washington University

Introductions of Meeting Participants

8:30 **Brief Review of Bosnia and SWA Morbidity Data**
COL Jose Sanchez-Bosnia
Lt Col Don Thompson-SWA

9:15 **CENTCOM Perspective on Deployment Surveillance**
Col Bruce Green, CENTCOM/SG

9:30 **Discussion of Pre-Deployment Preventive Medicine and Protective Measures**
What has been the experience in Bosnia, SW Asia, or other recent deployments for:
- pre-deployment questionnaires
- risk communication issues
- degree of automation
- psychological factors

10:30 **Break**

10:45 **Preventive Medicine and Protective Measures During Deployment**
- medical surveillance—through weekly DNBI and other means
- medical record keeping—degree of automation and other issues
- risk communication

- psychological factors
- vaccination/prophylactic drugs

12:15 **Working Lunch—Continued Discussion**

1:00 **Preventive Medicine and Protective Measures Following Return from Deployment**

- post-deployment questionnaires and follow-up
- post-deployment serum draws
- health surveillance following deployment
- risk communication
- reintegration issues

2:30 **Break**

2:45 **General Issues in Preventive Medicine and Risk Reduction for Deployed Forces**

- buy-in of line commanders
- medical record keeping—logistics of data collection
- medically unexplained physical symptoms
- interaction of PM and mental health docs/caregivers
- risk communication

4:15 **Summary Comments and Suggestions from Military Participants**

4:45 **Adjourn**

AGENDA CONTINUED
March 24, 1999

At Skyline Buildings in Northern Virginia

8:00 **Demonstration of Public Health Care Application (PHCA)**

9:30 **Briefing by Office of Information Management for the Military Health System**
Mr. James Reardon
Director, Information Management, Technology, and Reengineering

10:30 **Adjourn Open Session**

APPENDIX F

Commissioned Papers

Unexplained Physical Symptoms in Primary Care and the Community: What Might We Learn for Prevention in the Military? (June 1999)

LTC Charles Engel, M.D., M.P.H.
Medical Corps, U.S. Army
Chief, Gulf War Health Center
Walter Reed Army Medical Center

Wayne Katon, M.D.
Professor and Vice Chair
Department of Psychiatry and Behavioral Sciences
University of Washington Medical School

Medically Unexplained Symptoms After Community Disasters: A Review of the Literature (August 1998)

Carol North, M.D.
Associate Professor of Psychiatry
Washington University School of Medicine

Neuroendocrine Responses and Susceptibility and Resistance to Inflammatory and Infectious Diseases: Implications for Unexplained Symptoms (November 1998)

Esther Sternberg, M.D.
Chief, Section on Neuroendocrine Immunology and Behavior
National Institute of Mental Health
Bethesda, MD

Treating Medically Unexplained Symptoms: The Real and Potential Contributions of Cognitive-Behavior Therapy (July 1998)

Arthur Nezu, Ph.D.
Professor and Chair, Department of Clinical and Health Psychology
Associate Dean for Research, School of Health Professions
Allegheny University of the Health Sciences

What Does the Research on Informational Interventions to Reduce the Stress of Medical Procedures Tell Us About Communicating to Troops the Risks of Deployment? (July 1998)
Jean Johnson, Ph.D., R.N., F.A.A.N.
University of Rochester School of Nursing

Strategies to Protect the Health of U.S. Deployed Forces: Surveillance in the Military (September 1998)
Lee H. Harrison, M.D.
Associate Professor
Department of Epidemiology
University of Pittsburgh

Robert Pinner, M.D.
Special Assistant for Surveillance
Office of the Director
National Center for Infectious Diseases
Centers for Disease Control and Prevention
Atlanta

Role of Registries after Military Deployments (June 1998)
Arthur K. McDonald
Director, Division of Hazard and Injury Data Systems
U.S. Consumer Product Safety Commission
Washington, DC

Paper on the G-CPR Project (December 1998)
W. Edward Hammond, Ph.D.
Professor, Division of Medical Informatics
Duke University Medical Center

Review of the GCPR Project for the Institute of Medicine (December 1998)
Clement J. McDonald, M.D.
Distinguished Professor of Medicine
Regenstrief Institute for Health Care

APPENDIX G

Acknowledgments

The study team is grateful to the following individuals who provided information and assistance to the project through presentations at meetings and workshops, technical review, or other means.

Robert Alonso
1st Marine Division
Camp Pendleton, Calif.

Nancy Bakalar
Office of the Assistant Secretary of Defense (Health Affairs)

Jane Banard
U.S. Army Reserve Command

Courtney Banks
Office of the Special Assistant for Gulf War Illnesses

Natalie Bassett
Air Force Reserve

Catherine Beck
U.S. Army Medical Research and Materiel Command

Robert (Todd) Bennett
ADAPT Program
Mountain Home AFB, Id.

Linza Bethea
U.S. Indian Health Service (Uniband)

James Bolton
U.S. Army Medical Command

Catherine Bonnefil
U.S. Army Center for Health Promotion and Preventive Medicine

Robert Borowski
Joint Program Office for Biological Defense

Sheila Brackett
Office of the Assistant Secretary of Defense for Reserve Affairs

Dana Bradshaw
Air Force Medical Operations

Kelley Brix
SRA International, Inc.

Evelyn Bromet
SUNY Stony Brook

John Brundage
Henry M. Jackson Foundation

Spencer Campbell
Walter Reed Army Institute of Research

Tom Cardella
Office of the Special Assistant for Gulf War Illnesses

Suzanne Chiang
Office of the Assistant Secretary of Defense (Health Affairs)

Gary Christopherson
Office of the Assistant Secretary of Defense (Health Affairs)

George Chrousos
National Institute of Child Health and Human Development

Kathryn Clark
Walter Reed Army Institute of Research

Tom Clines
Medical Readiness, The Joint Staff

Daniel Clauw
Georgetown University Medical Center

David Conner
Navy Personnel Command

David Cowan
Exponent Health Group

Michael Cowan
Medical Readiness, The Joint Staff

Angela Coyle
11th Wing Personnel and Family Readiness
NCO-Family Readiness Program
11th Mission Support Squadron/ DPF

Maureen Coyle
U.S. Department of Veterans Affairs

Stephen Craig
U.S. Army Center for Health Promotion and Preventive Medicine

Samar DeBakey
Birch & Davis Associates, Inc.

Robert DeFraites
U.S. Army Center for Health Promotion and Disease Prevention

Kevin Delaney
U.S. Army Center for Health Promotion and Preventive Medicine

Benedict Diniega
Office of the Army Surgeon General

Bruce Dohrenwend
New York State Psychiatric Institute and Columbia University

Mike Dove
Defense Manpower Data Center

David Edman
Persian Gulf Veterans Coordinating Board

Debbie Eitelberg
Defense Manpower Data Center

Charles Engel, Jr.
Walter Reed Army Medical Center
Uniformed Services University of the Health Sciences

Charles Figley
Florida State University

Roy Flowers
Army Medical Department Center and School

Len Fogelsonger
Birch & Davis Associates, Inc.

Vincent Fonseca
U.S. Air Force Office for Prevention and Health Service Assessment

Jeffrey Gambel
Walter Reed Army Medical Center

Hank Gardner
U.S. Army Center for Environmental Health Research

Joel Gaydos
Henry M. Jackson Foundation

Tim Gerrity
U.S. Department of Veterans Affairs

John Graham
British Liaison Office

Ollie Gray
PKC Corporation

Bruce Green
Central Command

Kevin Hall
Office of the Command Surgeon
Langley AFB

Samuel Hall
U.S. Air Force Office for Prevention and Health Service Assessment

Edward Hammond
Duke University Medical Center

Kevin Hanson
Uniformed Services University of Health Sciences

Lee Harrison
University of Pittsburgh

Konrad Hayashi
United States Atlantic Fleet

Harry Holloway
Uniformed Services University of the Health Sciences

Elizabeth Holmes
Uniformed Services University of the Health Sciences

Craig Hyams
Naval Medical Research Institute

Imelda Idar
Office of Naval Training

James Jackson
U.S. Army Community and Family Support Center

Jean Johnson
University of Rochester

Bruce Jones
U.S. Army Center for Health Promotion and Preventive Medicine

Edgar Jones
University of London

Dale Kasab
Birch & Davis Associates, Inc.

Wayne Katon
University of Washington

Terry Keane
Veterans Affairs Medical Center, Boston

Patrick Kelley
Walter Reed Army Institute of Research

Douglas Kempf
Naval Medical Center

Michael Kilpatrick
Office of the Special Assistant for Gulf War Illnesses

Sheila Kinty
U.S. Department of Defense
Deployment Surveillance Team

Dan Kohner
Office of the Assistant Secretary of Defense for Reserve Affairs

Robert Kolodner
U.S. Department of Veterans Affairs

Mark Kortepeter
U.S. Army Medical Research Institute for Infectious Diseases

Margot Krauss
Walter Reed Army Institute of Research

James LaMar
II Marine Expeditionary Force
Camp Lejeune, N.C.

Robert Landry
U.S. Army Medical Command

James Little
U.S. Army Medical Research Institute of Chemical Defense

Max Lum
National Institute of Occupational Safety and Health

Mark Lyford
Theater Medical Information Program

Gina Marchi
Defense Manpower Data Center

David Marlowe
Uniformed Services University of the Health Sciences

John Mateczun
U.S. Naval Hospital, Charleston, S.C.

Wayne McBride
Navy Bureau of Medicine and Surgery

Arthur McDonald
U.S. Consumer Product Safety Commission

Clement McDonald
Regenstrief Institute for Health Care

Kelly McKee
U.S. Army Medical Research Institute of Infectious Diseases

Brian McMaster
Birch and Davis Associates, Inc.

Kathleen McPhaul
University of Maryland

Barbara Melamed
Yeshiva University

Jane Meyer
Office of the Assistant Secretary of Defense (Health Affairs)

Mary Meyer
FDA Center for Biologics Evaluation and Research

Mary Ann Morreale
Office of the Assistant Secretary of Defense (Health Affairs)

Thomas Mundie
U.S. Military Academy

Frances Murphy
U.S. Department of Veterans Affairs

Arthur Nezu
Allegheny University of the Health Sciences

Carol North
Washington University School of Medicine

Ann Norwood
Uniformed Services University of the Health Sciences

Frank O'Donnell
Office of the Special Assistant for Gulf War Illnesses

Dorothy Ogilvy-Lee
National Guard Bureau

Michael Ostroski
Directorate for Accession Policy

Lynn Pahland
Office of the Assistant Secretary of Defense (Health Affairs)

Deborah Page
CHCS II Program Office

Gerald Parker
U.S. Army Medical Research Institute of Infectious Disease

John Parker
U.S. Army Medical Research and Materiel Command

Jane Parsons
U.S. Department of Veterans Affairs

Noel Perry
Defense Manpower Data Center

Lizette Peterson
University of Missouri

Robert Pinner
Centers for Disease Control and Prevention

Matthew Puglisi
American Legion

Randy Randolph
Office of the Army Surgeon General

Bill Ray
Navy Personnel Command

Lynn Ray
CHCS II Program Manager

James Reardon
Chief Information Officer, Military Health System

William Rice
Uniformed Services University of the Health Sciences

James Riddle
Office of the Assistant Secretary of Defense (Health Affairs)

Pedro Riviera
PKC Corporation

Mark Rubertone
U.S. Army Center for Health Promotion and Preventive Medicine

Bruce Ruscio
U.S. Army Center for Health Promotion and Preventive Medicine

José Sánchez
U.S. Army Center for Health Promotion and Preventive Medicine

Scott Sherman
I Marine Expeditionary Force

Norma St. Claire
Office of the Secretary of Defense for Personnel and Readiness

Esther Sternberg
National Institute of Mental Health

James Stokes
Army Medical Department Center and School

Cathy Stokoe
Naval Family Service Center

Theresa Thibodeau
ACS Government Solutions

Donald Thompson
Force Health Protection and Surveillance Branch
Brooks Air Force Base, Tex.

Robert Thompson
Medical Readiness, The Joint Staff

Paul Tibbets
Military Health System Information Technology

Glenna Tinney
Navy Bureau of Medicine and Surgery

Roberto Torres, Jr.
Office of the Special Assistant for Gulf War Illnesses

David Trump
Office of the Assistant Secretary of Defense (Health Affairs)

Janet Viola
1984th Reserve Hospital
Tripler Army Medical Center
Suburban Pavillion
Cleveland, Ohio

Steve Williams
Office of the Special Assistant for Gulf War Illnesses

John Wilson
University of Kentucky

Jessica Wolfe
Veterans Affairs Medical Center, Boston

Kathleen Woody
Office of the Assistant Secretary of Defense for Reserve Affairs

Tina Wortzel
Office of the Army Surgeon General

APPENDIX H

Department of Defense Directive 6490.2: Joint Medical Surveillance

---

Available on line at: **www.amsa.army.mil.**

Department of Defense
DIRECTIVE

August 30, 1997
NUMBER 6490.2

SUBJECT: Joint Medical Surveillance

References: (a) DoD Directive 5136.1, "Assistant Secretary of Defense for Health Affairs," May 27, 1994
(b) DoD Directive 4715.1, "Environmental Security," February 24, 1996
(c) DoD Directive 1332.18, "Separation or Retirement for Physical Disability," November 4, 1996
(d) DoD Instruction 1400.32, "DoD Civilian Work Force Contingency and Emergency Planning Guidelines and Procedures," April 24, 1995
(e) through (h), see enclosure 1

A. PURPOSE

This Directive:

1. Establishes policy and assigns responsibility, under references (a) and (b), for routine joint medical surveillance of all Military Service members during active Federal service, especially military deployments.

2. Designates the Secretary of the Army as the DoD Executive Agent for the medical surveillance for deployments for the Department of Defense and for the maintenance of the Armed Forces Serum Repository consistent with this Directive.

B. APPLICABILITY AND SCOPE

This Directive:

1. Applies to the Office of the Secretary of Defense, the Military Departments, the Chairman of the Joint Chiefs of Staff, the Combatant Commands, the Defense Agencies, and the DoD Field Activities (hereafter referred to collectively as "the DoD Components"). The term "Military Service" as used herein, refers to the Army, the Navy, the Air Force, and the Marine Corps.

2. Encompasses all aspects of military preventive medicine under reference (b) that pertain to medical surveillance for major deployments identified by the Chairman of the Joint Chiefs of Staff in coordination with the Assistant Secretary of Defense for Health Affairs (ASD(HA)). Personnel attached to joint forces during deployments, such as members of the Coast Guard when it is operating as a Military Service in the Navy, will be included in the surveillance system. Technical representatives are not included.

C. DEFINITIONS

1. *Medical Surveillance* . The regular or repeated collection, analysis, and dissemination

of uniform health information for monitoring the health of a population, and intervening in a timely manner when necessary. It is defined by the Centers for Disease Control and Prevention as the ongoing, systematic collection, analysis, and interpretation of health data essential to the planning, implementation, and evaluation of public health practice, closely integrated with the timely dissemination of these data to those who need to know. The final link of a military medical surveillance system is the application of these data to military training, plans and operations to prepare and implement early intervention and control strategies. A surveillance system includes a functional capacity for data collection, analysis and dissemination of information linked to military preventive medicine support of operational commanders.

2. *Military Preventive Medicine* . The anticipation, prediction, identification, prevention, and control of communicable diseases (including vector-, food- and water-borne diseases), illnesses, injuries and diseases due to exposure to occupational and environmental threats, including non-battle injury threats, combat stress responses, and other threats to the health and readiness of military personnel and military units, including such fields as epidemiology, clinical preventive medicine, medical entomology, occupational medicine, industrial hygiene, environmental health sciences and engineering, health promotion and wellness, community health, mental health disciplines, and toxicology and laboratory support sciences (environmental, occupational and radiological chemistry and microbiology) and risk communication.

3. *Risk Communication* . A process used to discuss risks, their impacts and how they should be communicated. Risks and their management decisions must be credibly communicated to help ensure that messages are constructively formulated, transmitted and received in a meaningful manner.

D. POLICY

It is DoD policy under DoD Directive 1332.18 (reference (c)) that:

1. All Service members, Active, National Guard and Ready Reserve be physically and mentally fit to carry out their missions.

2. Medical and personnel information systems be designed, integrated and utilized compatible with military medical surveillance to maintain, assess, and protect the physical and mental health of Service members throughout their Military Service.

3. Such systems be continuously in effect throughout the Service member's period of Military Service and be specifically configured to assess the effects of deployment on the health of Service members.

4. Before and during deployment, Service members be made aware of significant health threats and corresponding medical prophylaxis, immunization and other unit and individual countermeasures for the Area of Operations. Commanders shall provide their personnel the appropriate medical support and training, equipment and supplies to implement unit and individual countermeasures. Once deployed, personnel shall be provided updates to health threats and countermeasures based upon need and situations encountered.

5. Medical surveillance shall encompass the periods before, during, and after deployment:

    a. To monitor environmental, occupational and epidemiological threats and diverse stressors;

b. To assess disease and non-battle injuries, stress-induced casualties, and combat casualties, including those produced by chemical and biological and nuclear weapons; and,

c. To reinforce command directed and individual preventive countermeasures and the provision of optimal medical care during and after deployment.

6. Commanders shall be kept informed before, during and after deployment of the health of the force, health threats, stressors, risks, and available countermeasures.

7. There shall be a serum repository for medical surveillance for clinical diagnosis and epidemiologic studies. The repository shall be used exclusively for the identification, prevention and control of diseases associated with operational deployments of military personnel.

8. The DoD Components conduct comprehensive, continuous and consistent medical surveillance to implement early intervention and control strategies using joint technologies, practices and procedures before, during, and after deployments in a manner consistent across the Military Services.

9. To the extent applicable, medical surveillance activities will include essential DoD civilian and contractor personnel directly supporting deployed forces, consistent with plans established under DoD Instructions 1400.32 and 3020.37 (references (d) and (e)).

10. The serum repository operated pursuant to subsection D. 7. (above) and other systems of records pursuant to this Directive shall comply with all requirements of the Privacy Act, under DoD Directive 5400.7 (reference (f)).

E. **RESPONSIBILITIES**

1. The *Assistant Secretary of Defense for Health Affairs* , under the *Under Secretary of Defense for Personnel and Readiness* , shall have overall responsibility for joint medical surveillance, shall issue Instructions as necessary to implement the policies of this Directive, and shall monitor the implementation of this Directive and implementing Instructions.

2. The *Assistant Secretary of Defense for Reserve Affairs,* under the *Under Secretary of Defense for Personnel and Readiness,* shall ensure that policies for health surveillance for the Ready Reserve are consistent with the policies established for the active component.

3. The *Secretaries of the Military Departments* shall:

   a. Ensure compliance with this Directive and implementing Instructions; and

   b. Evaluate and recommend changes or improvements to the overall medical surveillance program to the Secretary of Defense through the ASD(HA).

4. The *Chairman of the Joint Chiefs of Staff* , in consultation with the Commanders of the Combatant Commands and the Chiefs of Staff of the Military Services, shall monitor the implementation of the policies of this Directive and implementing Instructions.

5. The *Commanders of the Combatant Commands,* with the coordination of the Chairman

of the Joints Chiefs of Staff, shall ensure that the policies of this Directive and implementing Instructions, including DoD Instruction 6490.3 (reference (g)) are executed during all operations.

6. The *Assistant Secretary of Defense for Command, Control, Communication and Intelligence* shall ensure that the Director, Defense Intelligence Agency, through the Armed Forces Medical Intelligence Center, under DoD Directive 6420.1 (reference (h)), shall provide information for use in health threat assessments for medical surveillance purposes.

7. The *Secretary of the Army* shall serve all of the Department of Defense for medical surveillance for deployments consistent with this Directive. As Executive Agent, the Army shall provide the work force located at the Armed Forces Serum Repository at the U.S. Army Center for Health Promotion and Preventive Medicine (USACHPPM). Funding shall be provided through the centralized Defense Health Program. Although no routine reporting is required, periodic epidemiological studies at the USACHPPM shall include analysis of data derived from the Armed Forces Serum Repository.

F. EFFECTIVE DATE

This Directive is effective immediately.

John J. Hamre
Deputy Secretary of Defense

Enclosure
References

REFERENCES, continued

(e) DoD Instruction 3020.37, "Continuation of Essential DoD Contractor Services During Crises," November 6, 1990
(f) DoD Directive 5400.7, "DoD Freedom of Information Act Program," May 13, 1988
(g) DoD Instruction 6490.3, "Implementation and Application of Joint Medical Surveillance for Deployments," August 7, 1997
(h) DoD Directive 6420.1, "Armed Forces Medical Intelligence Center, (AFMIC)," September 30, 1996

[Top]
Last update: 9/18/1998

APPENDIX I

Department of Defense Instruction 6490.3 Implementation and Application of Joint Medical Surveillance for Deployments

---

Available on line at: **www.amsa.army.mil.**

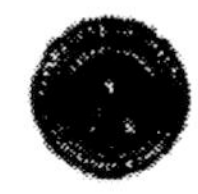

Department of Defense
INSTRUCTION

August 7, 1997
NUMBER 6490.3

SUBJECT: Implementation and Application of Joint Medical Surveillance for Deployments

References: (a) DoD Directive 6490.2, "Joint Medical Surveillance," August 30, 1997
(b) DoD Directive 5400.7, "DoD Freedom of Information Act Program," May 13, 1988
(c) Joint Staff Memorandum J-4A 00106-93, "Medical Surveillance Report," January 28, 1993
(d) Title 32, Code of Federal Regulations, Part 219, "Protection of Human Subjects," January 1, 1996
(e) through (g), see enclosure 1

A. PURPOSE

This Instruction:

1. Implements policy, prescribes procedures, and assigns responsibilities under reference (a) for joint military medical surveillance in support of all applicable military operations. Medical surveillance of all Military Service members during active Federal service, including Reserve components, especially before, during and after military deployments, is mandated. The identification of health threats and the routine, uniform collection, analysis, and rapid dissemination of information relevant to troop health has proven of inestimable value in recent operations. The intent of this Instruction is to expand the concept of joint deployment medical surveillance to a more comprehensive approach to monitoring and assessing health consequences related to participation of Service members in deployments.

2. Describes routine military medical surveillance activities during major deployments, or for deployments in which there is a significant risk of health problems, as identified by the Chairman of the Joint Chiefs of Staff in coordination with the Assistant Secretary of Defense for Health Affairs (ASD(HA)).

B. APPLICABILITY AND SCOPE

This Instruction:

1. Applies to the Office of the Secretary of Defense (OSD), the Military Departments, the Chairman of the Joint Chiefs of Staff, the Combatant Commands, the Defense Agencies, and the DoD Field Activities (hereafter referred to collectively as "the DoD Components"). The term "Military Service" as used herein, refers to the Army, the Navy, the Air Force, and the Marine Corps. Personnel attached to joint forces during deployments, such as members of the Coast Guard when it is operating as a Military Service in the Navy, will be included in the military medical surveillance system. Technical representatives are not included.

2. Encompasses all aspects of a joint medical surveillance program that is operated in the context of a full military preventive medicine program for the collection and analysis of health status and threat information supporting military operations during the full cycle of pre-deployment, deployment, employment and post-deployment activities.

3. Aside from emphasizing the development of automated recordkeeping and linkage of personnel and medical databases, preserves the value of timely collection, analysis, and dissemination of information to guide public health policy and practice using those collection methods available and appropriate for the operational situation.

C. **DEFINITIONS**

Terms used in this Instruction are defined in enclosure 2.

D. **POLICY**

It is DoD policy under DoD Directive 6490.2 (reference (a))that:

1. The Military Departments shall conduct joint comprehensive medical surveillance. Medical surveillance is essential to ensure a fit and healthy force and to prevent illness, disease, adverse stress responses, and injuries from degrading mission effectiveness and warfighting capabilities. These activities shall be in effect continuously for individual Service members throughout their entire period of military service in a manner consistent across the DoD active and reserve Components. Although wide-ranging in scope, some of the most significant surveillance activities can be categorized according to before, during, and after deployment phases of military operations. (See enclosure 3, table 1.)

2. The military surveillance process shall be configured to assess the effects of deployment on the health of Service members. Medical surveillance records, including the Armed Forces Serum Repository, shall be maintained in accordance with DoD Directive 5400.7 (reference (b)).

3. Medical surveillance is the continuous responsibility of the DoD Components for their individual Service members. During a deployment, this responsibility becomes shared with the joint task force (JTF) commander and the commander in chief (CINC) of the appropriate Combatant Command.

E. **RESPONSIBILITIES**

1. The *Assistant Secretary of Defense for Health Affairs* , under the *Under Secretary of Defense for Personnel and Readiness* , shall monitor the implementation of this Instruction and reference (a).

2. The *Assistant Secretary of Defense for Reserve Affairs* , under the *Under Secretary of Defense for Personnel and Readiness* , shall ensure that policies for Health Surveillance of the Ready Reserve are consistent with the policies established for the active component.

3. The *Deputy Under Secretary of Defense for Program Integration,* under the *Under Secretary of Defense for Personnel and Readiness* , shall track deployed personnel by developing and maintaining databases that are compatible with pertinent medical surveillance databases.

4. The *Chairman of the Joint Chiefs of Staff* , in consultation with the Commanders of the Combatant Commands and the Chiefs of Staff of the Military Services, shall monitor the implementation of the policies of this Instruction.

5. The *Commanders of the Combatant Commands* , with the coordination of the Chairman of the Joint Chiefs of Staff, shall ensure that the policies of this Instruction are executed during all applicable operations.

6. The *Secretaries of each Military Department* , in coordination with the other Military Departments, shall ensure compliance with this Instruction and evaluate and recommend changes or improvements to the overall medical surveillance program to the Secretary of Defense through the ASD(HA).

7. The *Secretary of the Army* shall ensure that the U.S. Army Center for Health Promotion and Preventive Medicine (USACHPPM) shall operate and maintain a repository of serum samples for medical surveillance. The DoD Serum Repository shall be subject to the rules and procedures to protect privacy interests of members and ensure exclusive use of specimens for the identification, prevention, and control of injuries and diseases associated with military operations. USACHPPM will also maintain a medical surveillance system to integrate, analyze, and report data from multiple sources relevant to the health and readiness of military personnel.

F. **PROCEDURES**

1. *General* . The routine determination of unit-specific rates of illnesses and injuries of public health significance is the foundation for any medical surveillance program. Categories of illness and injury described in the Joint Staff Memorandum J-4A 00106-93 (reference (c)) have been used in recent operations and provide a framework for the collection of morbidity data. In the future, several new systems and procedures will be required to initiate a comprehensive medical surveillance program for monitoring mental and physical health status, the occurrence of illness, injury, and disease as well as the identification and assessment of potential hazards and actual exposures to environmental contaminants and stressors. Innovative technology shall be used, such as an automated medical record device for documenting field and fixed-facility patient encounters (inpatient and outpatient) that can archive the information for local recall and format it for an injury, illness, and exposure surveillance database. Included, as innovative technologies to be developed and used, will be better inpatient and outpatient electronic medical records; devices, systems, and procedures to monitor mental and physical health status, devices, systems, and procedures to identify and assess potential hazards and evaluate and document actual exposures; and the electronic transmission and fusion of medical surveillance data to produce the minimum information for command and medical decisions in near-real time. Surveillance information shall be made available in a timely fashion to JTF surgeons and field medical facilities and shall be transmitted to central data repositories. Devices used and the format of data collected shall be compatible with the medical data system used by fixed-facility units. A geographical information system shall be used to conduct the necessary spatial analyses of environmental and disease exposures of company-sized and larger units, and shall be capable of being linked to individual Service members' medical records. Any research activities conducted as part of medical surveillance shall be consistent with 32 CFR 219 (reference (d)). To the extent applicable, military medical surveillance will include essential DoD civilian and contractor personnel directly supporting deployed forces, consistent with plans established under DoD Instructions 3020.37 and 1400.32 (references (e) and (f)).

2. Pre-deployment (Baseline Readiness)

a. The ASD(HA), under the Under Secretary for Personnel and Readiness, shall:

(1) Field, through DoD Executive Agents, DoD medical data systems that provide uniform data fields allowing the consistent capture of personnel identifiers, health profile and/or status, diagnoses and other outcomes, combat or operational stress briefings; and other preventive measures (including immunizations and prophylaxis), disposition, and disability. Exposure data systems shall include geographical, environmental and occupational information. Centralized repository (ies) of these preventive medical and exposure data will be established. These data bases will be linked through shared data fields. Examples of systems include but are not limited to the Composite Health Care System, Geographical Information Systems, Comprehensive Clinical Evaluation Program, Defense Occupational Health Readiness System (DOHRS), health risk appraisal systems, and other military inpatient and outpatient data tracking systems. These systems shall be used on deployments and in the garrison or non-deployment setting, be compatible among the DoD Components and eventually be capable of linking deployment and non-deployment environmental and occupational exposure and health hazard and/or health risk assessments to individual medical records and medical outcome databases. Automation of routine medical data collection will be necessary for the full development of these systems.

(2) Charter a Joint Preventive Medicine Policy Group (JPMPG) to:

(a) Draft recommendations for joint policy on preventive medicine and health promotion issues and staffing and equipment requirements related to the three principal preventive medicine functions of assessing the health threat, identifying and recommending preventive countermeasures to include immunizations and stress briefings, and conducting medical surveillance.

(b) Develop uniform preventive medicine policies and educational materials.

(c) Serve as an information and coordination exchange among the Military Departments' preventive medicine leadership.

(d) Monitor operational and organizational changes within the Services to assess the ability to keep a joint force healthy.

(e) Advise the J-4 (Medical Readiness Division) on the content of the Preventive Medicine Appendix of the Medical Annex of Joint Operation Plans.

(f) Evaluate joint preventive medicine programs and policies.

(g) Recommend manpower and equipment needs for fully operational teams for epidemiological, and environmental and occupational exposure missions.

(h) Recommend research priorities relevant to military public health.

(i) In coordination with the Armed Forces Medical Intelligence Ce (AFMIC), reference develop and maintain country- or region-specific Armed Forces preventive medicine recommendations for joint operations. The group shall review and update these recommendations annually.

(3) CINC and/or JTF Surgeons shall identify and report illnesses, injuries,

and diseases of military significance during deployments and inform the cognizant JTF or Theater Commander concerning appropriate countermeasures. Support deployment data collection through the Deployment Surveillance Teamwhich will provide overprinted forms and/or requirements, aggregate the data and forward the database to the Deployment Surveillance Team analyst, United States Army Center for Health Promotion and Preventive Medicine (CHPPM). The DST, in collaboration with medical surveillance agencies in each Service, shall collect, analyze, report and archive data collected in Service-specific and Joint operations.

b. The Deputy Under Secretary of Defense for Program Integration, under the Under Secretary of Defense for Personnel and Readiness, shall collect and maintain individual Service member data, such as, dates of deployment, redeployment or evacuation, and unit of assignment while deployed.

c. The Military Services shall institute standard military medical surveillance systems capable of operation during all phases of military deployment cycles. They shall maintain records of personal medical readiness, to include levels of compliance, limitations of duty, immunizations, prophylaxis and examinations provided in preparation for deployment. They shall ensure that such records are protected in accordance with DoD Directive 5400.7 (reference (b)) and that appropriate disclosure accounting entries are made in such records.

d. The Military Services and the Commanders of the Combatant Commands, with the coordination of Chairman of the Joint Chiefs of Staff, shall:

(1) Integrate health promotion, medical surveillance, and the prevention of illness, non-battle injury and disease, to include combat stress in the training of individual Service members, in the training of military units, and in military exercises.

(2) Assure that troop commanders inform Service members about all potential health threats to include: illness, injuries, and disease, to include combat stress, climatic and other environmental health threats in the area of operations and emphasize preventive medicine countermeasures.

(3) Ensure that troops complete pre-deployment processing, including requirements pertaining to the Armed Forces Repository of Specimen Samples for the Identification of Remains.

(4) Conduct pre-deployment health screening assessments, which are documented on standardized forms for inclusion in individual medical r accordance with Service and Chairman of the Joint Chiefs of Staff direc These forms, at a minimum, shall include pertinent information as direc Office of the Assistant Secretary of Defense for Health Affairs. A copy of each form or an electronic data record generated during the health screening process shall be sent to the Deployment Surveillance Team. The health screening shall include a mental health assessment.

(5) Ensure that personnel support functions, such as family advocacy services and combat stress control resources, are developed and available before deployment.

(6) For certain deployments, upon the direction of the ASD(HA), include additional medical screening requirements and guidance in Operation Plans. This guidance must include uniform data collection forms and procedures. This

guidance will be submitted to the TRICARE Readiness Executive Committee through the JPMPG for approval by ASD(HA).

e. Each Military Service, in coordination with the other Military Services shall:

(1) Appoint designated medical officers or proponents to develop and coordinate, through the Joint Preventive Medicine Policy Group, joint surveillance procedures implementing the policies described in this Instruction.

(2) Prepare, in coordination with the JPMPG, tailored troop medical information.

(3) Recommend, in coordination with the JPMPG, appropriate countermeasures.

(4) Support special preventive medicine activities in all phases of deployment.

(5) Maintain specific or consolidated serum bank(s) to aid in the assessment of illnesses.

(6) Unless a serum specimen has been obtained and forwarded to the Armed Services Serum Repository within the 12 months preceding deployment, obtain serum from 7-10 cc of blood from each Service member to be deployed and forward it to the repository designated by CHPPM.

f. The Defense Intelligence Agency, through AFMIC, shall develop and distribute assessments on environmental health factors and endemic infectious diseases of operational importance to allow the development of joint preventive medicine recommendations.

g. CINC Surgeons and JTF surgeons shall use the Armed Forces preventive medicine recommendations as distributed by AFMIC in planning scenario-specific medical requirements including requirements for combat stress control and determining appropriate preventive countermeasures. JTF surgeons shall identify specific diseases and conditions of military significance in the Area of Operation.

h. J-4 (Medical Readiness Division), as the CINC proponent, will work closely with each of the Combatant Commands to monitor implementation of a comprehensive military medical surveillance program across the strategic, operational, and tactical warfighting spectrum. J-4 shall ensure that joint medical surveillance doctrine is integrated into deployment medical planning.

3. During a Deployment

a. The Defense Manpower Data Center, under the Under Secretary for Personnel and Readiness, shall provide, for any deployed force, collective data such as daily strength by unit and total, grid coordinate locations for each unit (company size and higher), and inclusive dates of individual Service members' deployment. Such data shall be linkable to collective medical surveillance data and to individual Service members' medical records.

b. The Surgeons General of the Military Departments shall support unique medical surveillance activities during deployment, including early deployment of specialized environmental and occupational exposure and epidemiology teams to assist the Theater or JTF Surgeon concerned in identifying and assessing threats, and recommending countermeasures to the Theater Commander.

c. The CINC surgeon and JTF surgeon shall:

(1) Ensure accurate and thorough medical recordkeeping and documentation of health-related events occurs during deployment consistent with Department policies.

(2) Ensure that medical surveillance data are collected and analyzed, in accordance with Joint Staff Memorandum J-4A 00106-93 (reference (c)), and this information made available on a weekly basis to the Service Surgeons General.

(3) Identify and report illnesses, injuries and diseases, to include combat stress responses of military significance and inform the cognizant JTF or Theater Commander concerning appropriate countermeasures.

(4) Provide troop commanders with appropriate information on troop health status, illness, injury and disease threat analyses, and redeployment health concerns.

(5) Collect and, through the Chairman of the Joint Chiefs of Staff, report deployment data to the Deployment Surveillance Team, U.S. Army Center for Health Promotion and Preventive Medicine, unless otherwise designated.

(6) Record the physical and mental health status of personnel at time of redeployment or within 30 days of final departure from theater, in accordance specific guidance and data forms template provided by the ASD(HA).

(7) Deploy technically specialized units with capability and expertise in the conduct of surveillance for occupational and environmental illnesses, injuries, and diseases, health hazard assessments, and advanced diagnostic testing. Examples of these units are the Navy Forward Deployable Laboratory, the 520th Theater Army Medical Laboratory, and the Air Force Tactical Reference Lab. These specialized units may be deployed to meet the requirements of the deployed force through surveillance for occupational and environmental illnesses, injuries, and diseases, application of preventive medicine, use of advanced diagnostic testing, and coordination with combat stress control personnel. These units shall conduct health assessments of potential exposure to biological, chemical, or physical agents that threaten the health and safety of the command.

(8) Deploy combat stress control personnel and units to meet the mental health requirements of the deployed force. Medical staff, chaplains, and other assets with expertise in the assessment and management of stress shall participate in the stress control program.

d. Troop commanders shall:

(1) Inform troops of illness, injury, and disease threats, the risks associated with those threats, and the countermeasures in place, or to be used, to minimize those risks while deployed.

(2) Ensure compliance with preventive medicine guidance.

(3) Promote combat stress control programs and policies.

(4) Ensure completion of pre and post deployment questionnaires.

4. Upon Return from Deployment

a. The CINC Surgeons and JTF Surgeons shall:

(1) Through the Service Surgeons, ensure that all personnel complete health screening assessments prior to leaving the areas of operation. The health screening shall include a mental health assessment. Where certain situations may not allow screening prior to departure, commanders of the Service member's parent organization or command will ensure that redeployment medical surveillance is completed and submitted to local medical treatment facility commander within 30 days of return. Post-deployment assessments of Reserve component personnel must be completed prior to release from active duty. These assessments are to be documented on standardized form DD 2697, for inclusion in individual medical records in compliance with Service and Chairman of the Joint Chiefs of Staff directives. These screening forms, at a minimum, shall include pertinent information as directed by the ASD(HA). A copy of each form or an electronic data record generated during the health screening process shall be sent to the Deployment Surveillance Team.

(2) When directed by the Assistant Secretary of Defense for Health Affairs, and in coordination with the Surgeons General and the Chairman of the Joint Chiefs of Staff, obtain serum from 10 cc of blood from each redeploying service member and submit such serum to the Tri-Service serum repository.

(3) Collect and forward redeployment processing data.

(4) Develop and forward medical lessons learned to the Joint Uniform Lessons Learned System and to other appropriate Service Lessons Learned systems to improve subsequent preventive medicine support of operations.

b. The JPMPG shall reassess uniform preventive medicine policies and staffing guidance based on lessons learned during the deployment and recommend improvements to the medical military medical surveillance system and requirements for needed countermeasures.

c. The Military Services and the Defense Manpower Data Center, under the USD (P&R), shall, in collaboration with medical surveillance agencies in each Service, provide data and databases for post-joint deployment medical surveillance aggregation to the Deployment Surveillance Team. When aggregated, the data will then be forwarded to CHPPM for analyses.

d. The Military Services shall:

(1) Support combat stress control and personal support and family advocacy programs.

(2) Ensure that troop commanders support post-deployment preventive countermeasures, such as redeployment stress debriefings and malaria prophylaxis.

e. The Surgeons General of the Military Departments shall:

(1) In coordination with the ASD(HA), CINC surgeon, the JTF surgeons and the Chairman of the Joint Chiefs of Staff, provide scenario-specific screening of Service members and appropriate, targeted, medical evaluations as indicated.

(2) Forward screening and medical evaluation data to the Deployment Surveillance Team. Appropriate data shall be aggregated and forwarded to CHPPM.

(3) When directed, obtain serum from 10 cc of blood from each redeployed Service member and submit to the serum repository designated by CHPPM.

(4) Develop and support tailored post-deployment data collection and analyses. For certain deployments, the Chairman of the Joint Chiefs of Staff and CINC Surgeons in collaboration with the ASD(HA), may require additional screening within 30 days after return from deployment. This may include mental health assessments, if not previously accomplished, collection of additional laboratory specimens, and surveys of unique exposures or health outcomes. Special attention must be paid to ensure collection of additional post-deployment assessments from Active or Reserve component personnel prior to their release from active duty.

f. The Defense Intelligence Agency, through AFMIC, shall update assessments on occupational and environmental health factors and infectious diseases of operational importance.

G. INFORMATION REQUIREMENTS

The Joint Medical Surveillance data collected for the purposes of monitoring the individual and collective health of the military population prior to, during and following deployment operations is exempt from licensing in accordance with paragraph E.4.i. of DoD 8910.1-M (reference (g)).

H. EFFECTIVE DATE

This Instruction is effective immediately.

Rudy F. de Leon
Under Secretary of Defense
(Personnel and Readiness)

Enclosures - 3
1. References
2. Definitions
3. Table of Medical Surveillance Components Related to Deployment

---

REFERENCES, continued

(e) DoD Instruction 3020.37, "Continuation of Essential DoD Contractor Services During Crises," November 6, 1990

(f) DoD Instruction 1400.32, "DoD Civilian Work Force Contingency and Emergency Planning Guidelines and Procedures," April 24, 1995

(g) DoD 8910.1-M, "DoD Procedures for Management of Information Requirements", November 28, 1986, authorized by DoD Directive 8910.1, June 11, 1993

DEFINITIONS

1. **Combat Stress Control**. Encompasses actions taken by military personnel to prevent, identify and treat adverse combat stress responses which impair duty performance and Service member well being. It includes primary prevention through monitoring and control of personnel selection, stressors, and increasing stress tolerance of individual units; secondary prevention through early identification and far forward treatment of combat stress cases and tertiary prevention through treatment in rear echelons to minimize or prevent chronic disability.

2. **Disease**. An interruption, cessation, or disorder of bodily functions, systems, or organs.

3. **Endemic Diseases**. Those diseases that may be expected to occur in a specific population.

4. **Environmental Risk Assessment**. The science and art of predicting the frequency of disease in a population based on actual or projected (modeled) environmental exposures.

5. **Health Hazard Assessment**. An assessment that characterizes the possible health risks of occupational exposures of Service members during the course of their normal duties.

6. **Illness**. Disease or functional disorder.

7. **Injury**. The damage or wound of trauma.

8. **Medical Surveillance**. The regular or repeated collection, analysis, and dissemination of uniform health information for monitoring the health of a population, and intervening in a timely manner when necessary. It is defined by the Centers for Disease Control and Prevention as the ongoing, systematic collection, analysis, and interpretation of health data essential to the planning, implementation, and evaluation of public health practice, closely integrated with the timely dissemination of these data to those who need to know. The final link of the military medical surveillance system is the application of these data to prevention and control. A military medical surveillance system includes a functional capacity for data collection, analysis, and dissemination of information linked to public health programs.

9. **Military Preventive Medicine**. Encompasses the anticipation, prediction, identification, prevention, and control of preventable diseases, illnesses and injuries caused by exposure to biological, chemical, physical or psychological threats or stressors found at home stations and during deployments. Epidemiology, clinical preventive medicine, occupational medicine, industrial hygiene, environmental health sciences and engineering, medical entomology, health promotion and wellness, community health, mental health disciplines, toxicology and laboratory support sciences (environmental, occupational and radiological chemistry and microbiology) form military preventive medicine's core disciplines.

10. **Preventive Medicine**. The branch of medical science concerned with the prevention of disease and the promotion of physical and mental health through study of the etiology and epidemiology of disease processes. As used in this document, it is global in scope and

encompasses not only traditional preventive medicine functions, but also these of occupational medicine and industrial hygiene. Couples with this is the recognition of the role of surveillance efforts in the identification, control and prevention of not only diseases, but occupational and environmental illnesses and injuries.

11. **Risk Communication.** The process of adequately and accurately communicating the magnitude and nature of potential environmental and occupational health risks to commanders and to Service members.

	Pre-deployment	During Deployment	Post-deployment
Identify population at risk.	Field a seamless DoD ambulatory health data system. Ensure deployment readiness of individual Service members, using automated record system.	Collect data on unit strength, locations, and traumatic stressors on individual Service members' deployment histories.	Archive deployment information related to units and individual Service members.
Identify exposures	Prepare and distribute threat assessments for potential area of operations.[1] Identify threats for area of operations during planning for specific operations.	Special assessments of occupational and environmental exposures, including traumatic stressors. Analyze disease/injury/combat stress incidence data.	Update threat intelligence based upon special assessments and disease/injury/combat stress data.
Protective Measures	Determine countermeasures and incorporate into specific Op-Plans. Execute pre-deployment countermeasures (train, equip, supply, combat stress brief, immunize).	Reinforce or introduce added, protective countermeasures based upon analysis of disease/injury/combat stress data.	Identify requirements for new countermeasures.
Assess health	Perform continuous health status surveillance [1] and tracking of deployability status,[1] (includes human immunodeficiency virus,[1] dental,[1] immunizations,[1] deoxyribonucleic acid). Maintain Serum Bank.	Capture disease/injury/combat stress events (medical surveillance). Analyze data on disease/ injury/combat stress occurrence.	Perform scenario-specific screening and targeted medical evaluation of Service members. Perform continuous medical surveillance as follow-up. Disseminate findings.

1. Continuous readiness requirements, independent of deployment.

Table 1: **MEDICAL SURVEILLANCE COMPONENTS RELATED TO DEPLOYMENT**

[Top]
Last update: 9/21/1998

This page intentionally left blank.

APPENDIX J

Joint Chiefs of Staff Memorandum on Deployment Health Surveillance and Readiness, December 1998

Available on line at: **www.amsa.army.mil.**

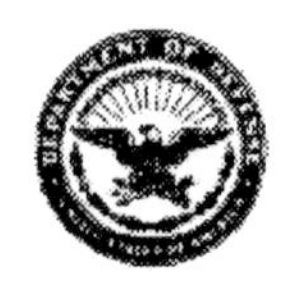

OFFICE OF THE CHAIRMAN
THE JOINT CHIEFS OF STAFF
WASHINGTON, D.C. 20318-9999

Reply ZIP Code:
20318-0300

MCM-251-98
04 December 1998

MEMORANDUM FOR: Under Secretary of Defense for Personnel and Readiness
Chief of Staff, US Army
Chief of Naval Operations
Chief of Staff, US Air Force
Commandant of the Marine Corps
Commander in Chief, US Atlantic Command
Commander in Chief, US Central Command
Commander in Chief, US European Command
Commander in Chief, US Pacific Command
Commander in Chief, US Southern Command
Commander in Chief, US Space Command
Commander in Chief, US Special Operations Command
Commander in Chief, US Strategic Command
Commander in Chief, US Transportation Command
Commander in Chief, US Forces Korea

Subject: Deployment Health Surveillance and Readiness

1. Force health protection (FHP) provides a conceptual framework for optimizing health readiness and protecting Service members from all health and environmental hazards associated with military service. A robust health surveillance system is a critical component of FHP. Deployment health surveillance includes identifying the population at risk (through, but not limited to, pre- and post-deployment health assessments), recognizing and assessing hazardous exposures (medical, environmental, and occupational), employing specific countermeasures, and monitoring health outcomes (through weekly disease and non-battle injury reporting). This memorandum provides routine, standardized procedures for assessing health readiness and conducting health surveillance in support of the Joint Chiefs of Staff and unified command deployments. General guidance is provided at Enclosure A and specific guidance is at enclosures B through E.

2. Effective 1 February 1999, the uniform and standardized health surveillance and readiness procedures described in this memorandum will be adhered to for all deployments (as defined at Enclosure A). This memorandum

supersedes the medical surveillance reporting procedures contained in the Joint Staff memorandum J-4A 00106-93,[1] and supports the implementation of DODD 6490.2,[2] DODI 6490.3,[3] and ASD-HA policy memorandum.[4]

3. Blank forms for the pre- and post-deployment health assessment and the weekly DNBI report are available for download under Deployment Surveillance at the following web site: http://cba.ha.osd.mil. The Deployment Surveillance Team (DST) maintains this section of the web site. The DST points of contact are Captain Lenny Denaro, DSN 761-7153 ext 4727, commercial (703) 681-7153 ext 4727, or Staff Sergeant Mark Carter, DSN 761-7153 ext 4742, or commercial (703) 681-7153 ext 4742. The fax number for the DST is DSN 761-5920 or commercial (703) 681-5920.

4. The Joint Staff point of contact is Lieutenant Colonel Bob Thompson, J4, DSN 223-5105 or commercial (703) 693-5105.

For the Chairman of the Joint Chiefs of Staff:

DENNIS C. BLAIR
Vice Admiral, U.S. Navy
Director, Joint Staff

Enclosures

References:

1 Joint Staff memorandum, J-4A 00106-93, 28 January 1993, "Medical Surveillance Report"
2 DODD 6490.2, 30 August 1997, "Joint Medical Surveillance"
3 DODI 6490.3, 7 August 1997, "Implementation and Application of Joint Medical Surveillance for Deployments"
4 ASD-HA memorandum, 6 October 1998, "Policy for Pre- and Post-Deployment Health Assessments and Blood Samples"

ENCLOSURE A

GENERAL GUIDANCE

1. **Deployment Defined.** For the purpose of joint health surveillance, a deployment is defined as a troop movement resulting from a JCS/unified command deployment order for 30 continuous days or greater to a land-based location outside the United States that does not have a permanent US military medical treatment facility (i.e., funded by the Defense Health Program). Routine shipboard operations that are not anticipated to involve field operations ashore for over 30 continuous days are exempt from the requirements for pre- and post-deployment health assessments.

a. Weekly DNBI reporting is strongly encouraged on a routine basis, whether in garrison or deployed, to facilitate a seamless transition to joint operations.

b. If the duration of deployment is uncertain, then the surveillance requirements described in this enclosure (pre- and post-deployment health assessments, health readiness, and DNBI reporting) will be adhered to.

c. The baseline surveillance requirements described in this enclosure should be augmented as necessary based upon health threat assessments.

2. **Predeployment.** The unified command, through deployment orders and/or separate instructions, will require the Services and supporting CINCs to accomplish the following at the home station or processing station of the deploying Service member:

a. Health Threat/Countermeasures. Inform Service members on all known potential health threats, to include endemic diseases; injuries; nuclear, biological, or chemical (NBC) contaminants; toxic industrial compounds; combat and deployment-related stress; climatic extremes; and other environmental health threats (such as use of non-approved pesticides). Proven preventive medicine countermeasures will be employed, to include appropriate personal protective measures and use of personal protective equipment.

b. Health Readiness. Complete individual health readiness processing, including the following:

(1) Immunizations

(a) DOD Minimum Requirements. Must be current in tetanus-diphtheria, influenza, hepatitis A, MR/MMR, and polio.

(b) Service-specific Requirements. Refer to AFJI 48-110, AR 40-562, BUMEDINST 6230.15, and CG COMDTINST M6230.4E, "Immunizations and Chemoprophylaxds," 1 November 1995 (examples include yellow fever, hepatitis B, typhoid, and plague).

(c) Deployment-specific Requirements. Based upon the geographical location, the unified command will determine additional immunizations, chemoprophylactic medications, and other individual personal protective measures (such as insect repellent, bednetting, and uniform impregnation).

(2) Medical Record. Update the Service-specific medical record with:

(a) Blood type.

(b) Medication/allergies.

(c) Special duty qualifications.

(d) Immunization record.

(e) Pre-deployment health assessment form.

(f) Summary sheet of past medical problems.

(3) HIV within previous 12 months (serves dual purpose: HIV screening and predeployment serum sample).

(4) Tuberculosis skin test within 24 months. For previous PPD converters, handle IAW Service policy.

(5) DNA sample on file. To confirm the unit/individual status of DNA specimens on file, contact the DOD DNA Specimen Repository (voice 301-295-4379, fax 301-295-4380, or e-mail afrssir@afip.osd.mil).

(6) Current physical exam or assessment IAW Service policy.

(7) Dental Class I/II.

(8) 90-day supply of prescription medications.

(9) Required medical equipment (glasses, gas mask inserts, hearing aids, dental orthodontic equipment, etc.).

(10) Personal occupational health equipment (respiratory protection, hearing protection, and personal exposure dosimeters).

(11) No unresolved health problems (P-4 profile, limited duty status, pregnancy).

c. Health Assessment. Conduct predeployment health assessments using the form and processing instructions at Enclosure B.

3. **During Deployment**. The unified command will provide guidance and support to:

a. Ensure DNBI surveillance data is collected and analyzed using the form and instructions at Enclosure C.

b. Establish procedures for documenting and reporting those reportable medical events listed at Enclosure D. Refer to the US Army Medical Surveillance Activity (AMSA) publication, "Tri-Service Reportable Events," version 1.0, July 1998, for guidelines and case definitions. Report on presumptive as well as confirmed reportable medical events.

c. Ensure Service-specific procedures are maintained for appropriate archiving of health documents (DNBI, pesticides, and environmental surveillance data) and records (individual health treatment provided).

d. Provide troop commanders with appropriate and timely health status information.

e. Based upon the threat assessment and guidance provided in the Services joint implementation instructions to DODI 6490.3, "Implementation and Application of Joint Medical Surveillance for Deployments," conduct a systematic and comprehensive program of surveillance, assessment, and prevention of occupational and environmental health hazards.

f. Ensure the integrity of occupational health and safety programs.

g. Conduct pest control operations using the integrated pest management (IPM) program described in DODI 4150.7, "DOD Pest Management Program," 22 April 1996. When pesticides are employed ensure the use of only DOD approved pesticides.

4. **Post-Deployment**.

a. The unified command will provide guidance and support to:

(1) Conduct post-deployment health assessments using the form and processing guidance at Enclosure E.

(2) Identify Service members in need of medical evaluation upon return to home/processing station based on review of medical treatment received in theater, the post-deployment health assessment form, and other pertinent health surveillance data.

(3) Conduct medical debrief to deployed Service members on all significant health events and exposures.

(4) Document environmental exposures in after action reports (AARs).

(5) Develop and forward health lessons learned to the Joint Uniform Lessons Learned System (JULLS).

b. The Services and supporting CINCs are requested to accomplish the following at the home station or processing station of the redeploying Service member:

(1) Conduct tuberculosis screening within 1 year of redeployment or sooner IAW Service-specific requirements.

(2) Collect, when indicated by Service policy, a serum sample for HIV testing and storage in the serum repository.

(3) Conduct additional health assessments and/or health debriefs if indicated by health threats or events occurring in theater.

ENCLOSURE B

PRE-DEPLOYMENT HEALTH ASSESSMENT FORM PROCESSING GUIDANCE

1. Service members must complete or re-validate the health assessment form at their home station or processing station within 30 days of their deployment.

2. The form must be administered and then immediately reviewed by a health care provider. The provider can be a medic or corpsman for administering and initially reviewing the questionnaire. However, positive responses to questions 2-4 and 7-8 must be referred to a physician, physician assistant, nurse, or independent duty medical technician.

3. Copies of the completed form must be placed in the Service members' permanent medical record. The originals will be immediately forwarded to the Deployment Surveillance Team (DST), 5113 Leesburg Pike, Suite 701, Falls Church, Virginia, 22041, DSN 761-7153 (ext. 4727 or 4742) or commercial 703-681-7153 (ext. 4727 or 4742).

4. The DST provides the U.S. Army Center for Health Promotion and Preventive Medicine (USACHPPM) with a predeployment health assessment database on a monthly basis for inclusion in the Defense Medical Surveillance System (DMSS).

5. USACHPPM provides the Joint Staff, unified commands, and the Services with periodic trend analysis reports on the completed predeployment health assessment forms.

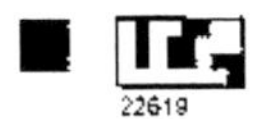

22619

PRE-DEPLOYMENT Health Assessment

INSTRUCTIONS **PRIVACY ACT OF 1974**

Please read each question completely and carefully before marking your selections. Provide a response for each question. If you do not understand a question, ask the administrator.

Demographics

Location of Operation / Deployment:

- O Europe
- O SW Asia
- O SE Asia
- O Asia (Other)
- O South America
- O Other ______
- O Australia
- O Africa
- O Central America
- O Unknown

List country (IF KNOWN): [ ]

Name of Operation: [ ]

Today's Date (mm/dd/yyyy) [ ][ ] / [ ][ ] / [ ][ ][ ][ ]

Last Name [ ]

Social Security Number [ ][ ][ ] - [ ][ ] - [ ][ ][ ][ ]

First Name [ ] MI [ ]

DOB (mm/dd/yyyy) [ ][ ] / [ ][ ] / [ ][ ][ ][ ]

Pay Grade/Rank

- O E1 O E2 O E3 O E4 O E5 O E6 O E7 O E8 O E9
- O O1 O O2 O O3 O O4 O O5 O O6 O O7 O O8 O O9 O O10
- O W1 O W2 O W3 O W4 O W5 O Other

Gender

- O Male
- O Female

Service Branch

- O Air Force
- O Army
- O Coast Guard
- O Marine Corps
- O Navy
- O Other

Component

- O Active Duty
- O National Guard
- O Reserves
- O Civilian Government Employee
- O Non-Government (Contract) Employee
- O Other

Health Assessment

1. Would you say your health in general is: O Excellent O Very Good O Good O Fair O Poor
2. Do you have any medical or dental problems? O Yes O No
3. Are you currently on a profile, or light duty, or are you undergoing a medical board? O Yes O No
4. Are you pregnant? (FEMALES ONLY) O Don't Know O Yes O No
5. Do you have a 90-day supply of your prescription medication or birth control pills? O N/A O Yes O No
6. Do you have two pairs of prescription glasses (if worn) and any other personal medical equipment? O N/A O Yes O No
7. During the past year, have you sought counseling or care for your mental health? O Yes O No
8. Do you currently have any questions or concerns about your health? O Yes O No

Please list your concerns: ______

I certify that responses on this form are true.

Service Member Signature [ ]

End of Questions

22619

Pre-Deployment Health Assessment Questionnaire
ASD (HA) APPROVED SEPTEMBER 1998

22619

Pre-Deployment Health Provider Review (For Health Provider Use Only)

After interview/exam of patient, the following problems were noted and categorized by Review of Systems. More than one may be noted for patients with multiple problems. Further documentation of problem to be placed in medical records.

REFERRAL INDICATED

- ○ None
- ○ Cardiac
- ○ Combat/Operational stress reaction
- ○ Dental
- ○ Dermatologic
- ○ ENT
- ○ Eye
- ○ Family Problems
- ○ Fatigue, Malaise, Multisystem complaint
- ○ GI
- ○ GU
- ○ GYN
- ○ Mental Health
- ○ Neurologic
- ○ Orthopedic
- ○ Pregnancy
- ○ Pulmonary
- ○ Other ____________________

Indicate the status of each of the following

Yes	No	N/A	
○	○	○	Medical threat briefing completed
○	○	○	Medical information sheet distributed
○	○	○	Serum for HIV drawn within 12 months
○	○	○	Immunizations current
○	○	○	PPD screening within 24 months

FINAL MEDICAL DISPOSITION: ○ Deployable ○ Not Deployable

Comments: (If not deployable, explain)

____

____

____

____

I certify that this review process has been completed.

Provider's signature and stamp:

Date (mm/dd/yyyy) ☐☐ / ☐☐ / ☐☐☐☐

End of Health Review

Pre-Deployment Health Assessment Questionnaire
ASD (HA) APPROVED SEPTEMBER 1998

22619

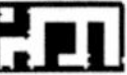

ENCLOSURE C

WEEKLY DISEASE AND NON-BATTLE INJURY REPORT INSTRUCTIONS

Disease and Non-Battle Injury Rates - The Vital Signs of the Unit

The main reason for tracking disease and non-battle injury (DNBI) rates is that they are an important tool at the unit level. They are the "vital signs of the unit," an early warning system for trouble. Abnormal rates serve to focus medical attention on a problem area immediately. They are the ultimate outcome measure of how well a command's preventive medicine program is working. The data can be used by the medical staff to identify and highlight feasible means of reducing the incidence of preventable disease and injury. The data must be reported up the medical chain so that a "big picture" of disease patterns can be assembled to localize problems and quickly intervene with appropriate preventive medicine countermeasures. Additionally, the data must be reported on a weekly basis (ending Saturday 2359 hrs local) through command channels to the JTF Surgeon, CINC Surgeon, Joint Staff, Service Surgeons, and the U.S. Army Center for Health Promotion and Preventive Medicine (USACHPPM). USACHPPM provides the Joint Staff, unified commands, and the Services with periodic DNBI trend analysis reports for current deployments.

The DNBI report summarizes weekly DNBI rates and provides baseline rates for comparison. This system depends on a proper sick call logbook (or its electronic equivalent), which MUST record at a minimum the following information on EVERY patient encounter:

1. Patient's name, SSN, gender, unit, unit identification code (UIC), and duty location.

2. Type of visit - new, follow-up, or administrative.

3. Primary compliant.

4. Final diagnosis.

5. For injuries, a classification into recreation/sports, motor vehicle accident (MVA), work/training, or other.

6. Final disposition into one of the following categories:

   - Full duty.
   - Light duty (estimated number of days).
   - Sick in quarters (estimated number of days).
   - MTF in-patient admissions.

7. DNBI category (case definitions are provided at the end of this enclosure).

Sick call logbooks or their electronic equivalents must be retained by the medical unit at the conclusion of the deployment.

To fill out the weekly DNBI report, follow these steps:

1. Record the administrative data in the spaces provided at the top of the form. The troop strength refers to the number of troops being taken care of by the reporting medical unit. Obtain average troop strength for the reporting period from the S-1/J-1.

2. Review the sick call log and add up the total number of new cases (excluding follow-ups) seen during the entire week in each DNBI category. Fill in the appropriate block. Add up the total DNBI and record the number in the space provided.

3. To calculate DNBI rates, divide the total number of patients seen in each category by the average troop strength, and multiply by 100. For the gynecologic category, the FEMALE troop strength must be used to calculate the rate, not the total troop strength. Remember to calculate an overall DNBI total rate.

   Example. If there were 20 dermatological cases this week in 500 troops, the percent would be calculated as follows:

   $\frac{\text{20 dermatological cases}}{\text{500 Troops}} = 0.04$ then $0.04 \times 100 = 4\%$

4. Next, add up the total number of estimated light duty days, lost duty days, and MTF in-patient admissions in each category, and fill in the appropriate block.

5. Compare calculated rates for each category with the suggested reference rate for that category (comment is required under the section "Problems Identified - Corrective Actions" for all categories where rates are above the suggested reference rate). When comparing rates, keep the following information in mind:

   a. The suggested reference rates are only approximate and should be used as a rough guide only. The CINC Surgeon or JTF Surgeon may modify the "Suggested Reference Rates" based upon theater specific trends.

   b. Exceeding a rate by 0.1% is not necessarily an indication of a significant problem. However, going from half the suggested rate to twice the suggested rate probably indicates that there is a health problem needing immediate attention.

   c. The individual suggested reference rates are not intended to add up to the total DNBI suggested reference rate. An individual category could have a high rate without causing the total rate to exceed the reference rate - attention to the individual category is appropriate and necessary in this situation. Alternatively, the total DNBI rate could be high without causing individual categories to exceed their reference rates – attention to systemic problems causing general sick call visits to rise is appropriate and necessary in this situation.

   d. Use common sense in interpreting the DNBI rates. Track DNBI rates over time and compare current DNBI rates with your unit's past DNBI rates for comparable situations.

6. Report weekly DNBI data to the unit commander and to medical personnel at higher echelons (as noted in the first paragraph of these instructions).

CASE DEFINITIONS

Notes: 1. Count only the initial visit. Do not count follow-up visits.
2. All initial sick call visits should be placed in a category.
3. If in doubt about which category, make the best guess.
4. Estimate days of light duty, lost work days, or admissions resulting from initial visits.

Combat/Operational Stress Reactions - Acute reaction to stress and transient disorders which occur without any apparent mental disorder in response to exceptional physical and mental stress. Also includes post-traumatic stress disorder which arises as a delayed or protracted response to a stressful event or situation of an exceptionally threatening or catastrophic nature.

Dermatological - Diseases of the skin and subcutaneous tissue, including heat rash, fungal infection, cellulitis, impetigo, contact dermatitis, blisters, ingrown toenails, unspecified dermatitis, etc. Includes sunburn.

Gastrointestinal, Infectious - All diagnoses consistent with infection of the intestinal tract. Includes any type of diarrhea, gastroenteritis, "stomach flu", nausea/vomiting, hepatitis, etc. Does NOT include non-infectious intestinal diagnoses such as hemorrhoids, ulcers, etc.

Gynecological - Menstrual abnormalities, vaginitis, pelvic inflammatory disease, or other conditions related to the female reproductive system.

Heat/Cold Injuries - Climatic injuries, including heat stroke, heat exhaustion, heat cramps, dehydration, hypothermia, frostbite, trench foot, immersion foot, and chilblain.

Injuries, Recreational/Sports - Any injury occurring as a direct consequence of the pursuit of personal and/or group fitness, excluding formal training.

Injuries, Motor Vehicle Accidents - Any injury occurring as a direct consequence of a motor vehicle accident.

Injury, Work/Training - Any injury occurring as a direct consequence of military operations/duties or of an activity carried out as part of formal military training, to include organized runs and physical fitness programs.

Injury, Other - Any injury not included in the previously defined injury categories.

Ophthalmologic - Any acute diagnosis involving the eye, including pink-eye, conjunctivitis, sty, corneal abrasion, foreign body, vision problems, etc. Does not include routine referral for glasses (non-acute).

Psychiatric, Mental Disorders - Any conventionally defined psychiatric disorder as well as behavioral changes and disturbance of normal conduct which is either out of normal character, or is coupled with unusual physical symptoms such as paralysis.

Respiratory - Any diagnosis of the: lower respiratory tract, such as bronchitis, pneumonia, emphysema, reactive airway disease, and pleurisy; or the upper respiratory tract, such as "common cold", laryngitis, tonsillitis, tracheitis, otitis and sinusitis.

Sexually Transmitted Diseases - All sexually transmitted infections including such diseases as chlamydia, HIV, gonorrhea, syphilis, herpes, chancroid, and venereal warts.

Fever, Unexplained - Temperature of 100.5ºF or greater for 24 hours, or history of chills and fever without a clear diagnosis (this is a screening category for many tropical diseases such as malaria, dengue fever, and typhoid fever). Such fever cannot be explained by other inflammatory/infectious processes such as respiratory infections, heat, and overexertion.

All Other, Medical/Surgical - Any medical or surgical condition not fitting into any category above.

Dental - Any disease of the teeth and oral cavity, such as periodontal and gingival disorders, caries, and mandible anomalities.

Miscellaneous/Administration/Follow-up - All other visits to the treatment facility not fitting one of the above categories, such as profile renewals, pregnancy, immunizations, prescription refills, and physical exams or laboratory tests for administrative purposes.

Definable - An additional category established for a specific deployment based upon public health concerns (e.g. malaria, dengue, airborne/HALO injuries, etc.).

WEEKLY DNBI REPORT

Unit/Command: ____________________ Troop Strength: __________
Dates Covered: ________ (Sunday 0001) Through ________ (Saturday 2359)

Individual Preparing Report: ______________________________
Phone: ______________ E-Mail: ______________________________

CATEGORY	INITIAL VISITS	RATE	SUGGESTED REFERENCE RATE		DAYS OF LIGHT DUTY	LOST WORK DAYS	ADMITS
Combat/Operational Stress Reactions			0.1%				
Dermatologic			0.5%				
GI, Infectious			0.5%				
Gynecologic			0.5%				
Heat/Cold Injuries			0.5%				
Injury, Recreational/Sports			1.0%				
Injury, MVA			1.0%				
Injury, Work/Training			1.0%				
Injury, Other			1.0%				
Ophthalmologic			0.1%				
Psychiatric, Mental Disorders			0.1%				
Respiratory			0.4%				
STDs			0.5%				
Fever, Unexplained			0.0%				
All Other, Medical/Surgical							
TOTAL DNBI			4.0%				

Dental		XXXXXXX					
Misc/Admin/ Follow-up		XXXXXXX					
Definable							
Definable							

Problems Identified:
____
____
____

Corrective Actions:
____
____
____

DNBI Reporting Form for Joint Deployments
JOINT STAFF APPROVED – DECEMBER 1998

ENCLOSURE D

TRI-SERVICE REPORTABLE MEDICAL EVENT LIST

- Amebiasis
- Anthrax
- Biological Warfare Agent Exposure
- Botulism
- Brucellosis
- Campylobacter
- Carbon Monoxide Poisoning
- Chemical Agent Exposure
- Chlamydia
- Cholera
- Coccidioidomycosis
- Cold Weather Injury (All)
    - Frostbite
    - Hypothermia
    - Immersion Type
    - Unspecified
- Cryptosporidiosis
- Cyclospora
- Dengue Fever
- Diphtheria
- E. Coli 0157:H7
- Ehrlichiosis
- Encephalitis
- Filariasis
- Giardiasis
- Gonorrhea
- H. Influenzae, Invasive
- Hantavirus infection
- Heat Injuries
    - Heat Exhaustion
    - Heat Stroke
- Hemorrhagic Fever
- Hepatitis A
- Hepatitis B
- Hepatitis C
- Influenza
- Lead Poisoning
- Legionellosis
- Leishmaniasis (All)
    - Leishmaniasis, Cutaneous
    - Leishmaniasis, Mucocutaneous
    - Leishmaniasis, Unspecified
    - Leishmaniasis, Visceral
- Leprosy
- Leptospirosis
- Listeriosis
- Lyme Disease
- Malaria (All)
    - Malaria, Falciparum
    - Malaria, Malariae
    - Malaria, Ovale
    - Malaria, Unspecified
    - Malaria, Vivax
- Measles
- Meningococcal Disease
    - Meningitis
    - Septicemia
- Mumps
- Pertussis
- Plague
- Pneumococcal Pneumonia
- Poliomyelitis
- Q Fever
- Rabies, Human
- Relapsing Fever
- Rheumatic Fever, Acute
- Rift Valley Fever
- Rocky Mountain Spotted Fever
- Rubella
- Salmonellosis
- Schistosomiasis
- Shigellosis
- Smallpox
- Streptococcus, Group A, Invasive
- Syphilis (All)
    - Syphilis, Congenital
    - Syphilis, Latent
    - Syphilis, Primary/Secondary
    - Syphilis, Tertiary
- Tetanus
- Toxic Shock Syndrome
- Trichinosis
- Trypanosomiasis
- Tuberculosis, Pulmonary
- Tularemia
- Typhoid Fever
- Typhus Fever
- Urethritis, Non-Gonococcal
- Vaccine, Adverse Event
- Varicella, Active Duty Only
- Yellow Fever

ENCLOSURE E

POST-DEPLOYMENT HEALTH ASSESSMENT FORM PROCESSING GUIDANCE

1. Service members must complete the health assessment form in theater, preferably, within 5 days prior to redeployment back to their home station.

2. The form must be administered and then immediately reviewed by a health care provider. The provider can be a medic or corpsman for administering and initially reviewing the questionnaire. However, positive responses must be referred to a physician, physician assistant, nurse, or independent duty medical technician.

3. Copies of the completed form must be placed in the Service member's permanent medical record or in the deployed medical record for transfer to their permanent medical record upon redeployment to their home station. The originals will be immediately forwarded to the Deployment Surveillance Team (DST), 5113 Leesburg Pike, Suite 701, Falls Church, Virginia, 22041, DSN 761-7153 (ext. 4727 or 4742) or commercial 703-681-7153 (ext. 4727 or 4742).

4. The DST provides the US Army Center for Health Promotion and Preventive Medicine (USACHPPM) with a post-deployment health assessment form data base on a monthly basis for inclusion in the Defense Medical Surveillance System (DMSS).

5. USACHPPM provides the Joint Staff, the unified commands, and the Services with periodic trend analysis reports on the completed post-deployment health assessment forms.

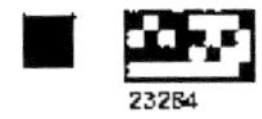

23284

POST-DEPLOYMEN Health Assessment

INSTRUCTIONS | **PRIVACY ACT OF 1974**

Please read each question completely and carefully before marking your selections. Provide a response for each question. If you do not understand a question, ask the administrator.

Demographics

Location of Operation / Deployment:

○ Europe ○ Australia
○ SW Asia ○ Africa
○ SE Asia ○ Central America
○ Asia (Other) ○ Unknown
○ South America
○ Other ________

List country (IF KNOWN): [ ]

Name of Operation: [ ]

Today's Date (mm/dd/yyyy) [ ][ ] / [ ][ ] / [ ][ ][ ][ ]

Date of arrival in theater (mm/dd/yyyy) [ ][ ] / [ ][ ] / [ ][ ][ ][ ]

Date of departure from theater (mm/dd/yyyy) [ ][ ] / [ ][ ] / [ ][ ][ ][ ]

Last Name [ ]

Social Security Number [ ][ ][ ] - [ ][ ] - [ ][ ][ ][ ]

First Name [ ] MI [ ]

DOB (mm/dd/yyyy) [ ][ ] / [ ][ ] / [ ][ ][ ][ ]

Pay Grade/Rank

○ E1 ○ E2 ○ E3 ○ E4 ○ E5 ○ E6 ○ E7 ○ E8 ○ E9
○ O1 ○ O2 ○ O3 ○ O4 ○ O5 ○ O6 ○ O7 ○ O8 ○ O9 ○ O10
○ W1 ○ W2 ○ W3 ○ W4 ○ W5 ○ Other

Gender

○ Male ○ Female

Service Branch

○ Air Force ○ Army ○ Coast Guard ○ Marine Corps ○ Navy ○ Other

Component

○ Active Duty ○ National Guard ○ Reserves ○ Civilian Government Employee ○ Non-Government (Contract) Employee ○ Other

Health Assessmen

1. Would you say your health in general is: ○ Excellent ○ Very Good ○ Good ○ Fair ○ Poor
2. Do you have any unresolved medical or dental problems that developed during this deployment? ○ Yes ○ No
3. Are you currently on a profile or light duty? ○ Yes ○ No
4. During this deployment have you sought, or intend to seek, counseling or care for your mental health? ○ Yes ○ No
5. Do you have concerns about possible exposures or events during this deployment that you feel may affect your health? ○ Yes ○ No

   Please list your concerns: ________

6. Do you currently have any questions or concerns about your health? ○ Yes ○ No

   Please list your concerns: ________

I certify that responses on this form are true.

Service Member Signature [ ]

End of Questions

23284

Post-Deployment Health Assessment Questionnaire
ASD (HA) APPROVED SEPTEMBER 1998

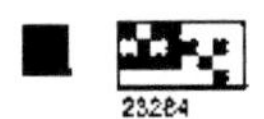
23284

Post-Deployment Health Provider Review (For Health Provider Use Only)

After interview/exam of patient, the following problems were noted and categorized by Review of Systems. More than one may be noted for patients with multiple problems. Further documentation of problem to be placed in medical records.

REFERRAL INDICATED

- O None
- O Cardiac
- O Combat / Operational Stress Reaction
- O Dental
- O Dermatologic
- O ENT
- O Eye
- O Family Problems
- O Fatigue, Malaise, Multisystem complaint
- O GI
- O GU
- O GYN
- O Mental Health
- O Neurologic
- O Orthopedic
- O Pregnancy
- O Pulmonary
- O Other ______________

EXPOSURE CONCERNS (During deployment)

Provider see questions 5 & 6 on the reverse of this form

- O Environmental
- O Occupational
- O Combat or mission related
- O None

Indicate the status of each of the following

Yes	No	N/A	
O	O	O	Medical threat debriefing completed
O	O	O	Medical information sheet distributed
O	O	O	Post-Deployment serum specimen collected, if required

Comments: ______________

I certify that this review process has been completed.

Provider's signature and stamp:

Date (mm/dd/yyyy) __ __ / __ __ / __ __ __ __

End of Health Review

23284

Post-Deployment Health Assessment Questionnaire
ASD (HA) APPROVED SEPTEMBER 1998